NEW DIMENSIONS IN PSYCHIATRY:
A WORLD VIEW

NEW DIMENSIONS IN PSYCHIATRY:
A WORLD VIEW

Volume 2

Edited by

Silvano Arieti, M.D. *and*
Gerard Chrzanowski, M.D.

A Wiley-Interscience Publication

JOHN WILEY & SONS, New York • London • Sydney • Toronto

Copyright © 1977 by John Wiley & Sons, Inc.

Library of Congress Cataloging in Publication Data (Revised)

Arieti, Silvano.
    New dimensions in psychiatry.

    "A Wiley-Interscience publication."
    Includes bibliographies.
    ISBN 0-471-03317-0
    1. Psychiatry.   2. Psychotherapy.   3. Psychiatry,
Transcultural.   [DNLM: 1. Psychiatry—Periodical.
2. Psychotherapy—Periodical.   W1 NE373]

RC454.A68   616.8'9   74-16150
ISBN 0-471-03318-9

Printed in the United States of America

10 9 8 7 6 5 4 3 2 1

AUTHORS

Canada

Ferdinand Knobloch, M.D. The University of British Columbia, Department of Psychiatry, Vancouver, British Columbia

Jirina Knobloch, M.D. The University of British Columbia, Department of Psychiatry, Vancouver, British Columbia

India

Erna M. Hoch Superintendent, Government Mental Hospital, Srinagar, Kashmir

J. S. Neki, M.A., D.P.M., F.R.C.Psych, F.A.M.S. Department of Psychiatry, All-India Institute of Medical Sciences, New Delhi

Israel

A. R. Bodenheimer, M.D. H. Sheba Medical Center, Department of Psychiatry and Psychotherapy, Tel Hashomer

Italy

Adriano Marino Università di Bari, Instituto di Farmacologia, Piazza Giulio Cesare, Bari

Japan

Akihisa Kondo, M.D. Yakumo, Meguro-Ku, Tokyo

Norway

Christian Fangel, M.D. Asgard Sykehus, Asgard, Tromso

Spain

Marina Prado de Molina, A.S.   Serrano Jover, Madrid

Francesco Simone   Hospital for Nervous and Mental Disorders, Faculty of the University of Naples, Naples

Switzerland

R. Battegay   Psychiatrische Universitätspoliklinik, Basel

Hans Heimann   Universitäts-Nervenklinik, Tübingen

Magdalena Schmocker,

Eckart Straube,

United States

John B. Calhoun   Unit for Research on Behavioral Systems, Laboratory of Brain Evolution and Behavior, National Institute of Mental Health, Bethesda, Maryland

Robert Cancro, M.D.   Med.D.Sc., University of Connecticut Health Center, Farmington, Connecticut

Ferruccio Di Cori, M.D.   New York, New York

Jan Ehrenwald, M.D.   New York, New York

Vladimir G. Levit, Dr. Med. Sci.   Research Center, Rockland State Hospital, Orangeburg, New York

Paul D. MacLean, M.D.   Chief, Laboratory of Brain Evolution and Behavior, National Institute of Mental Health, Bethesda, Maryland

Ashley Montagu   Princeton, New Jersey

Anthony Pietropinto, M.D.   Lutheran Medical Center, Brooklyn, New York

Leon Roizin, M.D.   New York State Psychiatric Institute, New York

E. Paul Torrance   The University of Georgia, College of Education, Department of Educational Psychology, Athens, Georgia

West Africa

Tolani Asuni   Neuro-Psychiatric Hospital, Aro, Abeokuta, Nigeria

This is the second volume in the present series under our coeditorship that follows a series initiated by one of us and first published by Basic Books in the fall of 1970 under the title "The World Biennial of Psychiatry and Psychotherapy."

Our principal aim in *New Dimensions in Psychiatry* is to offer an overview of present day psychiatric directions in various parts of the world. Emphasis is placed on recent contributions from numerous foreign countries as well as on some current work done in the United States. We address ourselves to psychiatrists, psychotherapists, psychoanalysts, and people working in a number of related specialties. The information contained in the book highlights some unusual, extraordinary aspects otherwise not found under one cover or in conventional textbooks. Much of the material presented here will be of interest to the priviate practitioner, to clinicians working in hospitals, to researchers, and to all who wish to stay in touch with what goes on in the psychiatric world at large. No attempt was made to collect papers on a single theme, but rather to bring together what is new, promising, and not easily accessible.

Authors from 11 countries cover a wide range of topics from sociocultural aspects, to novel therapeutic modalities, to biological and clinical studies. The material is divided into four sections in keeping with the tradition of this series. Part I deals with psychiatric issues in relation to the social environment, including sociogenic brain damage, cultural transformations, psychotherapy for the illiterate, the role of women analysts in Latin cultures, and changing conditions in Norway, Sardinia, and Nigeria. New therapies and related issues are discussed in Part II, with contributions on creativity and mental health, poetry therapy, folklore therapy in Japan, extrasensory perception, and psychodrama. In focusing on biological research Part III addresses itself to advances in pharmacotheraphy, psychophysiology, neuropathology, and the evolution of three mentalities. In Part IV are papers on clinical contributions ranging from work with schizophrenic patients, to group therapy and communication by means of drawing and painting, to advances in residential and day-care treatment.

We hope that the present collection of papers offers useful and stimulating material that will appeal to a broad group of readers.

GERARD CHRZANOWSKI
SILVANO ARIETI

December 1976
New York, New York

CONTENTS

NEW DIMENSIONS IN PSYCHIATRY:
A WORLD VIEW

PART ONE

PSYCHIATRIC ISSUES IN RELATION TO THE SOCIAL ENVIRONMENT

SOCIOGENIC BRAIN DAMAGE

CROWDING AND SOCIAL VELOCITY

PSYCHOLOGICAL ADAPTATION IN A CHANGING ENVIRONMENT

PSYCHOPATHOLOGY AND CULTURAL TRANSFORMATIONS IN A PASTORAL-AGRARIAN SOCIETY IN INDUSTRIAL EVOLUTION: EXPERIENCES IN SARDINIA

PSYCHOTHERAPY FOR THE ILLITERATE

DEPENDENCE: CROSS-CULTURAL CONSIDERATION OF DYNAMICS

PSYCHIATRY AND THE PSYCHIATRIST IN MODERN INDUSTRIALIZED NORWAY

THE IMPACT OF LATIN CULTURE ON THE WORK OF A WOMAN ANALYST

AFRICA WITH SPECIAL REFERENCE TO NIGERIA

CHAPTER ONE

SOCIOGENIC BRAIN DAMAGE

ASHLEY MONTAGU

When the functions of the brain are disordered in neuromuscular, structural, chemical, electrical, or other observable ways, the tendency has been to seek the organic causes of the disorder or malformation. Function is the other face of structure. Functions are dependent upon organic structures, hence the obvious, though not necessarily accurate, conclusion is customarily drawn that disordered function must be caused by disordered structures, and frequently we tend to look no further. We tend, in our thinking, to be limited to the idea that physical factors such as genetic, viral, bacterial, parasitic, chemical, iatrogenic, complications of pregnancy, prematurity, and postmaturity are the kind of factors that must be involved in the brain damage that causes the observable malfunction. This is often quite true, but it is also quite frequently not the whole story. No more the whole story than that pellagra is due to a deficiency of vitamins of the B complex, especially niacin (nicotinic acid) and its amide. It is quite true that under any conditions a diet deficient in nicotinic acid and other vitamins of the B complex will result in pellagra. In fact, however, under ordinarily normal socioeconomic conditions the diet is likely to be more than adequate in B complex vitamins. Hence the question must be asked whether or not the socioeconomic conditions in most cases constitute the principal factor in the causation of pellagra? Ever since 1915, we have known, thanks to the work of Goldberger, that pellagra is a disorder of extreme poverty, most unlikely to occur among those who can afford an adequate diet.

While it should be obvious that no matter how inadequate the socioeconomic conditions may be, if the diet is adequate, pellagra will not develop; nevertheless, it is almost exclusively under poor socioeconomic conditions that pellagra is encountered. In 1917–1918 there were over 200,000 cases of pellagra in the United States, and deaths from the condition numbered 10,000 annually. Between 1929 and 1949 the decrease in mortality in the southern states, where pellagra most frequently occurred, was striking: from 22.4 to 5.1 per 100,000. The number of acute cases and deaths from this disorder is today very low, largely as the result of a limited improvement in the dietary intake of people living in socioeconomically depressed environments. So it was not really the deficiency in niacin intake that was the principal cause of pellagra, but a socioeconomic environment which led to that deficiency.

Indeed, it would appear that many, if not most, disorders are to a significant extent due to social conditions resulting from an environment impoverished in the elements necessary for the maintenance of health.

From *Amer. Anthropol.* **74** (5), 1045–1061, October 1972. Reprinted by permission. Reprinted with additions by the author.

There is a class of brain damage of sociogenic origin to which, it seems to me, insufficient attention has been paid. Functional expressions of this class of brain damage are the deficits in behavior, and especially in motivation, learning ability, and intelligence which are produced by malnutrition.

It is generally agreed that the most important factor in the healthy development of the conceptus is nutrition—not merely the nutrition derived from the mother, but also the nutrition of the mother's mother, and probably also of the mother's father, not to mention the child's own father.[2]

At 20-week fetal age to 30-week fetal age in the human female there are about seven million oocytes present in the ovary which, by about 40-week fetal age become enveloped by granulosa cells, forming follicles containing ova which are already in the prophase of meiotic division. During later fetal life and childhood, these follicles undergo successive waves of development and atresia, the number of primordial follicles falling from a maximum of two million just before birth to about 300,000 in the adult.[40] Should the fetus suffer from inadequate nutrition, these egg-cells, like all tissues of the fetus, may be detrimentally affected. The process of mitosis, from interphase, through prophase, metaphase, anaphase, to telophase, takes about 18 hours, and meiosis almost as long.[75] During those fundamental phases of genetic development, almost anything can happen to the cellular structures as a consequence of inadequate nutrition. Not only the female, but also the male who has himself suffered from malnutrition during his postnatal life may also have suffered some damage to his gonadal tissues. These are not conjectures. We know them to be very real possibilities. For a detailed discussion of the effects of malnutrition upon offspring, reference may be made to the excellent book on disadvantaged children by Herbert B. Birch and Joan Dye Gussow.[6] Morbidity, mortality, and teratogenic rates are significantly higher in the children of malnourished pregnant women than in those who were adequately nourished. Height, weight, and intelligence are also lower in the children of malnourished mothers. These are important facts, and they have long been known, even though the relation of fetal and childhood malnutrition to lowered intelligence does not seem to have stirred those who should have been most impressed by it. The physicalistic or biogenic bias seems to have been largely responsible for the failure to recognize the role played by social conditions in the causation of physical and behavioral deficiencies.

Maternal malnutrition in relation to impairment of the offspring has received some attention, but the role of paternal malnutrition in producing deficits in his offspring has been largely neglected. Stieve has shown, both in other animals and in man, that malnutrition may severely injure the sexual tissues in both male and female. Stieve found that stressful conditions of any kind may damage the development of sperm, and that such sperm fertilizing a normal ovum may jeopardize the healthy development of the conceptus. Stieve also found that at the very moment the female undergoes a stressful experience "and there is in the ovary a follicle ready to emerge or almost so, it does not erupt, but instead collapses and the whole follicle degenerates."[37, 69-71] Stress in the mother may have a more or less damaging effect upon the ovary as a whole or upon specific ova in it. Selye and others have produced abundant evidence that in rats the characteristic response of the female sex organs to systemic stress manifests itself mainly by ovarian atrophy and more or less permanent suppression of the female sex cycle (anestrus).[67] Physiologically these changes are known to be due to decreased gonadotrophin production from the anterior lobe of the pituitary. It is highly probable that a similar mechanism, under similar conditions, is at work in the human female.[26, 75] To malnutrition, and as a factor entirely apart from it, resulting from the pressures of a disadvantaged socioeconomic environment must be added stress. It is known that stress alone is capable of exerting all sorts of unfavorable effects upon the developing conceptus and child. Interaction of stress with the genotype is discussed in Joffe's book *Prenatal Determinants of Behaviour*[39] and in my own book *Prenatal Influences.*[53] Stott, in his book *Studies of Troublesome Children,*[74] has stated the case for prenatal neural damage to the fetus of the stressed pregnant mother. The harm may vary from actual damage to brain tissue to abnormalities of metabolism impinging on brain tissue. Göllnitz has proposed a syndromic axis with the milder forms including overreactivity, distractibility, stimulus domination, variability of mood, of motivation, and of bodily function, and general behavior disturbance. The more severe forms comprise emotional explosiveness, rage responses, passivity, loss of insight, slowing up of thought processes, and general personality disintegration.[28] Birch speaks of brain damage as referring to a behavior syndrome and not to the fact of brain damage as such,[5] and this may well apply to dysfunctional behavior resulting from temporary impairments of brain function, such as the conditions he describes, namely, development lag, behavior disturbance, motor awkwardness, minor perceptual disturbance, and distractibility. To these malfunctions Stott would add a number of symptoms indicative of inefficient neural control or regulation of the soma: poor vocal articulation, faults of homeostasis, enuresis, excessive sweating or salivation, choroid movements, restless or overheavy sleep, and "hysterical" pains and disabilities.[74]

It would be quite misleading to suggest that we understand the nature of the morphological or metabolic counterparts of these phenomena. We do not. In the absence of firm evidence of brain damage in behavioral impairments of disorders, the inference can at best be presumptive only. Stott[74] therefore suggests that we use the less tendentious term neural impairment or neural dysfunction in preference to brain damage. The suggestion has merit for some of the less severe deficits or impairments to which Stott refers and which were characteristic of his disadvantaged troublesome children. My purpose here, however, is to suggest that there exists a whole range of behavioral deficits caused by brain damage which, though not irreversible, constitutes, while it exists, a more or less severe impediment to learning and social development, all of which is sociogenic in origin. Hence while agreeing with Stott that neural impairment or dysfunction may be a better term for the milder forms of behavioral disorders he has considered, I shall here be discussing the disorders which I believe are due to sociogenic brain damage.

EARLY MALNOURISHMENT

There is a universal embryogenic law to the effect that the earlier the noxious influences to which the organism is exposed the more severe is the developmental damage. This law extends to the whole developmental period, and especially to the earlier stages of prenatal development. The living organism is so sensitive that even after it has achieved full growth and development, unfavorable environmental influences may severely adversely affect the organism at any time during later life. This was tragically demonstrated by what happened to many concentration-camp victims of the Nazis during World War II. For example, among a group of Norwegians who had been prisoners of the Nazis, those who had been in the concentration camps the longest, and had suffered the severest deprivations and abuses, presented the most serious evidence of impairment of brain function and structure. "Late sequelae of the suffering and misery," writes Wolff, "were major behavior disturbances and even degenerative changes in the brain. . . . Defects were roughly proportional to the duration and intensity of the abuse" (Ref. 84, p. 209). Such were the effects of stress on fully developed adults. It would hardly be a bold speculation to suggest that similar stresses may be transmitted, in humoral and metabolic forms, through the placenta to the tissues of the developing conceptus and especially to the brain. Man's total number of cortical brain cells, 13 billion, appears to be established by 25 fetal weeks of age. On experimental animals, the evidence indicates that behavior disturbances as a consequence of damaging environmental effects may be irreversible.[8] There is good evidence that chromosomal structure may be so affected, even to the extent of disturbing chromosomal mechanisms and resulting in such disorders as Down's syndrome.[22, 53, 73] Recent research indicates that behavior may be seriously affected as a result of metabolic disturbances in the monoamines of the brain, the catecholamines, norepinephrine and dopamine, and the indole amine, serotonin, acting differentially in the different parts of the brain in which they are mostly found.[65, 45]

That socioeconomic environmental factors may determine the conditions which directly affect the very elements that influence the constitutional development of the individual, long before that individual is even conceived, and substantively after conception, is now no longer disputable.

In the 14 largest cities of the United States in 1950, approximately 1 child out of 10 was culturally underprivileged or deprived. By 1960, this figure had risen to one in three.[58] In 1970, this figure approached almost one in two enrolled in the public schools of these large cities.[58] In the Santiago slums, in Chile, Dr. Fernando Mönckeberg found that 45% of the preschool children were mentally deficient, while between 60 and 70% were malnourished.[50,51] There can be very little doubt that much the same conditions prevail in the slums of other impoverished regions virtually everywhere in the Americas. Throughout the Americas there is a high positive correlation between poor socioeconomic conditions and malnutrition—low per capita income, illiteracy, low cultural level, bad sanitary conditions, low intellectual performance of the underprivileged groups, and, finally, racial and religious prejudices. Faced as we are with a coming world situation in which there will be less and less food for more and more people, a world in which the complexities of the social and political conditions thus exacerbated will render even more difficult the problems which will confront us, the challenge presented becomes urgently more pressing each hour, and with each hour the time grows shorter.

It has been conservatively estimated that the total number of malnourished children in the world between the ages of 1 and 6 years reached 269 million in 1966, 276 million in 1967, 329 million in 1968,[48] well over 400 million in 1969, and well over 460 million in 1970. By the end of this century, when world population is expected to double to over seven billion, it is more than likely, if present trends continue, that there will be more than a billion malnourished children on this earth, and that 80% of all inhabitants will be living in those parts of the world in which hunger is now a predominant everyday fact of life.

Dr. Mönckeberg's findings in Santiago present a shocking example of conditions that are not only widespread throughout the Americas but are also reported from many other parts of the world.[30] Furthermore, those findings present something of a forecast of the shape of things to come should we fail to take the proper measures in time. Hence it is important to set out Dr. Mönckeberg's findings, and to reflect upon their meaning.

Dr. Mönckeberg found that only 51% of his malnourished preschool children had a normal development quotient of over 85. The percentage of adequately nourished children rated as normal from the slums (95%) was very similar (97%) for the children from middle-class homes in Santiago.

In 150 preschool children from a very low-class homogeneous population, in which malnutrition was prevalent, Dr. Mönckeberg found a marked difference in intellectual capacity in children whose weights were under the third percentile on a standard scale and had a marked growth retardation, as compared with those children whose weights were over the tenth percentile and were considered nutritionally normal. A very significant relationship was found between the degree of growth retardation, when outside the normal limits, and psychomotor development.

In addition to growth retardation, these children had smaller heads than those of 500 adequately nourished middle-class children. These deficits in cranial growth were significantly correlated with decreased IQ. In infants with severe marasmus during the first months of life, not only is the head smaller, but the brain is disproportionately smaller than the head. In normal children, transillumination of the skull with a beam from a 500-W bulb directed at the top of the head will show a zone of illumination approximately 2 cm wide around the point of contact between the light and the child's head. In children with marasmus, a much larger portion of the skull is illuminated, and in many cases, the entire skull, thus dramatically indicating the massive retardation of brain growth in these children.

In order to determine whether the early effects of malnutrition could be reversed, Dr. Mönckeberg conducted a follow-up study on 14 children admitted to a hospital with severe malnutrition beginning during the first months of life. Following long periods of treatment in the hospital, the children continued to make outpatient visits and received 20 liters of free milk per month. At 3 to 6 years of age, the clinical appearance and biochemical index of these children appear to be normal. Weight is within normal limits, but the children are short for their age. Head circumference is below normal, and the average IQ is only 62, significantly below the average of Chilean preschool children from low socio-economic areas. In no case was a child's IQ above 76. Since it is well established that brain growth, consisting largely of protein synthesis, takes place early in the life of the child, Dr. Mönckeberg concluded "it is logical to assume that the effects of malnutrition during this critical period are permanent" (Ref. 50, pp. 30–31).

Cravioto, summarizing the results of many studies on the relation of malnutrition to development, concludes "that the existence of an association between protein-calorie malnutrition in infancy and retardation in mental development has been established beyond reasonable doubt. It can also be stated that there is a high probability that this lag in mental development may have long lasting consequences if severe malnutrition is experienced at a very early age in the life of the child" (Ref. 13, p. 12). In a similar survey, Eichenwald and Fry conclude: "Observations on animals and human infants suggest that malnutrition during a critical period of early life results in short stature and may, in addition, permanently and profoundly affect the future intellectual and emotional development of the individual" (Ref. 25, p. 648).

Since in malnutrition it would be expected that the lack of adequate protein and the vitamin and calorie deficiencies which are so often its accompaniments would affect the DNA and RNA that directs the formation of proteins, this has recently become the subject of inquiry. Winick and Rosso determined the amount of DNA in the brains of children who died of malnutrition as compared with the amount in the brains of normally nourished children. They found the amount of DNA in the brains of the malnourished children to be significantly less, thus indicating the presence of a substantially smaller number of brain cells. Head circumference, brain weight, and protein content were all reduced.[80-83] The protein-vitamin-calorie deficiencies may so affect DNA or RNA or both so that the mechanisms for incorporating amino acids into body proteins either cease to operate fully or function in abnormal ways.

Zamenhof and his co-workers have shown that deficient diets administered to female rats before and during pregnancy result in offspring that exhibit a substantial reduction in total brain DNA, and hence, presumably, in a reduction in the total number of brain cells. Such offspring also show behavioral deficiencies.[85, 86]

Myelination, cellular differentiation, development of arborizing collaterals between neurones,[15, 18-21, 64, 68] lipid production, and chemical structure of the nervous system[2,3] may all be seriously affected in the malnourished child with more or less serious consequences for its ability to learn or develop into a normally competent human being.[17, 30, 36, 57]

Stress factors of every sort are of the very essence of the life of the poor: physical illness, broken homes, malnutrition, emotional strain, and almost every kind of social deprivation. Every investigation that has ever been conducted on this subject has agreed that poverty or the poverty of emotional involvement is the principal cause of most of the developmental retardation encountered in human beings.[35, 62]

SOCIAL DEPRIVATION

Let us now turn our attention to a direct retardative influence on the development of the brain which is entirely the result of unfavorable social conditions. It has been known for many years that health, intelligence, achievement, and socially adequate behavior are highly correlated with socioeconomic factors: the better the socioeconomic environment the higher the scores achieved on all these parameters.[44] But more than that, the evidence is clear that the growth and development of the nervous system and the sense organs are greatly influenced by the social experience of the organism. One of the earliest, and now classical, experimental demonstrations of the effect of environmental experience on the development of the nervous system was George Ellett Coghill's investigation of the development of the salamander *Amblystoma punctatum,* set out in many papers and in his classic book *Anatomy and the Problem of Behaviour.*[11] Coghill showed that neuronal development was markedly more developed in stimulated than in nonstimulated animals. Axon terminals and the growth of collaterals was much more active in the stimulated than in the nonstimulated animals. Coghill concluded his book with the memorable words: "The real measure of the individual . . . whether lower animal or man, must include the element of growth as a creative power. Man is, indeed, a mechanism, but he is a mechanism which, within the limitations of life, sensitivity and growth, is creating and operating himself" (p. 110). The individual deprived of the stimulations necessary for the development of sensitivity and growth simply fails to develop in these modalities, and in the ability to create and operate himself.[1, 49, 78] For human beings, this is the greatest of all disasters. The greatest evil and the most enduring of all tragedies for the individual and his society lies in the difference between what he was capable of becoming and what he has in fact been caused to become.

It is of such sociogenically induced tragedies that I speak here. These tragedies and the mechanism of their production are of more than clinical interest, for there have always been those among us who have been eager to claim a genetic causation for such misfortunes, and to make such presumed and unsubstantiated genetic causes the basis for social policy. This has been especially so in connection with the problem-solving form of behavior we call intelligence, especially as allegedly measured by IQ tests.

Intelligence is something which develops as the result of the interaction of brain potentials with experience, nutritional and social. Fundamentally and functionally, intelligence is both a special and general ability resulting primarily from the social organization of brain potentials for the making of adaptive responses to the particular challenges of the environment. At birth, the brain is continuing the accelerated rate of growth which began during the last 2 months of intrauterine development, gaining weight at the rate of between 1 and 2 mg/minute, a rate which is continued throughout the first 6 months. By the end of this period, the brain has virtually doubled in size, from a weight of 350 to 656 g, a gain of 306 g. The size of this increment exceeds by far anything ever achieved this way again (see Table 1). By the end of the first year, the rate of increase has decelerated to half the rate of the first 6 months, when the brain attains a weight of 825 g. The same

TABLE 1. GROWTH OF THE HUMAN BRAIN

Fetus Lunar Months[a]	Weight (g)	Gain (g)	Percentage of Gain	
5	62.5	25.5	40.0	
6	88.0	25.5	29.0	
8	277.0	189.0	68.6	A threefold increase in weight in this two-month period.
9 birth	350/392	73/115	29.3	An increment of about a third the previous month's weight.
½ year	656.0	306.0	46.7	Almost doubles in weight in first six months.
1	825.0	169.0	20.5	Reduction to half rate of increase of first six months.
2	1010.0	185.0	18.3	Reduction to half rate of increase of first six months.
3	1115.0	105.0	9.4	Reduction to one-third rate of increase of first six months.
4	1180.0	75.0	6.4	Gradual deceleration of rate of growth.
6	1250.0	70.0	5.6	
9	1307.0	57.0	4.3	
12	1338.0	31.0	2.3	
20–29	1396.0	58.0	4.1	

[a] Lunar month = 29½ days.

decelerated rate is maintained during the whole of the second year, with the brain achieving a weight of 1010 g. During the third year, there is a further deceleration to one-third the rate of the first 6 months. And by the end of the third year, the brain of the average 3-year-old has achieved more than four-fifths of its maximum adult size. At the end of the third year, the child's brain weighs, on the average, 1115 g. When the brain attains its maximum size, at between 20 and 29 years, it will have added, in the additional 17 or so years, no more than 281 g to the grand total of 1396 g.

All the evidence suggests that during the long period of brain growth, and especially during the first critical 3 years, it is probably the first 6 months, when the brain in its most rapid phase of growth and when cell number is also increasing, that are the most critical.

CRITICAL PERIODS IN BRAIN DEVELOPMENT

The evidence further suggests that at birth the human neonate is only half gestated, and that he completes his gestation, like the little marsupial, outside the womb. This latter developmental period I have called *exterogestation*. It terminates when the infant begins to crawl about for himself, at about 9 or 10 months.[52] The infant of humankind is much more precariously poised in relation to the environment than we have been accustomed to think. He is born biologically premature in every respect, and it is during the first 6 months of postnatal life that the brain, continuing its fetal rate of growth, accomplishes all that packaging of cellular materials which will serve it for the rest of its life. The whole of the first 3 years of postnatal life will constitute the period of the experiential, the social, organization of those nervous tissues. The early first 3 years of rapid brain growth coincide with the fundamental learning period of the child, of the individual. Upon learning, that is, upon the social organization of his brain, almost the whole of the individual's later integrative behavioral abilities will depend. It is during this critical period that purely social environmental deficiencies may seriously and detrimentally affect the organization of the brain.

Such deficiencies often result in what may be termed the *social deprivation syndrome*. This syndrome is principally characterized by a short attention span and learning difficulties resulting in poor test performance. This is usually measured in a lower than normal IQ test score, in poor school and poor social performance. Such deficits are commonly attributed to genetic inadequacies. The difficulty is, indeed, that the social deprivation syndrome mimics the genetically influenced condition. Such mimicked conditions are known as phenocopies; that is to say, the apparent condition resembles the genetic one, but is in fact due to nongenetic causes. Much ink has been spilled and many a reputation lost in the sinuous convolutions of this difficult subject in the endeavor by many writers to show that such behavioral deficits are principally due to genetic factors.

There can be not the least doubt that there exist many behavioral deficits of this sort that are due to genetic deficiencies.[45] It is, therefore, of great importance to be able to distinguish the genetic conditions from the phenocopies. We cannot, at present, do much to prevent the birth of genetically influenced poor learners, but we can do a great deal to prevent the development of poor learners who owe their disability to nothing more nor less than a poor social environment.

With rather monotonous regularity there appear, at almost predictable intervals, elaborate studies which purport to show that certain racial or ethnic or social groups of other kinds are, on the whole, poorer learners and achievers and score significantly lower on IQ tests than the group to which the investigator happens to belong. Such reports invariably suffer the same eventual fate. They are lauded by those who prefer to believe what these studies purport to demonstrate, and are severely criticized and condemned by the experts. Following a period of perfervid discussion in the press, and partisan misuse in legislatures, the brouhaha generally dies down, and the entire incident is finally consigned to the archives in which such incidents are eventually preserved. In the meantime, aid and comfort has been given to racists, segregationists, those who perhaps should know better, and serves to fortify in their citadels of infallibility the half-educated and the many who have been "educated" beyond their intelligence.

The latest work of this kind is by Arthur R. Jensen, Professor of Educational Psychology at the University of California, Berkeley. In a study entitled "How much can we boost IQ and scholastic achievement?" published in the Winter 1969 issue of the *Harvard Educational Review,* Jensen argues that it is "a not unreasonable hypothesis that genetic factors are strongly implicated in the average Negro-White intelligence difference" (Ref. 38, p. 82). Jensen then proceeds to show what everyone has known since the initiation of intelligence testing, namely, that blacks on the average do not do as well on such tests as whites. As others have done before him, Jensen attributes this difference largely to the operation of genetic factors, believing as he does that the IQ test constitutes the best available method of measuring the genetic contribution to intelligence. As Lee Edson, an expositor of Jensen's claims, put it, intelligence, which Jensen "equates with the ability measured by IQ tests, is largely inherited, a matter of genes and brain structure, and therefore no amount of compensatory education or forced exposure to culture is going to improve it substantially" (p. 11). In brief, whatever it is that intelligence tests measure is, according to Jensen, intelligence. This is, of course, a circular definition, and therefore no definition at all. Furthermore, he holds that intelligence is largely genetically determined. It has been suggested that the only thing IQ tests really measure is the intelligence of the intelligence tester. I think there is more to be said for this suggestion than for that which proposes that IQ tests largely measure genetic intelligence, for the facts, derived from innumerable studies, indicate that what IQ tests measure is very far removed from the genetic potentials for intelligence: that what IQ tests measure represents the expression of the interaction between those genetic potentials and the nutritional, socioeconomic, emotional, motivational, and schooling experience of the individual.[34]

One wonders whether those who are so ready to settle for the genetic factor as the principal cause of the differences in IQ between blacks and whites would also hold that the enormous overall differences, at every age level, in morbidity and mortality rates, between those two groups are also due to genetic factors? Or that Messrs. Maddox of Georgia and Wallace of Alabama are where they are because of genetic factors, while no black has ever occupied a similar office in those states for similar "genetic" reasons? Whatever their views might be the evidence is overwhelming that these differences are principally due to social factors.[62]

Why is it that these racial ideologists refuse to acknowledge, even to consider, that social factors may be the principal causes responsible for the differences in learning abilities of different "racial" groups? Learning ability is highly correlated with social class within the same ethnic group.[14, 35, 44] What racists fail to understand is that in man "race" is, for all practical purposes, a social concept and an institutionalized way of behavior, a special form of social class, a caste status, and that as such it is subject to all the influences and consequences that flow from such facts.

The best answer to Jensen's equation, "How much can we boost IQ and scholastic achievement," is provided by the studies contained in the two volumes published by the Department of Health, Education and Welfare, entitled *A Report on Longitudinal Evaluations of Preschool Programs*. The first volume reports eight different Head Start programs[61]; the second volume deals with the importance of early intervention.[9] Both volumes demonstrate the enormous importance of the environment in influencing IQ test performance, and what amazing improvements can be achieved in this manner. The two volumes make the most dramatic and impressive reading.

That a significant genetic element contributes to the basic intelligence potential of every individual is beyond dispute. It should, however, be clear that, like every other genetic potential, the development of intelligence is perhaps more than any other trait dependent on the kind of environmental stimulations to which it is exposed. Instead of dismissing such environmental factors as unimportant in order to sustain even the veriest semblance of his claims, Jensen should have carefully investigated the possible effects of such environmental factors upon IQ test results. This he conspicuously failed to do, and for this reason alone his claims would have to be wholly rejected. To assign, as he does, a good 80% of an individual's intelligence to genetic factors and a mere 20% to environmental influences constitutes not only a scientifically groundless assumption but also a wholly indefensible one. For there exists a vast body of scientific evidence which indicates not that genetic potentials or environmental ones are more important than the other, but that both are of the greatest importance for the adequate development of intelligence. I have already made reference to some of the evidence indicating the damage that malnutrition can do to genetic potentials for intelligence. The evidence indicating the damage capable of being done by unfavorable socioeconomic conditions to the development of intelligence is even more extensive and conclusive. This evidence is set out in hundreds of independent studies ranging from Gladys Schwesinger's 1933 volume *Heredity and Environment* to the most recent publication on the subject, namely Cancro's symposium on *Intelligence: Genetic and Environmental Influences,*[10] Birch and Gussow's book on *Disadvantaged Children,*[6] and Hurley's book on *Poverty and Mental Retardation,*[36] not to mention many others.

The universal conclusion to which these researches point is that no matter what the quality of the genetic potentials for intelligence may be in any individual, the expression of those potentials will be significantly influenced by his total environment. Poverty as such is not necessarily either a necessary or a sufficient condition in the production of intellectual deficits, for if nutrition and the home cultural environment are adequate, the child will suffer no handicapping effects. But if nutrition is poor, health care deficient, housing debasing, family income low, family disorganization prevalent, discipline anarchic, ghettoization more or less complete, personal worth consistently diminished, expectations low, and aspirations frustrated, in addition to numerous other environmental handicaps, then one may expect the kind of failures in intellectual development that are so often gratuitously attributed to genetic factors. Those who make such attributions fail to understand how dependent the development of intelligence is upon the reduction of such conditions of privation, frustration, and hopelessness.[79] When the effects of such postnatal environmental factors are combined with the adverse effects of prenatal ones, there emerges a continuum of psychosocial, as well as psychophysical casualty, which renders it utterly nonsensical to compare casualties of such environments with the products of average middle class environments by whom and on whom IQ tests were devised. It is not simply the culture of poverty or even the poverty of culture or any other one single factor, but the combination of many socioenvironmental factors, which produces the sociogenic deficits so irresponsibly attributed to genetic factors. As Gladys Schwesinger pointed out at the conclusion of her book on *Heredity and Environment* in 1933, "the problem of heredity and environment is not a general problem, but is specific to each individual, to each of his characteristics, and to each environment" (Ref. 66, p. 465). In the development of so complex an ability as intelligence, making every allowance for possible differences in genetic endowment, the environment is of paramount importance. Just as the individual learns to speak, with vocabulary, imagery, and accent according to environmental influences that have been operative upon him, so he learns, within the limits of his genetic capacities, the vocabulary, imagery, and accent of intelligence, according to the environmental influences with which he has interacted. As Bodmer and Cavalli-Sforza have put it, "any given test . . . depends on the ability acquired at a given age, which is inevitably the result of the combination of innate ability and the experience of the subject. Intelligence tests are therefore at most tests of achieved ability" (Ref. 7, p. 19). And that is precisely the point. If seriously handicapping impediments are placed in the way of the individual's development of any capacity he will to that extent simply fail to achieve that ability, for abilities are trained capacities. Limiting environments place limits upon the development of abilities. In the matter of problem-solving, that is to say, intelligence, Harlow found that rhesus monkeys subjected to ambiguous rewards for tasks performed, so that no specific perceptual clues were available to the animals, were not nearly as effective problem-solvers as those in the control group who were consistently rewarded. Harlow thus showed that the learning sets which make insight possible do not come ready-made, but must be acquired, and that once acquired they increase the capacity of the organism to solve certain problems.[30, 32] Thompson and Heron have shown that pet-reared dogs in a variety of situations behave more intelligently than their litter-mates who have been caged for the first 8 months of their lives.[77] All animals thus far studied show the effects of early experience or its deprivation in much the same ways.[8]

Bennett, Rosenzweig, and Diamond have shown that exposure of rats to different environments—enriched, colony, or impoverished—leads to characteristic changes in wet and dry weight of samples of rat brain, in enzymatic activity, and in depth of cerebral cortex. Impoverished animals were caged singly, colony animals 2 or 3 per cage, and enriched animals 10 or 12 per larger cage including toys. In every case, dry weight depth of cerebral cortex, enzymatic activity, and problem-solving behavior were increased by exposure to enriched environment as compared with standard colony and impoverished conditions.[4, 60] In mice, Henderson found that an enriched environment resulted in an increase in brain weight.[33]

Since the internal consistency of the evidence for other animals fully agrees with that obtained in studies of man, there can remain little doubt that for the development of innumerable behavioral traits, but especially for the development of intelligence the stimulation of certain kinds of social experience is indispensable.[47, 70] It is, in a word, experience of an encouraging kind, as contrasted to experiences of a discouraging kind, the experiences of an advantaging kind that count, as contrasted with experiences of a disadvantaging kind.

When we consider the complexity of the factors operating upon the child the sociogenic brain damage done in man must be very considerable indeed, for there can be no question that brain damage is involved when size, weight, failure of cortical development, quantity and size of brain cells, and enzymatic activity of the brain are the effects of a socially impoverished environment.

Jensen so completely fails to understand the nature of socially disadvantaging conditions he actually believes that the children of blacks and whites of similar income level enjoy equal cultural and other environmental advantages. Hence, since these children, according to Jensen, enjoy similar environmental experiences, the differences in IQ test results must be due to genetic factors. What Jensen fails to understand is that income level alone does not determine the quality of cultural background, and that it is quite unsound to equate the two. There is no income level at which blacks enjoy the same basic opportunities as whites. By basic opportunities I mean a sustaining cultural background of stimulation which encourages the growth and development of aspirations for achievement, a cultural background in which one does not suffer from malnutrition of the body or the mind, in which one has not suffered severe emotional, economic, social, and educational privations, but to which, in most of these respects, a positive rather than a negative sign is attached.[56]

The truth is that at no time have blacks of any income group enjoyed anything approaching equal basic opportunities with whites.[55] It is, therefore, quite unsound to attribute to genetic factors what may well be due to environmental ones.[42]

What is quite certain is that IQs vary with environmental experience. It is, for example, well known that American Indians generally test out at about 80 IQ points. But, interestingly enough, when oil is discovered on Indian land and the Indians are permitted to share in the accruing profits, there is a spectacular rise in Indian IQs. There is nothing mysterious about this. The oil simply facilitates the lubrication of intelligence potentials by making the conditions available which enable Indian children to enjoy a social and economic environment similar to that enjoyed by white children. Under such conditions, among the Osage Indians of Oklahoma, for example, Rohrer found that on one test, the Goodenough "Draw-a-man" test, the white children obtained an average IQ of 103, and the Indian children an average of 104. On a second test, using language, the Indian children scored 100 and the white children scored 98.[59]

Similarly, Garth found that a group of Indian children living in white foster homes obtained an average IQ of 102, which is a quite significant improvement over an IQ of 80. The brothers and sisters of this group still living on the reservation obtained an average IQ of 87.5[27]

Clearly, the environmental differences were principally responsible for the differences in the scores of these children. There is no question of brain damage being involved here—simply a difference in environment. Nor, for that matter was a difference in genetic intelligence involved, for clearly that is not what these test results reflected; what they reflected was a difference in environmental experience acting upon genetic potentials for the ability to respond to IQ tests. It is not that the lower testing siblings were any less intelligent than their higher testing siblings, but that they were less experienced in the requirements necessary to meet the challenges of those tests.

Since genetic factors are involved in virtually all forms of behavior, there can be little doubt that such factors play a significant role in performance on IQ tests. But that is a very different thing from claiming that IQ tests measure the genetic contribution to intelligence. Scarr-Salapatek has published a study in which she found differences in heritability of IQ scores in black and white and in social and class groups.[63] The differences are in the expected directions and could have been predicted. Scarr-Salapatek sees the variance in performance as difference, *not* as deficit, and she welcomes these differences as contributing to the greater enrichment and variety of humanity. "To the extent," she writes "that better, more supportive environments can be provided for all children, genetic variance and mean scores will increase for all groups" (p. 1295). Indeed, "equality of opportunity" will lead "to bigger and better genotype-phenotype correlations" (p. 1295), but meanwhile, it needs to be emphasized, so long as the inequalities in opportunities remain, so long will the misery and poor performance on IQ tests and in life situations remain for millions of the socially deprived.

There are many flaws in IQ tests, and among those usually overlooked by those who administer and evaluate these tests is the fact that a difference of as much as 20 points can be produced in IQ scores depending upon the mood or attitude of the testee. Feelings toward the person administering the test can be an important factor in influencing performance on tests. Katz, Heuchy, and Allen[41] found that Negro boys of grade-school age performed better on verbal learning tasks with Negro examiners than with white examiners. Watson found that West Indian students in a London secondary school in a working class neighborhood scored an average of 10 points less on IQ tests than when the same tests were falsely described as an experiment to help curriculum. Watson, who is white, also found that when the tests were given by his assistant, a "very black" West Indian, the scores typically climbed.[79]

Similarly, Katz has found that Black students did better on IQ tests when they were deceived into believing that their intelligence was not being tested. Black students, when they were freed of anxiety about intellectual performance, achieved higher IQ scores under a white investigator than a black one.[17]

With little expectation of overcoming the judgment of their intellectual inferiority, which they knew to be held by many white Americans, the students' motivation was low, and so were their scores. But when the IQ test was disguised as something else, human ambition soared. As long as their intelligence was not being evaluated, they felt more challenged to show the white examiner what they could do than one of their own kind.

The expectation of inadequate performance on IQ tests undoubtedly contributes to the lower performance of blacks on these tests. Conversely, confidence bolstered by some successes raises scores by 5 to 10 points.

I am not aware that either Jensen or Scarr-Salapatek made any allowance for such factors.

Cooper and Zubek in an interesting experiment have shown how in different genetic lines different environments may serve either to develop or depress problem-solving capacities. These investigators used two lines of rats whose ability to find their way through a maze had been especially selected by selective breeding. When rats from the "bright" and "dull" lines were raised for a whole generation in a restricted environment which differed from the normal laboratory environment, no differences between the lines could be found. The bright and dull performed at the same level. When both were raised in the same stimulating environment, both did almost equally well. In a normal environment, bright rats made 120 errors, whereas the dull ones made 168. In a restricted environment, both made about 170 errors, but in a stimulating environment, the bright made 112 errors while the dull made 120.[12]

Levitsky and Barnes[46] found that early malnutrition and isolation in rats during the first 7 weeks of postnatal life led to various behavioral sequelae. Compared with the controls the experimental animals showed a significant increase in open field locomotion, an increase, but not statistically significant, in mutual grooming, a reduction in following response, an increase in fighting time, and a marked depression in exploratory behavior. These investigators found that in all the observed responses, except fighting, whatever effect early malnutrition produced it was always exaggerated by environmental isolation and depressed by environmental stimulation. They found, also, that the behavioral effects of the malnutrition were completely eliminated in most cases by additional stimulation early in life.

The theoretical mechanisms the authors suggest as possibly explaining the mechanisms through which malnutrition and environmental stimulation may interact to produce long term behavioral changes are two. This explanation applies with equal cogency to the social deprivation syndrome.

Malnutrition may alter the experience or perception of the environment during early development by rendering the organism physiologically less capable of receiving and/or integrating environmental information. Decreases in brain size, brain DNA, myelinization, cortical dendritic growth, brain cholinesterase content, and brain norepinephrine control have all been reported in malnourished animals. Environmental stimulation produces changes in brain norepinephrine, cholinesterase, as well as cortical dendritic growth. Hence malnutrition during a critical period of development may produce the changes that render inoperative the physiological mechanisms that are responsible for the long-term effects of early stimulation.

> Another mechanism through which early malnutrition and environmental variables may interact may be purely behavioral in nature. Malnutrition may produce behavior that is incompatible with the incorporation of environmental information necessary for optimum cognitive growth. In the case of a malnourished animal, the behavior may be primarily food oriented and in the case of a malnourished child, the behavior may be expressed as apathy and social withdrawal.[43]

Thus, specific kinds of information or specific behavioral responses which may be required for optimum cognitive development as reflected by test behavior or educational performance may be absent or depressed in the malnourished child as a result of a higher priority of responses elicited by the malnutrition.

> The demonstration of a behavioral interaction between early nutritional conditions and the environment of young animals not only demonstrates the complexity of understanding determinants of behavior, but also points out the profundity of early experience and early nutrition as major contributors to ultimate adult behavior (Ref. 46, pp. 70–71).

The power of the environment is clearly very considerable indeed, and the earlier it affects the developing organism the more substantive are its effects. The point I wish to make here is that brain damage is no less brain damage when the social stimuli necessary for mental development are inadequate or rendered ambiguous or confusing, than when the physical nutrition necessary for adequate cerebral development is insufficient. The brain damage done by social deprivation, even though it may be more occult, is, in its behavioral consequences, at least as substantial as that done by physical malnutrition.

To conclude, the evidence clearly indicates that during the first 3 years, when the basic foundations and organization of the brain are in the process of construction, inadequate provision and poor quality of experience may seriously affect the fabric of the brain, of which the mind is presumably a function. In such cases, the brain and mind are rendered incapable of later organization at levels of cognitive integration matching those achieved by others who have not suffered such sociogenic damage.

In such cases, the brain may not have been damaged in quite the same manner as it may be by physical malnutrition, but the damage done by social malnutrition is nonetheless real. This, we may postulate, consists in the disabling failure of organization which, both structurally and functionally, renders it extremely difficult if not impossible for individuals to respond appropriately to many of the challenges of the environment with the competence that their genetic potentials would, under the organizing stimulation of an adequate social environment, have permitted. Social malnourishment, both structurally and functionally, can be just as brain/ mind damaging as physical malnourishment. Such sociogenic malnourishment affects the brains of millions of human beings not only in the United States but all over the world. It is a form of brain damage which has received far too little attention. Yet it constitutes an epidemic problem of major proportions. What it calls for is, first, the recognition that the problem exists, second that it can only be solved by those improvements in the environment which will assure every newborn baby the realization of its birthright, which is development of its potentialities to the optimum.

We are each of us part of the problem. The question is whether we are going to remain parts of the problem or make ourselves part of the solution.

REFERENCES

1. Ambrose, A. (Ed.): *Stimulation in Early Infancy,* Academic Press, New York, 1969.
2. Bass, N. H., Netsky, M. G., and Young E.: Effect of neonatal malnutrition on developing cerebrum. *Arch. Neurol.* 23:289–302, 1970.
3. Bass, N. H., Netsky, M. G., and Young E.: Microchemical and histologic study of myelin formation in the rat. *Arch. Neurol.* 23:303–313, 1970.
4. Bennett, E. L., Rosenzweig, M. R., and Diamond, M. C.: Rat brain: Effects of environmental enrichment on wet and dry weights. *Science* 163:825–826, 1969.
5. Birch, H. G. (Ed.): *Brain Damage in Children: Its Biological and Social Aspects,* Williams & Wilkins, Baltimore, 1964.
6. Birch, H. G., and Gussow, J. D.: *Disadvantaged Children,* Harcourt, Brace & World, New York, 1969.
7. Bodmer, W. F., and Cavalli-Sforza, L. L.: Intelligence and race. *Sci. Am.* 223:19–29, 1970.
8. Bronfenbrenner, U.: Early deprivation in mammals: a cross-species analysis. In *Early Experience and Behavior,* G. Newton and S. Levene (Eds.), C. C. Thomas, Springfield, Illinois, pp. 627–764, 1968.
9. Bronfenbrenner, U.: Is early intervention effective? Department of Health, Education and Welfare Publication No. 74-24, 1974.
10. Cancro, R. (Ed.): *Intelligence: Genetic and Environmental,* Grune & Stratton, New York, 1971.

11. Coghill, G. E.: *Anatomy and the Problem of Behaviour,* Cambridge University Press, Cambridge, 1929.

12. Cooper, R. M., and Zubek, J. P.: Effects of enriched and restricted early environments on the learning ability of bright and dull rats. *Can. J. Psychol.* **12**:159-164, 1958.

13. Cravioto, J.: Complexity of factors involved in protein-calorie malnutrition. In *Malnutrition is a Problem of Ecology,* P. György and O. L. Kline (Eds.), Karger, Basel and New York, pp. 7-22, 1970.

14. Davidson, H. H.: *Personality and Economic Background,* King's Crown Press, New York, 1943.

15. Davison, A. N. and Dobbing, J.: Myelination as a vulnerable period in brain development. *Br. Med. Bull.* **22**:40-44, 1968.

16. Deutsch, M., and Associates: *The Disadvantaged Child,* Basic Books, New York, 1967.

17. Deutsch, M., Katz, I., and Jensen, R. (Eds.): *Social Class, Race, and Psychological Development,* Holt, Rinehart & Winston, New York, 1968.

18. Dobbing, J.: The influence of nutrition on the development of the brain. *Proc. R. Soc. Lond. Ser. B. Biol. Sci.* **159**:503-509, 1964.

19. Dobbing, J.: Effects of experimental undernutrition on development of the nervous system. In *Malnutrition, Learning and Behavior.* N. S. Grimshaw and J. E. Gordon (Eds.), M.I.T. Press, Cambridge, pp. 181-202, 1968.

20. Dobbing, J.: Undernutrition and the developing brain. *Am. J. Dis. Child.* **120**:411-415, 1970.

21. Dobbing, T.: Food for thinking. *New Sci.* **46**:636-637, 1970.

22. Drillien, C. M. and Wilkinson, E. M.: Emotional stress and mongoloid births. *Dev. Med. Child Neurol.* **6**:140-143, 1964.

23. Edson, L.: The theory that I.Q. is largely determined by the genes. *New York Times Magazine,* **August 31,** pp. 10-11, 40-41, 43-47, 1969.

24. Eells, K., and others: *Intelligence and Cultural Differences,* University of Chicago Press, Chicago, 1951.

25. Eichenwald, H. F. and Fry, P. C.: Nutrition and learning. *Science* **163**:644-648, 1969.

26. Gantt, W. Horsley: Disturbance in sexual function during periods of stress. In *Life Stress and Bodily Disease,* H. G., Wolff, S. G. Wolff, Jr., and C. C. Hare (Eds.) Williams & Wilkins, Baltimore, pp. 1030-1050, 1950.

27. Garth, T. R.: A study of the foster Indian child in the white home. *Psychol. Bull.* **32**:708-709, 1935.

28. Göllnitz, G.: Uber die Problematik der Neurosen im Kindesalter. *Ideggyogyaszat. Sz.* **16**:97-108, 1963-1964.

29. Grotberg, E. (Ed.): *Critical issues in Research Related to Disadvantaged Children,* Educational Testing Service, Princeton, New Jersey, 1969.

30. György, P. and Kline, O. L. (Eds.): *Malnutrition is a Problem of Ecology,* Karger, Basel and New York, 1970.

31. Harlow, H. F.: The formation of learning sets. *Psychol. Rev.* **56**:51-65, 1949.

32. Harlow, H. F.: Learning and satiation of response in intrinsically motivated complex puzzle performance by monkeys. *J. Comp. Physiol. Psychol.* **43**:289-294, 1958.

33. Henderson, N.D.: Brain weight increases resulting from environmental enrichment: a directional dominance in mice. *Science* **169**:776-778, 1970.

34. Hunt, J. McV.: *Intelligence and Experience,* Ronald Press Co. New York, 1961.

35. Hunt, J. McV.: *The Challenge of Incompetence and Poverty*, University of Illinois Press, Urbana, 1969.

36. Hurley, R. L.: *Poverty and Mental Retardation: A Causal Relationship*, Random House, New York, 1969.

37. Iagrashi, M., Tohma, K., and Ozama, M.: Pathogenesis of psychogenic amenorrhea and anovulation. *Int. J. Fertil.* **10**:311–319, 1965.

38. Jensen, A.: How much can we boost I.Q. and scholastic achievement? *Harv. Educ. Rev.* **39**:1–123, 1969.

39. Joffe, J. M.: *Prenatal Determinants of Behaviour*, Pergamon Press, New York, 1969.

40. Kase, N. G.: The ovary. In *Duncan's Diseases of Metabolism*, Vol. 2, P. K. Bondy (Ed.), Saunders, Philadelphia, pp. 1191–1226, 1969.

41. Katz, I., Heuchy, T., and Allen, H.: Effects of race of tester, approval, disapproval, and need on negro children's learning. *J. Pers. Soc. Res.* **8**:38–42, 1968.

42. Klineberg, O.: *Social Psychology*, Rev. ed., Holt, Rinehart & Winston, New York, 1954.

43. Latham, M. C.: In *Calorie and Protein Deficiencies*, R. A. McCance and E. M. Widdowson (Eds.), Cambridge University Press, New York and London, pp. 23–32, 1968.

44. Lesser, G. S., Fifer, G., and Clark, L. H.: Mental abilities of children from different social-class and cultural groups. *Monogr. Soc. Res. Child Growth Dev.* **30** 4, 1965.

45. Levitan, M., and Montagu, A.: *A Textbook of Human Genetics*, Oxford University Press, New York, 1971.

46. Levitsky, D. A. and Barnes, R. H.: Nutritional and environmental interactions in the behavioral development of the rat: long term behavior effects. *Science* **176**:68–71, 1972.

47. Light, R. J. and Smith, P. J.: Social allocation models of intelligence. *Harv. Educ. Rev.* **39**:484–510, 1969.

48. May, J. M. and Lemons, H.: The ecology of malnutrition, *J. A. M. A.* **207**:2401–2405, 1969.

49. Michael, R. P. (Ed.), *Endocrinology and Human Behavior*, Oxford University Press, New York, 1968.

50. Mönckeberg, F.: Mental retardation from malnutrition: 'irreversible . . .' *J.A.M.A.* **206**:30–31, 1968.

51. Mönckeberg, F.: Factors conditioning malnutrition in Latin America, with special reference to Chile. Advices for a volunteers action. In *Malnutrition Is a Problem of Ecology*, P. Gyorgy and O. L. Kline (Eds.), Karger Basel and New York, 23–33, 1970.

52. Montagu, A.: Neonatal and infant immaturity in man. *J.A.M.A.* **178**:56–57, 1961.

53. Montagu, A.: *Prenatal Influences*, C. C. Thomas, Springfield, Illinois, 1962.

54. Montagu, A.: *Man's Most Dangerous Myth: The Fallacy of Race*, 5th ed., Oxford University Press, New York, 1974.

55. Montagu, A.: Just what is "equal opportunity"? *Vista* **6**:23–25, 56, 1970.

56. Montagu, A. (Ed.): *Race and IQ*, Oxford University Press, New York, 1975.

57. Osler, S. F., and Cooke, R. E., (Eds.): *The Biosocial Basis of Mental Retardation*, The Johns Hopkins Press, Baltimore, 1965.

58. Reissman, F.: *The Culturally Deprived Child*, Harper & Row, New York, 1962.

59. Rohrer, J. H.: The test intelligence of Osage Indians. *J. Soc. Psychol.* **16**:99–105, 1942.

60. Rosenzweig, M. R., Krech, D., Bennett, E. L., and Diamond, M. C.: Modifying brain chemistry and anatomy by enrichment or impoverishment of experience. In *Early*

Experience and Behavior, G. Newton and S. Levine (Eds.), C. C. Thomas, Springfield, Illinois, pp. 258–298, 1968.

61. Ryan, S.: A report on longitudinal evaluations of preschool programs, Department of Health, Education and Welfare Publication No. 74-24, 1974.

62. Sanders, B. S.: *Environment and Growth,* Warwick & York, Baltimore, 1934.

63. Scarr-Salapatek, S.: Race, social class, and IQ. *Science* **174:**1285–1295, 1971.

64. Schapiro, S., and Vukovich, K. R.: Early experience effects upon cortical dendrites: a proposed model for development. *Science* **165:**293–294, 1970.

65. Schildkraut, J. J., and Kety, S. S.: Biogenic amines and emotion. *Science* **156:**21–30, 1967.

66. Schwesinger, G.: *Heredity and Environment,* Macmillan, New York, 1933.

67. Selye, H.: *Stress,* Acta, Inc., Montreal, 1950.

68. Sterman, M. B., McGinty, D. J., and Adinolfi, A. M. (Eds.): *Brain Development and Behavior,* Academic Press, New York, 1971.

69. Stieve, H.: Der Einfluss von Angst und psychischer Eregnung auf Bau und funktion der weiblichen Geschlechtsorgane. *Zentralbl. Gynäkol.* **66:**1698–1708, 1942.

70. Stieve, H.: Anatomisch nachweisbare Vorgänge im Eierstock des Menschen und ihre Umweltbedingte Steuerung. *Geburtshiffe Frauenheilk.* **9:**639–644, 1949.

71. Stieve, H.: *Der Einfluss des Nervens Systems auf Bau und Totigkeit der Geschlechtsorgane des Menschen.* Georg Thieme, Stuttgart, 1951.

72. Stinchcombe, A. L.: Environment: the cumulation of events. *Harv. Educ. Rev.* **39:**511–522, 1969.

73. Stott, D. H.: Mongolism related to emotional shock in early pregnancy. *Vita Hum.* **4:**57–76, 1961.

74. Stott, D. H.: *Troublesome Children,* Humanities Press, New York, 1966.

75. Swanson, C. P.: *The Cell,* 2nd ed., Prentice Hall, Englewood Cliffs, New Jersey, 1964.

76. Taylor, H. C.: Life situations, emotions and gynecologic pain associated with congestion. In *Life Stress and Bodily Disease,* H. G. Wolff, S. G. Wolff Jr., and C. C. Hare, (Eds.), Williams and Wilkins, Baltimore, pp. 1051–1056, 1950.

77. Thompson, W. R. and Heron, W.: The effects of restricting early experience on the problem-solving capacity of dogs. *Can. J. Psychol.* **8:**17–31, 1954.

78. Tobach, E., Aronson, L. R., and Shaw, E. (Eds.): *The Biopsychology of Development,* Academic Press, New York, 1971.

79. Watson, P.: How race affects I.Q. *New Society (London),* **July 16.** pp. 103–104, 1970.

80. Winick, M.: Nutrition and cell growth. *Nutr. Rev.* **26:**195–197, 1968.

81. Winick, M.: Fetal malnutrition and growth processes. *Hosp. Pract.* **May:** 33–41, 1970.

82. Winick, M. and Rosso, P.: The effect of severe malnutrition on cellular growth of the human brain. *Pediat. Res.* **3:**181–184, 1969.

83. Winick, M. and Rosso, P.: Head circumference and cellular growth of the brain in normal and marasmic children. *J. Pediat.* **74:**774–778, 1969.

84. Wolff, H. G.: *Stress and Disease,* 2nd ed. C. C. Thomas, Springfield, Illinois, 1968.

85. Zamenhof, S., Van Marthens, E., and Margolis, F. L.: DNA (cell number) and protein deficiency in neonatal brain: alteration by maternal dietary protein restriction. *Science* **160:**322–323, 1968.

86. Margolis, F. L.: DNA (cell number) in neonatal brain: second generation (F_2) alteration by maternal (F_0) dietary protein restriction. *Science* **172:**850–851, 1971.

CHAPTER TWO

CROWDING AND
SOCIAL VELOCITY

JOHN B. CALHOUN, PH.D.

$$W$$hen humans, or other social mammals, are studied in depth, it is commonly observed that members of groups vary widely with respect to the frequency of engaging in social interaction. At the lower range of participation in social life, individuals may be so withdrawn as to be essentially out of contact with the social milieu. Our studies of rodents have resulted in a formulation of this process of behavioral, psychological, and social differentiation. The purpose of this chapter is simply to describe this formulation concisely.

In our studies of mice (*Mus musculus*) and rats (*Rattus norvegicus*) we systematically record the frequency with which each individual is active or alert in public space. Individuals differ markedly in this measure of their kinetics, which is termed social velocity. It measures the physical distance traversed per unit of time and reflects the individual's movement through social space. High-velocity individuals are socially dominant and exhibit the full repertoire of behavior essential for species survival. As velocity decreases behavior becomes more simplified, aberrant, and fragmented, and the proportion of time spent in social interactions while active also declines.

OPTIMUM GROUP SIZE

Individuals of many species of mammals exhibit strong attachments to one or a few places near the center of their respective ranges. This is particularly true for those species with altricial young whose dependency on their mother requires that she return to the home site containing the young after each of her episodes of foraging. The evolved pattern of roaming through the terrain about a home site is one in which ever fewer trips are made to successively greater distances. As a consequence, resources are utilized more intensively nearer home than farther from it. Effective utilization of resources requires that the ranges of neighboring individuals overlap sufficiently to produce an equal impact on all portions of the habitat. When this degree of overlap occurs, each individual has contact with its 6 nearest neighbors and its 12 next-nearest neighbors. These contacts with neighbors culminate in loose social groups, even among fairly solitarily living mammals. Such groups have a mean size of 12. Gradually, through species evolution, such groups become more compact, until all members may live at the same place, or even travel together.

Twelve as the typical mean number of *adults* in a social group stands out as the central tendency of mammalian evolution. The human species arose out of such a lineage. Mice and rats tend to develop groups of about 12 adults in their natural habitat. Once a particular typical group size evolves, the behavioral capacities of individuals, expressed in a usual physical environmental context, produces a particular mean number of contacts between one individual and its associates. For each kind of social interaction there is some particular intensity or duration that optimizes gratification with respect to the number of contacts which transpire each day. Once this change in heredity culminates, a species may be said to be characterized by a particular optimum group size.

BEHAVIORAL DIFFERENTIATION

Every individual within a group is, from time to time, in a state of readiness to interact with some other individual. When two such individuals interact, each gains some satisfaction from the interaction that adds to its total gratification from social living. At the termination of such an interaction, each individual passes into a refractory state, whose duration is proportional to the intensity of the interaction. Should another individual, ready for social intercourse, meet one in a refractory state, the interaction will not prove satisfactory. It will then enter a frustrating or unsatisfying refractory period. The vagaries of chance encounters culminate in some individuals experiencing more frustration than others. As behavior toward another is less frequently reinforced by appropriate responses by the partner, behavior becomes more deviant, and the frustrated individual avoids contact with others. This avoidance takes such forms as reduced movement and alertness or avoidance of places inhabited by behaviorally more competent associates. All such differentiation takes place even in an optimal-sized group living under the most favorable circumstances.

BASIC ASPECTS OF SOCIAL VELOCITY

The theory of social velocity predicts that the variability of alertness and movement among the members of an optimum-sized group will have a particular expression. In a group of optimum size N_0, the velocity of the most active individual has a relative value of 1.0, and the least active individual will have a velocity of $1/N_0$. The difference in velocity between any two individuals, most similar to each other in velocity will also be $1/N_0$.

An empirical example involves a group of 8 hybrid male mice ($CXAF_1$) living in a closed physical environment (Figure 1), which we anticipated to be optimum for about 12 mice. We call such closed environments "universes." The study of a group of slightly less than expected optimum size permits determination of the optimum group size for a particular combination of heredity and physical environmental setting.

These eight mice had been living in this universe for 11 months after weaning. They were socially and physically at prime adulthood, of an age comparable to 35 years for humans. During each of 120 observation periods, the degree of alertness and movement for each mouse was noted. A weighting factor was applied to each observation to give higher scores to individuals seen active more often in socially more favored places. The sum of these scores was then converted into a crude measure of velocity v_c that

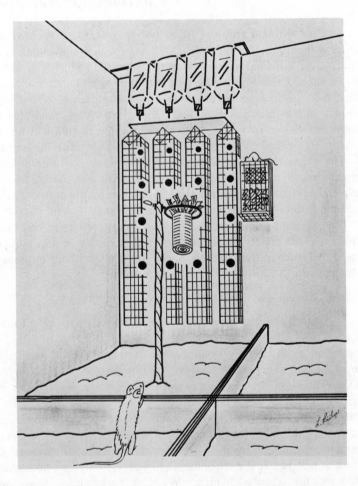

Figure 1. One cell of a four-cell mouse universe. A cell is a replicated configuration of the environment containing an abundance of all needed resources, including space. Wire vertical ramps provide access to nest boxes through holes in the wall. Mice climbing over the outside of the ramps gain access to food and water. The ring stand supporting a can permits animals to separate themselves from interaction below.

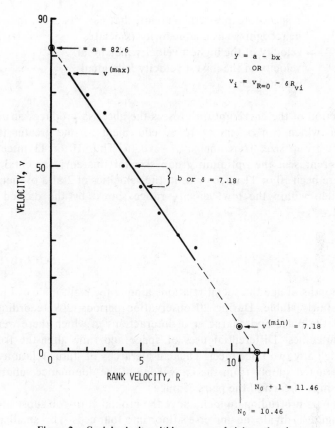

Figure 2.   Social velocity within a group of eight male mice.

reflects the proportion of time during the hours of most elevated activity that an individual is present, alert, and active in that portion of public space where status interactions more often occur. Figure 2 presents the results. "Crude" here is used in the sense that further analysis of behavior may provide more precise measures of social velocity.

The individuals were ranked from the highest to the lowest velocity individual and velocity plotted as a function of rank velocity. This treatment, of course, produces a curve with a negative slope. However, the theory predicted a straight-line curve when the data are presented on arithmetic scales of the ordinate and abscissa. Such a least-squares best-fit straight-line fits the data very well. Some points of terminology:

δ = difference in velocity between any two individuals ranked by velocity. δ implies a degree of "identity differentiation," with respect to expressed behavior, that permits every individual to be recognized as unique by its associates.

$v^{(max)}$ = velocity of the highest velocity individual.
$v^{(min)}$ = velocity of the lowest velocity individual.
R_v = rank velocity.

Projection of the curve until it crosses the abscissa produces an R_v value of 11.46, which can be shown to be equivalent to one greater than the optimum group size. Here then N_0 = 10.46. Thus 10 or 11 mice of this heredity represent the optimum group size for this environmental setting. Had there been 10 or 11 mice present, the velocities of 2 or 3 of them would have fallen within the low velocity range shown by the dashed line in Figure 2.

SOCIAL POWER

By 12 months of age the social relations among the eight mice of Fig. 2 had become fairly stable. During 20 observation periods, 209 recordings were made of the place and character of interactions in which there were clear status outcomes. Differential uses of space and time alter the frequency with which any two mice meet. Thus an hierarchy of status relations cannot be constructed simply from the knowledge of the dominance subordinance relationships of each of the pairs of mice.

Cross bars protruding an inch above the ground corn-cob substrate on the floor (Figure 1) divide the universe's floor into four cells. This small aspect of the environment sufficed to enable every mouse to distinguish one cell from the others. Each mouse spent most of its time in a single cell. Some never left the boundaries of one cell. Others invaded one or more of the other cells. Since each cell had a common boundary with only two other cells, most crossings from one cell to another were across these common boundaries. When two mice meet in one individual's cell, the winner of an encounter is more likely to be the resident of the cell where the encounter takes place.

Social power is here defined as the ability to control the place, time, character, frequency, and outcome of encounters with others. Six criteria, based on our data, permit an intuitive assessment of relative social power. They are as follows.

1.   Outcomes of status interaction: who wins and who loses.
2.   Place of interaction: cell of residence versus another cell.
3.   Ability to share residence in a cell with others, in the sense of binding others to self.

4. Ability to prevent others from entering self's cell of residence.

5. Ability to enter cells of major residence of others.

6. Ability to utilize preferred times: to maintain the normal bimodal nocturnal rhythm of activity. (This criterion was not included in the present analysis).

Figure 3 shows the spatial involvement in developed social power. Each mouse is there represented by a circled number to indicate the rank of its velocity. In the text they will be referred to as R1 to R8.

The highest velocity mouse R1 was the most dominant one. He incorporated three others into the major residence with him in Cell 1. His influence extended into Cell 4 where he more often dominated the resident dominant R5. At the time of the observations, R6 was clearly supplanting R2 in social power. This is the only instance in the analysis where social velocity and social power are not closely associated. R6 from Cell 1 also challenged R5 and R7 in Cell 4, but always lost out there, although he dominated them when they came into his Cell 1. Finally, R8 was extremely subordinate. Most of the time it huddled withdrawn in exposed public

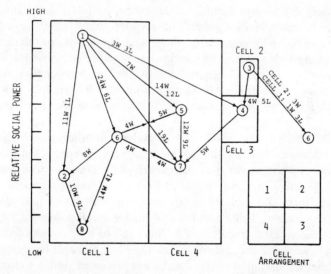

Figure 3. Social power structuring within a group. Circled numbers indicate rank velocity of the eight mice. Rank velocity 1 is the most active mouse. Arrows point toward the subordinate individual. The lower-right insert depicts the floor plan of the four-cell universe. Area of the cells in the main figure is proportional to the numbers of status interactions occurring in each cell. W = wins or dominant status, and L = losses or subordinate status for the dominant member of the pair. Number of W or L is posted in the cell where the encounters took place. Relative social power is an evaluation judgment, explained in part in the text. Data from Study 103, Universe 13, Run 4, $CXAF_1$ male mice.

TABLE I. OUTCOME OF STATUS
INTERACTIONS AMONG EIGHT MALE MICE
IN UNIVERSE 13, STUDY 103, RUN 4[a]

Social Power	Velocity Ranks	In Own Cell		In Other's Cell	
		Wins	: Losses	Wins	: Losses
Higher	1, 3, 4	54	: 17	28	: 43
		(.76)[a]	: (.24)	(.39)	: (.61)
Lower	2, 5–8	127	: 121	0	: 28
		(.51)	: (.49)	(0)	: (1.00)

[a] Proportions in parentheses.

space. At least one or two such extremely low-velocity individuals characterized by aberrant, fragmented behavior are normal for a socially fully structured group.

In Cell 4 R5 tended to dominate R7. The higher status of R5 is reflected by its greater number of relations with R1 from Cell 1. Somewhat anomalously R7 always dominated R1 when the latter came into Cell 4. This is in harmony with a general observation that high-status individuals often give in to, or ignore, those whose social power is considerably lower than their own. No status interactions took place between R1 when R7 invaded Cell 1. There R1 ignored R7. A similar phenomenon took place among the residents of Cell 1. R1 totally ignored R8. He left such interactions with R8 to his two associates with intermediate social power, R2 and R6.

Both R3 and R4 were nearly able to exclude all others from their cells of major residence. This ability to exclude others represented the major expression of their elevated social power. R3's greater social power was reflected in his ability to invade R4's Cell 3 and win nearly half the encounters there. R3 and R4 justify grouping with R1 as individuals with higher social power. Table 1 shows that higher social power individuals win relatively more status encounters in their cell of major residence and lose relatively fewer such encounters outside their cell of major residence.

This brief discussion of social structure is presented simply to indicate the complexities of which this species is capable. Adequate treatment of the relationship between social velocity and social power and structure would require a detailed treatment of the historical process as well as the differential usage of time of day by different individuals. It would also require examination of the many nonstatus interactions and individual behaviors, which fill up most of the life of any mouse.

IMPACT OF GREATER THAN OPTIMUM
GROUP SIZE ON SOCIAL VELOCITY

At the same time the study above was conducted, groups of 16 or 32 male mice were also studied in 4-cell universes. As noted above, 10 or 11 mice of this $CXAF_1$ strain represents the optimum group size for this 4-cell universe. Similar measures of social velocity were made of the mice in the larger groups when they were 12 months of age. Figures 4 and 5 give the results.

Only eight mice in the $N = 16$ group retained an approximately normal expression of velocity. However, identity differentiation δ increased 31% (from 7.18 to 9.39). Similarly the mean velocity of these eight most normal mice increased 39% from (50.0 to 69.55) over that of the eight mice in the $N = 8$ group. Despite these increases, changes from the normal, a projection of the slope of their velocity curve until it crossed the abscissa indicates that they had preserved their behavior compatible with an optimum group size of 10.9. For all practical purposes this is no different from the $N_0 = 10.46$ of the $N = 8$ group.

These relatively normal eight individuals in the $N = 16$ group retained this normality by rejecting the remaining eight mice, whose average low velocity is a reflection of their deviant and fragmented behavior, and their psychological and physical withdrawal from participation in social interactions. It is to be noted that the δ identity differentiation of these withdrawn mice decreased to 2.61, 36% of that characterizing the mice in the $N = 8$

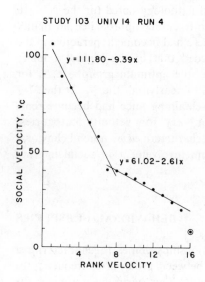

STUDY 103 UNIV 14 RUN 4

$y = 111.80 - 9.39x$

$y = 61.02 - 2.61x$

SOCIAL VELOCITY, vc

RANK VELOCITY

Figure 4. Social velocity within a group of 16 male mice.

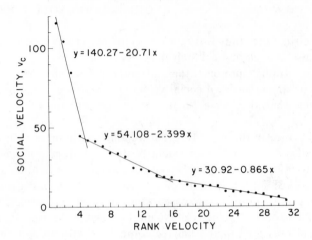

STUDY 103   UNIV. 15   RUN 4

Figure 5.   Social velocity within a group of 32 male mice.

group, and only 28% of their eight more normal associates. This lack of differentiation leads their more normal associates to react to these withdrawn
ones merely as equivalent representatives of a type, rather than as unique
individuals. This lack of individual uniqueness, in essence, makes nonmice
out of these rejected individuals. They no longer exist in the social field
inhabited by their more normal associates.

In the $N = 32$ group, all trends toward pathology noted for the $N = 16$
group became accentuated. No more than five mice approached normality
with respect to social velocity. Three of these had become hyperactive in the
sense that each of their velocities exceeded that of the highest velocity
mouse in the $N = 8$ group. Furthermore, the optimum group size N_0 for
these most normal mice had been reduced to nearly half the N_0 for the $N =
8$ group, that is from 10.46 to 5.8. The remaining mice had become reor-
ganized into either moderately low or very low-velocity categories.
Members of both of these categories were characterized by much behavioral
pathology, particularly by abstention from involvement in social interactions.

BEHAVIORAL SUBSPECIES

When a favorable pattern of stable relationships comes to characterize a
group of animals, a harmony will arise between group size, frequency of
interactions, and intensity of interactions.[2, 4] This harmony optimizes the

amount of gratification the average individual derives from participation in group life. When this harmony exists among individuals, they form an optimum sized group N_0. It may be shown that where i = intensity of one individual's behavior toward another:

$$i^2 = \text{intensity of an interaction}$$
$$= \frac{1}{N_0 - 1}$$

and i^2 is proportional to the duration of the refractory period following interaction. It may further be shown that the frequency of satisfactory social relations is proportional to $N_0 - 1$. That is to say, as the optimum group size decreases, there is an increase in intensity of interactions, and a decrease in the frequency with which two individuals, each of which is receptive to a social interaction, do interact.

The experimental evidence above indicates that a threefold increase in actual group size above the optimum reduced optimum group size in nearly half. The four or five most normal mice in the $N = 32$ group appear to have attained a new behavioral, and presumably physiological, harmony or stability. For them, intensity of interaction, calculated as $1/(N_0 - 1)$, had increased to a relative value of .209 from that of .106 for the $N = 8$ group. This doubling of intensity of social interaction, which accompanied a nearly halving of optimum group size, raises an important theoretical issue. Frequently in my examination of empirical data, or from related mathematical modeling of social process, a phase shift in dynamics often accompanies a doubling or halving of some important parameter. If the differences above in optimum group size and intensity of interaction had resulted from studies in natural habitats of animals, one would suspect that at least a subspecific genetic difference existed between the two populations. However, in the present experiment study, the F_1 cross between two highly inbred strains of mice made all subjects essentially identical genetically. Therefore, one must conclude that a threefold increase in group size above the optimum can produce biochemical and behavioral changes of a magnitude comparable to that accompanying subspecific differentiation through natural selection and gene drift. I shall apply the term behavioral subspecies to such marked nongenetic shifts in optimum group size and intensity (or character) of social interaction.

INFLUENCE OF GENETIC DIFFERENTIATION ON OPTIMUM GROUP SIZE

Experimental breeding has produced a wide range of inbred house mouse strains. Two of the most divergent strains are the C57 Black and the DBA.

Many physiological and behavioral measures support the judgment that the C57s represent an extremely stable strain. These same measures indicate that the DBAs are extremely unstable. The social behavior of these two strains were studied in habitats that were presumed to be optimum for 10 or 12 mice.[1] The C57s formed a stable social organization as expected. They were very successful in rearing young in a complex environmental setting despite the fact that they had lived for over 100 generations in the impoverished environment of a small cell. Most status interactions among males were muted and of low intensity. Gestures and mild threats usually sufficed to resolve status encounters. In contrast, the DBAs were never able to develop a stable, low-tension social organization. Nearly every status interaction between two males had to be acted out as if they were total strangers. This frequency of intense fighting among males affected reproductive performance. Most females were able to rear only a few of their progeny.

These studies were conducted before I developed the concept of social velocity. Fortunately a set of observations was made that provided an excellent measure of velocity. A "contact" was defined as two alert mice being within a distance from each other normally characterizing those approaches that culminated in a status interaction. Contacts, as a measure of social velocity, are plotted in Fig. 6 as a function of the mouse's rank by the number of its contacts with other males.

The 11 male C57 mice did form an optimum sized group, since the calculated N_0 from the contact velocity data is 11.3. In contrast, only five of the nine male DBA mice preserved a normality of velocity relationships, compatible with an N_0 of only 4.5. The other five rejected, low-velocity DBAs survived by altering their behavior so as not to challenge effectively the status of any associate. The five lowest velocity DBA mice exhibited only one-fifth of the capacity to express dominance in a social interaction as did the five lowest velocity C57s.

The C57 mice likely preserve as large a component of heredity of the wild type as does any inbred strain. In like fashion, the DBA mice represent as great a divergence from the wild type as it is possible to obtain from selective breeding, and still have the strain survive reproductively in a minimally complex environment. This degree of genetic divergence produced a strain having less than half the optimum group size as the stable one, and exhibiting three times the intensity of social interactions (i^2 = .286 for DBA, and .097 for C57). Thus behavioral differentiation from genetic causes slightly exceeds that produced by crowding to a threefold increase in density above the optimum. An inference from this line of reasoning is that overcrowding leads to a magnitude of nearly irreversible biochemical changes affecting behavior that are of a magnitude equivalent to genotype differentiation producing subspecies.

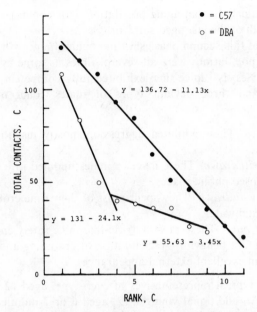

Figure 6. Comparison of social velocity between two strains of mice. The C57 is a physiologically and behaviorally stable strain. The DBA is an unstable strain. Number of contacts represent social velocity.

SEVERE LONG-TERM CROWDING

Another set of our studies involved populations of Balb C strain mice in 1, 2, 4, 8 and 16 cell universes.[6,8] Each population started with four males and four females. The history of each was marked by three major phases. During the first, the populations increased exponentially with few infant deaths. All progeny received relatively excellent maternal care. When each cell in a universe contained 10 to 12 socially adult individuals, the exponential growth rate of the population markedly declined. This change in rate of growth denoted a phase shift in social life. After this phase shift, infant abuse developed, as adults became stressed from the excess younger adults attempting, mostly unsuccessfully, to find a niche—a social role—in an established group. Some of the mice, who were abused as infants during this second population phase, in turn produced young. Partly as a result of these parents not relating effectively with their young, all of these later-born young became autistic-like. They never learned to relate sufficiently to others for these relations to culminate in conceptions by females after they had reached adulthood. Their failure to conceive brought a sudden shift from a reduced rate of population growth to a no-growth phase, which eventually culminated in an aging population with population extinction at the time of death of the last aged survivor.

At the time of this second phase shift in population growth and pattern of social life, the populations were all several times as large as that optimum for these universes. No mice then exhibited fully competent behavior. One quasi-normal and three deviant types of males could nevertheless be identified:

1. *Aggressive.* They exhibited aggression mostly just in the center of former territories.

2. *Pooled withdrawn.* These inactive males huddled in large aggregates in the most exposed public space.

3. *Solitary withdrawn.* They spent most of their time crouched near the source of food and water.

4. *Beautiful mice.* These most autistic-like mice rarely engaged in other than simple contact behavior. Accentuation of grooming and lack of fighting gave them an excellent external appearance.

Twelve most typical representatives of each type, aged 12 to 15 months, were selected. An additional younger 12, aged 6 or 7 months, was selected for types 2 and 4. Each of the six sets of males was then placed in a separate four-cell universe, where Dr. Halsey M. Marsden studied many aspects of their behavior, including social velocity. The objective of this study was to determine the extent that their differential histories, but long exposure to crowding might influence capacity to recoup normal behavior in a setting known to be quite ideal for 12 mice.

The analysis of the velocity data revealed a rigid, nearly identical, social structure in each universe. Five or six mice in each group preserved some modicum of normality. Little difference in velocity characterized the remaining very low velocity withdrawn individuals. In every case, the three highest velocity males maintained a single cell as their exclusive territory. The remaining nine mice lived in the fourth cell. Figure 7 depicts the average velocity analysis. For our present purpose, the most important conclusion that may be derived from this figure is that the mean optimum group size N_0 was only 5.5 [i.e., $(64.87/9.96) - 1$].

We believe that these six groups of males adequately represent an impact that generations of overcrowding had produced on all individuals. Their physiological stability had been so impaired that they no longer could tolerate the number of contacts per day appropriate to the optimum group size of 10 to 12 that had characterized this inbred strain during the first phase of population increase. It was "as if" there had been a massive change in genotype, through no more than five generations, that had made the terminal two generations resemble unstable DBA mice in comparison

STUDY 122 UNIV 12-19
MEAN v_c BY RANK

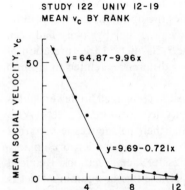

$y = 64.87 - 9.96x$

$y = 9.69 - 0.721x$

Figure 7. Mean social velocity of mice with long histories of exposure to overcrowding. The individual curves for the six groups of mice, contributing to this mean, were quite similar.

with their original selves which during phase one were more like stable C57 mice. We have little insight into the nature of the biochemical changes that must have occurred to transform a behaviorally stable strain into an unstable "behavioral subspecies." This transformation, if not irreversible, is at least not subject to return to the original condition by the simple expedient of placing animals in an uncrowded setting. For example, after many weeks of living in the uncrowded situation most males were essentially incapable of inducing receptive females to become pregnant, and the remaining few were rarely able to do so.

VITAMIN A AND SOCIAL VELOCITY

Rats living as members of a crowded group in a complex environment[3] exhibited certain physiological or anatomical pathologies that led us to suspect that the included increase in vitamin A content of the commercially produced diet that they were fed might have caused the pathologies. We further suspected that this elevation of dietary vitamin A might have influenced some of the abnormal social relations evidenced under crowded conditions. This led us to study two populations of Osborne-Mendel strain rats on synthetic diets. One contained vitamin A at a level comparable to that found in natural foods; that is at 3 IU/g of diet, a level comparable to 2500 IU/day for humans. The other diet contained 12 IU/g, the level in the commercial diet, which is comparable to 10,000 IU/day for humans.

The total universes in which the rats lived proved to be optimum for nine males and nine females. Studies of social velocity were made when the populations each included over 60 rats, 12 or 15 months of age, as well as

30 to 40 not yet socially mature rats, 6 months of age. At this time each population included approximately three times the optimum number of fully socially adult rats. In both populations the average social velocity had been suppressed, but much more so in rats on the 3-IU diet.[5, 6] Interpretation of this difference requires consideration of other differences related to vitamin A intake.

Male rats on the higher level vitamin A diet engaged in fewer status interactions, even though their higher velocity led to more contacts. As a result, they were wounded less frequently, and their pelage was less marred by scar tissue. Their hearts, kidneys, and adrenals were smaller, presumably as a consequence of lesser involvement in stressful social relations. Reduced engagement in status interactions by males on the higher vitamin A diet is interpreted as resulting from an impairment of perception by elevated vitamin A intake. This impairment of perception also influenced sexual behavior. Higher vitamin A intake males exhibited more homosexual behavior, and more often mounted inappropriate females—very young females or older ones not in estrous.

At both dietary levels, loading the male rats with tryptophan or methionine reduced the amount of inappropriate social behavior. This was particularly true of tryptophan. These two amino acids seem to counteract the action of elevated vitamin A in interfering with perception. As vitamin A intake increases, with accompanying elevation of amount stored in the liver and elevation of serum level of vitamin A, the rats seem to be less capable of interpreting a gestalt of stimuli emanating from an associate. As a result, they less frequently respond to an associate, or respond inappropriately. An example of the latter is the reduced ability to detect an appropriate sex partner. Among females, elevated vitamin A particularly disrupts maternal behavior.

Regardless of the level of vitamin A intake, the earlier in life crowded conditions impact on the individual, the higher the rate of vitamin A storage in the liver becomes, and thus the higher the level of circulating vitamin A in the serum. The third generation of rats in this study were born when the number of adults present was three times the optimum. These third-generation rats stored vitamin A at twice the rate of the first-generation rats. They had all the characteristics of the autistic-like beautiful mice born at times of comparable crowding. Like the beautiful mice, these third-generation rats, at both dietary vitamin A levels, were incapable of reproduction when placed in an uncrowded environment identical to the one they had matured in.

CONCLUSION

Members of an optimum-sized group become differentiated with respect to the amount of time each is alert and active in public space. This degree of alertness and activity measures social velocity. As velocity declines, behavior becomes more deviant and fragmented. A less than doubling of optimum group size culminates in a splitting of the total group into one half that preserves most of the attributes of an optimum group, and another half of rejected, deviant, withdrawn individuals with much reduced average velocity. When the group size more than doubles, most semblances of behavioral and social normality disappear. All members are transformed into what amounts to a different biochemical and behavioral strain or subspecies whose optimum size is reduced in half and whose intensity of interaction doubles. At these higher densities the population is fragmented into a very few hyperactive individuals, and a majority with extremely depressed velocity and marked deviance of behavior.

When a population has lasted through several generations of overcrowding, the rate of vitamin A storage increases. The increase of available circulating vitamin A enhances individual survival by blocking out of its awareness most of the events transpiring in the environment. This permits an elevation of velocity as it reduces social involvement. However, this reduced involvement by these autistic-like end-products of crowding is an expression of an incapacity to conduct those complex behaviors necessary for species survival.

REFERENCES

1. Calhoun, J. B.: A comparative study of the social behavior of two inbred strains of house mice. *Ecol. Monogr.* **26**:81–103, 1956.

2. Calhoun, J. B.: Social welfare as a variable in population dynamics. *Symp. Quant. Biol.* **22**:339–355, 1957.

3. Calhoun, J. B.: Population density and social pathology. *Sci. Amer.* **206**:32, 139–146, 1962.

4. Calhoun, J. B.: The social use of space. In *Physiological Mammalogy,* W. Mayer, and R. van Gelder, (Eds.), Academic Press, New York, 1963, Chapter 1, pp. 1–187.

5. Calhoun, J. B.: Ecological factors in the development of behavioral anomalies. In *Comparative Psychopathology,* E. Zubin (Ed.), New York, 1967, pp. 1–51.

6. Calhoun, J. B.: Space and strategy of life. In *Behavior and Environment*: The Use of Space by Animals and Men, A. H. Esser (Ed.), Plenum Press, New York, 1971, pp. 329–387.

7. Calhoun, J. B.: Disruption of behavioral states as a cause of aggression. *Nebraska Symp. Motivation* **1972**:183–260, 1973.

8. Calhoun, J. B.: Death squared: The explosive growth and demise of a mouse population. *Proc. Royal Soc. Med.* **66:**80–88, 1973.

9. Calhoun, J. B.: From mice to men. *Trans. Studies of the College of Physicians of Philadelphia* **41** (2):92–118, 1973.

AN INDEX

To *Calhoun's* writings relating to social velocity. (Numbers before colons correspond to the numbers preceding bibliographic entries. Numbers after colons refer to pages within references.)

CHAPTER THREE

PSYCHOLOGICAL ADAPTATION IN A CHANGING ENVIRONMENT

ROBERT CANCRO, M.D., MED. D. SC.

Long before the college campuses became concerned about the survival of the planet and its occupants, environmental scientists were deeply aware of the negative consequences of overpopulation and the massive industrial growth that sustained such an ecologically unsound number of people. The extraordinarily broad scope of the environmental sciences necessitated a relatively exclusive concentration on physical issues. Considerations of the health consequences of the environment also tended to focus on the physical. It is not a criticism that the environmental sciences failed to recognize their neglect of individual and group psychologic health. It is only relatively recently that even the behavioral sciences have begun to recognize and study these relationships. Despite the legitimacy of the various factors, historical and other, which have precluded a significant commitment of creative resources to the study of environmental-psychologic relationships, it is now necessary to improve these efforts. We must understand better the role of the environment—both physical and social—in determining the quality of a population's mental health.

The distinction between psychologic and physical has served science well but as with all cognitive devices, it is not an accurate approximation of reality, and therefore suffers from the danger of reification. We speak of adaptation in a manner that de-emphasizes this separation while returning to it later. In this way, we attempt to obtain the advantages of the distinction and to avoid the problems of overliteralness. Every organism is an improbable patterning of energy which exists in a nonequilibrium relationship to its environment on a transitory basis, that is, its lifetime.[1] It is advisable to think of this relationship in thermodynamic terms so as to work toward the goal of making behavioral models compatible with those used by other disciplines. Adaptation is the process whereby an organism achieves a dynamic steady-state with its environment which permits it to survive in that environment. Since all living creatures tend to revert to a patternless random state of matter, life can be defined as the struggle against and postponement of the return to this nonorderly condition. The regulation of mass-energy exchanges and the reduction of entropy serve to determine the effectiveness of any given dynamic steady-state. There are limitations inherent in this general formulation of man's adaptation to his environment. Clearly, it is applicable merely in a broad system sense in which individual details are obscured and only a general picture of the state of the system emerges.

If we accept the formulation that man lives in a dynamic steady-state with his environment, then disease and health can be operationally defined in terms of that steady-state. A relatively narrow range of the possible steady-states is considered health. Within this range, the adaptation of the organism to the environment is equally well optimized for a number of

48

variables, including, but not restricted to, those crucial for survival. Illness, from this point of view, consists of those dynamic steady-states outside this range wherein one or more important variables are no longer optimized but which are not inimicable to continued life. If the organism cannot establish a new steady-state within this larger range, equilibrium with the environment and death ensues. This formulation, at least in its major components, holds equally for psychologic or physiologic adaptation and leads us to conclude that the symptoms of disease are nothing more than the associated phenomena of a new steady-state. The new steady-state is an attempt to guarantee the continuation of the organism but at some cost. From this point of view, the so-called illness is both adaptive and maladaptive, since it sustains the existence of the organism in a new challenge situation while it reduces the efficiency of the adaptation in other ways. Illness can be viewed as a compromise in which the short-term existence of the organism takes precedence over the long-term quality or efficiency of that existence. We can view the acute phase of an illness as the period during which a new steady-state is being sought, and the chronic phase as the period in which it has been achieved.

Man differs from other animals in the degree to which he is aware of the adaptive process. This does not mean to imply that he consciously experiences the homeostatic adjustments of the concentration of various body substances. Rather, it means that he has some recognition of whether living is particularly difficult or easy at a given time. Even here his unique ability for self-deception tends to complicate matters. It is commonplace to find an awareness of the true degree of difficulty only after the stressful situation is over. This is particularly true of organismic adjustments that are made in response to gradual environmental changes. A sudden dramatic alteration of the environment with the concomitant necessity to find a new steady-state is almost always perceived as stressful, particularly if it must be done quickly and/or radically.

The quality of any human being's psychologic adaptation is a function not only of his individual, group, and social resources but also of the nature of the environment to which he must adapt. The term environment will be used hereafter to include both physical and nonphysical variables unless specified otherwise. The same person who functions effectively in one environment may decompensate in another. We have all had the opportunity to observe individuals who meet difficult demands quite successfully but at a different time are not able to cope with a set of circumstances of approximately equal duress. What makes the matter even more complex is an environment that is noxious for one person is not for another. Despite these individual differences, there are valid—albeit limited generalizations—that can be made. To put it another way, it is accurate to say there are environments to which most people can adapt successfully, and there are environments to which virtually no one can adapt successfully. Every environment falls some place on this spectrum of adaptational difficulty for the modal individual. It is biologically reasonable to assume that environments that are similar to those in which man evolved are likely to be more suitable for his present adaptation. Man developed historically in a relatively constant environment. His environment was constant not only in the pattern of sensory information being fed into his nervous system, but in a variety of other ways including seasonal variations, levels of physical activity, dangers, stability of social institutions, and such. This historic environment is radically different from today's.

ENVIRONMENTAL CONSIDERATIONS

We know very little about the effects of the physical environment on mental functioning. Yet what we know suggests that it plays an important role. A variety of physical factors either can or do affect psychologic adaptation. There have been dramatic changes over time in the sensory environment. The range of sounds, for example, impinging on the tympanic membrane of contemporary man bears little resemblance both in kind and intensity to those of the past. The experiments on sensory deprivation[2] and more recently on sensory overload[3] suggest that man's mental adaptation can be influenced through manipulation of sensory input to the nervous system. The presence or absence of trace minerals in the water supply can affect the prevalence of mania.[4] The periodicity of day and night produces regular variations in both physiologic and psychologic activity.[5] Vitamin levels in the available food supply, climatic effects on the endocrine system, and a host of other physical variables can contribute to the psychologic character and health of a given people. Obviously, as between-population physical environmental differences are reduced and populations become more geographically mobile, these effects will diminish in long-term importance. Nevertheless, over the short term, the physical differences may be more extensive than the health-range capacity of the population. The changes in the physical environment may also occur more rapidly than do the organism's compensatory mechanisms and thereby produce a situation in which health-range steady-states are difficult to achieve.

In addition to the obvious physical parameters of the environment such as the kind, duration, frequency, and intensity of sensory stimuli, we must also consider man's confidence in the physical environment. The reality of the environment is complicated by man's abstract reasoning capacity. He adapts in part to his conception of the environment, a conception that bears a variable resemblance to the environment in fact. If he strongly believes the physical environment to be noxious and perceives it as such, his adaptation will be influenced by this belief. When people are told that their food is adulterated by unseen chemical additives and their air and water are polluted by a variety of harmful agents, their confidence and trust in the environment are diminished. This kind of distrust and pervasive anxiety does not enhance the quality of human adaptation. The sense of helplessness in the face of these invisible and uncontrollable "dangers" is also psychologically injurious. Even if these environmental "dangers" were to be spurious in nature, this would not protect the population from the negative consequences of distrust and helplessness, but merely add a touch of irony. Obviously, the existence of man's abstract reasoning complicates his adaptative efforts beyond that found in simpler organisms. Yet this important consideration is often ignored and not included in our thinking. This realization leaves us with the possibility that the environment—physical and/or social—may be constant in fact but changing for an individual or a population. Certainly, many of the psychologic behaviors of mentally ill patients are quite appropriate to their perception of the social environment.

POPULATION CHARACTERISTICS

Other environmental considerations do not fit neatly into a physical-psychologic division. We consider certain characteristics that describe the human population as environmental variables.[6] It may be particularly useful to conceptualize population characteristics as environmental variables, since man has so outbred his ecologically appropriate niche. From the point of view of the stability of the biosphere, species diversification is the most desirable plan. Man has successfully disrupted this pattern and, thereby, contributed to the considerable threat that presently faces the planet. The current large number of homo sapiens is ecologically imbalanced. This source of disturbance to the biosphere only increases the necessity of our understanding population characteristics as environmental variables. The density characteristic of population has received considerable attention.[7] The broad spacing of a population is one of nature's major ways of reducing intraspecies conflict and increasing species diversification. This improves the stability of the biosphere by increasing the variety of populations to be found in any particular area and giving different subsets of each species slightly different microenvironments in which to adapt. Animal studies clearly demonstrate the importance of population density as an environmental variable. This line of research has related the density of a population to a variety of socially maladaptive behaviors including social withdrawal and violence. The work has been criticized on the interesting grounds that men are not mere animals. While it is wise to generalize carefully from animal models, it is unwise to reject their relevance in toto. Interestingly, this is something we only do when the finding displeases us. Certain human experiences, however, parallel the animal studies. Refugee-camp experiences clearly suggest under the type of stress that includes crowding, the veneer of civilization peels away quite quickly for some people. Every warden knows of the negative effect of overcrowding on selected prisoners. There is much evidence to suggest that population density is an important variable in determining the quality of the adaptation that man makes to his environment. Man is not likely to adapt successfully to every possible population density without paying an excessive price. Obviously, the rate as well as the degree of density change will determine the severity of the stress to man's adaptive resources.

While this particular population variable has been the most researched and publicized, many others are significant as well. Some of the important characteristics include the proportion of youth, the male-female ratio, the ratio of producers to consumers, the proportion of urban to rural, and the percentage of the population who are aged or infirm. All of these characteristics and others not listed are important features of the psychophysical environment to which man must adapt. These variables also play an important role in the establishment of his social organizations. The quality of the mental adaptation made by an individual or group to the environment is likely to be significantly altered by such population characteristics as those already cited.

SOCIAL ENVIRONMENT

The complete study of man's psychologic relationship to his environment must include the social environment as well. Man adapts to the group of which he is a member and its social institutions. The expectations, rewards, and values of his culture all make demands on his adaptive resources. The social environment is, however, unique in the sense that it requires and supports adaptive efforts simultaneously. Psychologic adaptation to the social environment not only involves the intrapersonal resources of the individual but also is supplemented by the psychosocial institutions that the group develops. These psychosocial institutions, therefore, serve to support man's individual adaptive resources although they also constitute part of the environment to which man must adapt. Once established these social organizations and institutions are transmitted through that society's culture. Culture changes slowly and, therefore, social organizations tend to remain operative for long periods of time in any given society. We make an assumption concerning the role of genetic factors in the development of psychosocial institutions. We are hypothesizing that the behaviors required by particular institutions and social organizations have a biologic as well as psychologic origin.[8] In other words, between-population differences in the choice of particular social organizations are in part because of genetic differences. If this is true, then each of these populations represents a unique biobehavioral experiment in which the environment operates on the genetic characteristics of that population not only to develop individual behavioral traits that are adaptive but also to develop social organizations consisting of a set of such behaviors that then become transmitted and reinforced through culture. Clearly, if the environment were to change rapidly and make these particular organizations obsolete, we could easily find that culture would perpetuate the now no longer adaptive organizations. A new class of problems emerges when the feedback from the environment stops acting as a selective mechanism. In this case, the genetic heterogeneity of the population for a variety of behavioral traits is increased without an associated diminution in the cultural transmission of the formerly adaptive organizations. Any adaptive individual behavior or social organization that has survival value that is both genetically loaded and culturally supported suffers from this potential difficulty if selective feedback is interrupted. As the behavior or social organization diminishes in adaptive value, the population becomes genetically more heterogeneous for that trait. Meanwhile, the culture supports the trait as if it were still adaptive. The result is social pressure for conformity in the face of biobehavioral diversity.

There have been several important points in the history of man when we can assume that selective feedback from the environment was markedly diminished. The development of agriculture was probably the first of these. With the advent of agriculture and the resulting increase in the stabilization of food production, man's numbers rose sharply. Social organization had to change drastically as well. The valuable behaviors of an agricultural people are quite different from those of a migratory hunting and food-gathering people. Agriculture also led to a more stable but less varied diet. The tending of crops and domesticated animals required a different kind of population than did the previous way of life. Many of the behavioral traits— including aggressiveness—which had survival value in the older society were maladaptive in the new. The lessons of this transitional period are of even greater importance for contemporary man.

More recently, the technology developed during the Industrial Revolution has led to powerful controls over death, infectious disease, and the environment. Technology and science have radically disrupted the balance that existed between man and his environment. The increased mobility and density of the population have led to a marked increase in genetic diversity. A far greater variety of individuals are available as breeding partners. Relatively small, geographically isolated tribes had far less opportunity to breed outward than does modern man. Geographic mobility and the richness of opportunity for mate selection have produced remarkable genetic diversity. While this diversity is the biologic hope for man's future, it does tend to undermine the validity of traditional social organizations.

SOCIAL ORGANIZATION

Contemporary man is the product of an age-old process of selection. While it is apparent that evolution selects the present representatives of a species in such a manner as to equip them best for adaptation to an environment most similar to that which was operative during the selection procedure, this does not mean that we must return to the prehistoric jungle to survive. It does mean, however, that as our environment differs increasingly from earlier ones, we are likely to find our traditional social organizations and institutions less effective in complementing man's individual reserves for satisfactory psychologic adaptation. Social organizations are quite effective so long as the environment of the next generation remains reasonably similar to the environment of the former.

An example may help to clarify this argument. The family is a ubiquitous social organization that has been found in all known human societies from the most primitive to the most advanced. The family has been remarkably effective in preserving the species. Through the family, man has protected and reared the young successfully. Through the differentiation of specialized roles, adult males and females have traditionally been able to take care of the psychologic and physical requirements of their offspring. The family is an effective medium for transmitting culture. With the advancement of technology, many of the historic functions of the family have been eroded. Formal education is now almost exclusively handled by professionals outside of the family group. Health care is increasingly the domain of other professionals again outside of the core family. Much of the entertainment and interpersonal sustenance of children derives from nonfamilial sources. The complaint of some middle-class suburbanite parents that they have been reduced to chauffeurs is not a total distortion. The increasing complexity of the society in which we live and the development of strangers to perform specialized and vital functions have weakened the validity of the family as a social mechanism for species survival. This does not mean that the family does not have other useful and even necessary functions, but simply that its historical role is changing.[8] This example also allows us to examine the problem of increasing genetic diversity. As the survival value of particular social organizations such as the family diminishes, the corrective feedback from the environment is removed. Returning to our earlier assumption of a genetic factor in some social organizations, we can argue then that genetic diversity relating to family formation is being encouraged. In other words, we should anticipate that there are an increasing number of individuals who are not disposed toward traditional family organization because of biologic as well as social factors. This in itself would not be a problem but for the fact that experimentation in substitute forms of social organization are poorly tolerated by the dominant culture and often labeled as illness.

COMPUTER-BASED AUTOMATION

In looking to the future, we can anticipate that computer-based automation will represent a quantum jump from industrialization.[9] In the past, technologic change has been at a sufficiently slow rate that man has had time, although limited, to somewhat accommodate himself psychologically to the changes. Automation does not promise to allow us this luxury. Another major consequence of automation is that it must, to an unprecedented degree, reshape society in its own image. In the past, technology has both followed man as the model and included him in its efforts. Tools were direct extensions of man, and technology often took what a man did by hand as its guiding principle. A power shovel digs a hole in precisely the same way as a man does with his hand. Up until very recently, it was even constructed in a manner that was quite similar to the anatomical joint structure of the human arm. The future of automation is such that man will no longer be the paradigm for and even may have to be designed out of the process. The ways of the machine, of necessity, must at times be shown preference over the ways of man. The problem of hand-wired circuits in electronic data processing is a clear example of this preference. The need for inexpensive, reliable, mass-produced wired circuits presented an important technical problem. Circuits had previously been hand-wired but this process was slow, costly, and produced oversized devices. The engineering approach to the problem was not to design a machine which automatically wired circuits as men do, but rather to design something which wired circuits as only a machine could.

Once the engineers set aside the conceptual restraints imposed by using hand-wiring as a model and the further constraints of including man in the activity, they were free to use their technology in a truly imaginative way.

The elaborate soldering machines used by men were replaced by the product of this new approach—the printed circuit. Printed circuits have had a major impact on a variety of industries. Ultimately, more important than the impact is the kind of thinking that went into their development. Machines were not designed that simulated or complemented man, but rather the engineers examined the problem from the point of view of what would be the best machine way of coming up with a device to perform the functions of hand-wired circuits. Despite our human pride, printed circuits are superior in almost every way. This example is meant to illustrate some actual conceptual consequences of automation which tend to distinguish it from previous technologic advances.

There will be a number of effects of automation on the environment in which man must adapt. It may be useful, therefore, to study the predictable effects of programmed machines on both social institutions and the physical environment to anticipate their probable consequences on man's efforts to adapt psychologically. Elsewhere a scenario has been described of the future effects of full-scale automation on work—a single social institution, important in psychological adaptation, that will be radically altered.[10] Obviously, the study of a single social institution will provide very limited insight into a complex problem. Nevertheless, the approach can serve as a paradigm for the study of others. There is a need to supplement the study of social structures by examining the probable effects of automation on energy consumption, pollution, water and air quality, population characteristics, and such. Automation threatens to disrupt the balance that exists between many people and their work. This balance may well be in need of change. Yet, it seems unlikely that economically motivated, psychologically unplanned interventions will be constructive. There are obvious inherent limitations to any scenario we can write. Many interactions will not be anticipated, and others will be estimated incorrectly. The models we construct will of necessity be inadequate and inaccurate, but they still are preferable to anything else available.

The environment to which we must adapt today is bizarre from the point of view of evolution. The moment-to-moment sensory data that we process have no resemblance to our historic sources of information. The kind, frequency, and intensity of stimuli are totally different from the environment in which the sensory systems developed. In every conceivable way, we are unprepared to deal with an environment that is remarkably synthetic and artificial. Increasingly foreign environments must be adapted to without the benefit of millions of years of biologic and social evolutionary selection. The more novel the environment, the greater the likelihood that there are only a few people who will successfully adapt to it. In a real sense, man's technologic success and its environmental impact have outstripped his adaptive psychologic reserves. It comes as little surprise that many people supplement their adaptive resources with tobacco, alcohol, marijuana, tranquilizers, sleeping pills, and such. Man is no longer biologically designed by the forces of evolution for a world that he rather than evolution has created. The success of man's cognitive apparatus has created the problem, and this is the only tool man has that may solve it as well. We cannot follow the nihilists who, recognizing that the problems have resulted from thought, believe that the solutions must come from an absence of thought. There is no substitute for reasoned planning, with all its limitations.

The key to the improved mental health of the population lies more in regulating the environment—both social and physical—in ways that match it to man's adaptive resources and less in hoping to deliver ever increasing amounts of psychiatric treatment. It is only in this way that we can reach the necessary numbers of people and prevent their decompensation into less adaptive steady-states. These formulations also highlight some important distinctions between the maintenance and the restoration of health. Many factors contribute to the maintenance of good health, and these of necessity must center on the facilitation of man's adaptation to the environment. This facilitation can take the form of alterations of the environment or complementing the capacity of man in various ways to establish a satisfactory steady-state—one within the health range. The restoration of health requires its prior loss. Psychiatric treatment represents a failure of health maintenance. While we must offer adequate levels of treatment, we cannot expect to meet the anticipated demand without improved methods of prevention. The only effective prevention foreseeable lies in a better understanding and regulation of the environment. The environmental sciences with their systems approach offer considerable potential for the prevention of human maladaptation—both physical and mental. Clearly, the very nature of the task requires an interdisciplinary effort. Sophistication in the methods of various environmental sciences must be supplemented by clinical competence. Yet if man as we know him is to survive, the disciplinary identities that separate us must be transcended. Behavioral, social, and environmental scientists must collaborate on the development of the necessary expertise that will make informed environmental options available.

REFERENCES

1. Lehninger, A. L.: *Bioenergetics*, Benjamin, New York, 1965.
2. Zubek, J. P. (Ed.): *Sensory Deprivation: Fifteen Years of Research*, Appleton-Century-Crofts, New York, 1969.

3. Ludwig, A. M.: "Psychedelic" effects produced by sensory overload. *Sci. Proc. 124th Ann. Mtg. APA* (abstract).

4. Gruenberg, E. M.: personal communication, 1973.

5. Stroebel, C. F.: Chronopsychophysiology. In *Comprehensive Textbook of Psychiatry,* Vol. II., A. M. Freedman, H. I. Kaplan, B. J. Sadock (Eds.) Williams & Wilkins, Baltimore, 1975.

6. Cancro, R.: Adaptational considerations of population characteristics. Unpublished manuscript.

7. Calhoun, J. B.: Population density and social pathology. *Sci. Amer.,* February 1962.

8. Cancro, R.: On monkeys, machines, and mothers. *Perspectives in Biol. Med.* **16**:312–322, Winter 1973.

9. Cancro, R.: Psychological adaptation in a world of programmed machines. *Ann. N.Y. Acad. Sci.* **184**:230–238, 1971.

10. Cancro, R.: Automation: The second emancipation proclamation. *Amer. J. Psychother.* **23**:657–666, 1969.

CHAPTER FOUR

PSYCHOPATHOLOGY AND CULTURAL TRANSFORMATIONS IN A PASTORAL-AGRARIAN SOCIETY IN INDUSTRIAL EVOLUTION: EXPERIENCES IN SARDINIA

FRANCESCO SIMONE

TRANSLATED BY CHERIDA LALLY

The Mediterranean island of Sardinia, with a population of a million and a half, currently offers a situation of socioeconomic and cultural change that results from its particular history and geography and, as such, is peculiar to Sardinia itself. These changes serve as models of the deep disturbances that can be caused by foreign industrialization of a static society with fixed cultural limits and a tradition of violent acculturation.

The mental health disorders that occur in the wake of rapid social and industrial transformations of countries with a traditionally pastoral-agrarian economy are very much the same in both the third-world countries and the underdeveloped areas of the West. Many psychic disorders can be seen to be in direct relationship with the conflicts that arise from the some-times contrasting coexistence of diverse levels of culture in a fixed society.

A situation of social disintegration is created by the impact on an inade-quately prepared and matured social structure of radically different behaviors and more advanced models of development. This markedly anxiety-producing situation is accompanied by a loss of traditional values and points of reference and the absence of any new ones to replace them. This situation, affecting in particular the young people, renders even more complex and acute the conflict between generations. The difficulties in com-munications between generations are accentuated in a way which creates even more broken homes. Furthermore, the diminution of traditional leader-and-followerships augments the hostility between different social groups.

These are stresses that are felt by all age groups and cause changes in the psychiatric situation which result in a larger number of people suffering from disturbances of personality and neuroses and psychoses.

Worldwide rapid changes are felt locally when the traditional boundaries that were created from an accumulation of social experiences over centuries and that were "always" used as points of reference are changed. This leads to a situation of profound existential insecurity and makes it impossible to confront oneself within the group. When manners, tastes, habits, abilities, and beliefs change all over the world, it destroys the traditional cohesion of a communal culture. Each member of the society elaborates on his new experience in a personal and sometimes dramatic way, but these experiences are not acquired and assimilated in the kind of stable manner that would create a new codified system of existence for the confrontation of reality, and as such, the confrontation of the new culture.

As Leighton has said, psychic disturbances ". . . are in part manifesta-tions of psychological strain derived from experiencing the world as a sea of frustrations, terrors, and disappointments. . . . Such conditions are due to the lack of shared values, lack of standards and codes of behavior, and lack of opportunity for satisfaction of such basic needs as freedom from fear, access to love and respect . . . and opportunity for the expression of spontaneity."[11]

Sardinia, where we have completed a study of almost 4 years, lends itself very well to observation of the changes caused by rapid industrialization and to direct research into those disturbances related to cultural transformations and social disintegration.

Infested by malaria until 1950, Sardinia was also characterized by a particularly ancient social, economic, and cultural situation with the most primitive and poor of shepherding and farming economies. Sardinia is also the Mediterranean island farthest from continental land.

A social order centering about the nucleus of the family and organized tribally corresponded with a subsistence economy that was limited by the narrow horizons of the island. This social order was governed by the respect for the laws laid down by the aged from their experiences and was influenced further by the island's isolation from the rest of the world. Between 1945 and 1950, malaria was almost completely wiped out. It was during this same period of time that the economic development of the island began by the formation of tourist sites, the installation of some of the major Mediterranean petroleum plants, and also a large industry of aluminum production.

These economic innovations were set up with the declared intention of creating "poles of development" for the economy of the island; their initial result during the decade of 1950 to 1960 was to end Sardinia's traditional isolation from the rest of the world through a close net of exchanges.

These more than summarial historical notes are necessary to demonstrate that Sardinia's rapid growth toward those patterns of life characteristic of an industrial society was in contrast to the gradual development in other areas. This economic transformation was followed by a total change in the habits and customs of the younger generation (in those cases where it was not opposed by the older generations and was observed from a distance). Changes in the habits of the young were also created by the arrival of the mass media and an intensive increase in education which has significantly reduced illiteracy on the island.

These changes have led to a marked increase in emigration, but have affected the whole population of the island as well. The push toward a change in patterns of life was not wholly the result of economic difficulties, but was created also by a fervert desire of the people to adapt their life-style to the kind of culture that began to be presented daily by the mass media and by direct confrontation with the "foreigners" who arrived with the new industry.

CULTURAL TRANSFORMATIONS AND PSYCHOPATHOLOGY

A new type of personality has been growing more delineated on the island (though not without confusion) for the last 20 years—a personality somewhere between the new myths of consumer society and the old myths of the previous culture. A consumer of goods—whenever he can be—who is reacting to constant deprivation and the continual discovery of new desires in a technical civilization, one who sees the new world rising around him both feared and desired as a liberating flight from the realities of the life that he is compelled to live.

In the introduction to the Fourth International Congress of Analytical Psychology (1974) Gerland Adler[1] questioned whether it is truly exact to speak of our civilization as a "civilization in transformation" as is often done. Are we really experiencing a critical nodal moment, or is this just a phenomenon common to all ages? Every civilization is always in flux and is a living organism that never stands still even in moments of stagnation.

Still Adler maintains that in this particular period the transformations we are experiencing *are* exceptionally significant, and he defines our present situation as being "different" from the others. Religion has lost most its force and meaning for most of the people who live in a technologically advanced society, he maintains, while family life, marriage, and relations between parent and child are full of explosive uncertainties; formerly stable social situations are now in dissolution. This kind of dissolution occurs violently and rapidly in those rural areas of archaic structure in which rapid changes happen as a result of factories being brought in from the outside, and can be observed the way Guntern did in 1975.[10] He was able to make interesting observations of the social and sociopsychiatric changes in an Alpine village in Switzerland which was transformed into a renowned vacation spot in just a few years by the opening of a new road.

As we have tried to show even in such a short summary, this kind of "extreme" transformation has happened in a particular and emphatic way on the Sardinian island, and it is remained for the large part marginal to the technological and cultural development of the rest of Italy.

The examples of life-styles set by the permanently residing foreigners or the seasonal visitors are the customs and habits of a leisure class and, as such, differ enormously from those of the shepherd. The hard life of being away from home for months on end following herds through extremely rough conditions and then returning to a poor village and a simple life reduced to the essentials becomes an unacceptable reality. The same rigid family structure based on a subsistence economy of preindustrial characteristics also comes to be radically contested, as it requires that boys be taken out of school and put to work at the age of 13 or 14. The young women are the most resolute in breaking with family ties; they are the ones who were deprived of even the most basic education that might have permitted them access to a different economic level than that to which they were born. Furthermore, one can see how the younger generations refute in body the cultural codes and authority of the old, and how they do this in their search for a new pattern of personal and group development and in-group communications that are not those of a rigid patriarchal and tribal system.

It is in this way that a process of cultural trend and sociocultural disintegration is formed. We are all subject to change, particularly in our epoch of rapid innovations and radical economic changes. To be valid, every change should be wanted and arranged by the whole social group, but, in fact, the introduction to the social scene of new facts and ideas is the fruit of elaborate programs of a small technocratic elite. This is happening in Sardinia where rapid acculturation was not adequately preceded by the "cultural diffusion" which is the natural prerequisite to every acculturation and transacculturation. It is felt in an ambivalent way, possibly even as deprivation, inasmuch as it takes away elements of cultural and social identity from the individual and leaves him in a void. We will be able to see that such a void can be experienced in a depressive, hallucinatory, or anguished way. The new values are understood in a confused and unclear manner, particularly by those who are not accustomed to the continual barrage of information and solicitation from the mass media. What becomes lacking is the one secure point of reference that was once supplied by the traditional culture. In a predominantly illiterate, and therefore oral, society, the teachings of the aged have always been the conducting line of the cultural message and have remained substantially unchanged for centuries. A split is created between old cultural information and the new. This distance is not just caused by the more or less confused instances of yielding to that which is considered "new" or "modern," but by the precise practical demands for manual labor in a technologically advanced society where the reference to the agrarian-pastoral and archaic experience of the forefathers is useless. It is a distance often felt as anguished laceration. Freud says, ". . . I would not know how to find another infantile need as strong as the one for protection by his father."[7] The anguish that results from feeling oneself alone and abandoned in the face of an inexorable external being and reality and being at the mercy of this very power is probably at the root of all the feelings of insecurity and privation that accompany such a process of violent acculturation. The youngest generations of women feel the crisis of religious sentiment with a sense of ulterior abandonment, solitude, and enormous insecurity, as women have traditionally been more religious than are men. They lack the firm point of reference that church practices and advice gave them, and they remember the infantile state of absolute dependence with the nostalgia for the father which this provokes.

The break with the traditional patriarchal culture in which the authority of the old was unquestioned brings with it strong feelings of guilt that are linked to the known ambivalences of feeling toward the father. It should be remembered that in almost all the cases we have observed, aggression against the father was not just on an unconscious level but was almost always manifested in family crises of considerable importance. Momentous guilt feelings accompany this aggression against the father as well as the unconscious confusion of feelings about the destruction of a determined cultural code and the destruction of the father figure along with unresolved Oedipal conflicts. Observing this "union of cultures" one recalls what Freud wrote in 1929:[7] "It could be one day that thanks to civilization this diffusion of guilt will reach such a high level that man will find it impossible to bear it."

Moreover, this sense of guilt can be connected to the imperatives of an ideally severe exigency of the superego: (Kultur Überich)—transgressions of the laws will be punished with anguish. In particular one observes[14-21] a problematic psychiatric interest quite similar to that described by other authors writing about different cases of subjects of diverse cultures who were exposed to the trauma of transacculturation and socioeconomic transformation.[3, 4, 8, 9, 12, 13] One can synthesize psychic disturbances along large lines under certain headings. (R. Terranova-Cecchini)

1. *Pathology of transacculturation.* That which is most immediately tied to the loss of traditional values and which manifests itself as extreme anxiety and a sense of inadequacy when the subject is faced with the new situations; with symptoms of depression, hypochondriacal states, magic-delirium defences, and symptoms of refusal.

2. *Pathology of transgressions of cultural models.* In a society like Sardinia, founded on the wisdom of the aged and characterized by their laws, with transgressions punished extremely severely (to the point of physical suppression of the offender), adapting oneself to the new cultural models, even those deemed both modern and necessary, brings feelings of guilt and fear. The condemnation of the group is particularly felt and feared and is often experienced in terms of *magic* and possibly punished by the "evil eye."

3. *Pathology tied to cultural violence.* Since communications become so difficult as to be almost impossible between the generations with the uncommunicative void existing between them, this inability to express oneself creates a sense of dehumanization and leads to apathy, ineffectuality, and hypochondriacal symptoms.

MODIFICATIONS IN SYMPTOMATOLOGY

It appears that we can enucleate some general observations from the various groups of disturbances that we have observed.

In the last few years a coexistence between hysterical phenomena, which are decreasing, and psychic disturbances, which are increasing, have been observed. Thus we can include as confirmation of this in a larger sphere Opler's observation that ". . . in general, most epidemiologists, myself included, feel that psychosomatic disorders increase in number in modern societies while the hysteriform illnesses diminish. A further point is that psychosomatic disorders are more disguised by body language, and hence more devious in terms of a psychological model including the emotional concomitants of organic states."[13]

Hysterical disturbances have been observed with a much greater frequency than might have been expected, for example, in Rome, where the types of behavior (and psychic disturbances) imposed by a large urban complex can be observed.

Besides "hysterical paralysis" we have observed *arc de cercle* hysterics, which are extremely rare in urban or industrial settings, those of the type described by Charcot. The conflict arises from having to decide whether to remain anchored to a world that is familiar as a protector and is profoundly a part of one, or to repudiate it to yield to newer behavioral examples of living and to become a stranger in a world that is an imposition. The conflict often explodes in a massive hysterical crisis. An intense desire for insensibility with its failure arises from this, along with a need for love and approval from the group and a strong tendency toward dramatizing the conflicting situation (in a theatrical sense) especially in illiterate cultures.

An example of what we could call the manner of reaction to conflicting situations of particular emotional resonance, according to a "traditional" pathology, can be found in one of our patients, 22-year-old Giovanna. She was admitted to the hospital after hysterical fits and convulsions diagnosed as right hemiplegia and total aphasia. The absence of any pyramidal signs and the normal results of all medical examinations convinced us absolutely that we were dealing with a case of hysterical paralysis. We were able to find out that Giovanna was engaged to be married to a young man from Northern Italy. Her family was opposed to this match and kept trying to force the son of neighbors on her instead. Her fiancé was insistently asking Giovanna to leave her family and come and live with him in Milan, but wanted to postpone actually getting married. If she wouldn't come, he said, he would be forced to leave her. Yet if she did go, she would be condemned violently by her family and her village, and would never be able to return.

It was then discovered from other family members that an old aunt to whom Giovanna had been very attached had died a month earlier of apoplexy with right hemiplegia and complete aphasia while in the same hospital where Giovanna was. After a series of sessions, the symptoms began to regress and were completely gone after a long stay in the hospital.

Suppressed desires, existential difficulties, deep-rooted or apparent conflicts, all find the most immediate means of relationship with others in body language. In hysterical disturbances the appeal to others is direct, and through theatricality finds the most exigent means of getting an answer from the group. In a society in which life is lived in a closed environment, and is exposed to a constant relationship with the extended family and clan, the entire life socially is conditioned by others. Observing, judging, controlling, they participate in even the most significant and intimate moments in the life of every individual. Whereas in urban settings, though a few of life's events are group-oriented—recognition communally of birth, marriage, and death still survives—the greater part of one's life is lived alone.

In regard to hysterical phenomena and group participation in each person's life, it is worth remembering that until 1948 a ritual of magic possession survived in Sardinia, which was related to a spider bite and which was called the ritual of "Argia." This was quite similar to other rituals of possession in North Africa (Sudan, Ethiopia, The Egyptian "Zor," the Tunisian "Bori") and the Afro-American cults of "Voodoo" in Tahiti, "Shango" in Trinidad, and the Brazilian cult of the "Santos." This ritual has been described very well in C. Gallini's book *The Rituals of the Argia.*[5] Here it is adequate to say that the bite of a certain poisonous spider is followed by reversible neuropsychic disturbances and is cured by a ritual dance lasting several days and executed by a group of exorcists. On some parts of the island it is the bitten person himself who dances, and is possessed (dressed as a woman if he is a man) along with the whole village.

It is important to note how the rite of the Argia furnished both patient and community with a metahistorical parenthesis for seeing things "as they are," and which permitted the reabsorption, understanding, and demystification of the patient's disturbances. Psychic disturbances were "understood" by being reduced to easily interpreted terms that the entire group could comprehend. In this way the group could separate and protect the disturbed one while keeping the specter of mental illness at bay.

The interchange of sexes (a man dances dressed as a woman) is extremely important. It symbolizes the complete negation of responsibility to the individual for what happens, for when a person discards his role, it means that whatever happened did not happen to that person but to someone radically different. The patient's disturbances are then interpreted in this light; if he has stomach pains, they are not his; it is the spider that has possessed him and wants to escape. If a person speaks in an incomprehensible tongue, it is not he who is talking, but someone else inside him. In this way, disturbances of one person are lived by the whole group collectively; "different" or "strange" behavior is demystified and interpreted as the result of connected facts and events that are considered normal by the group. A sick person is not excluded, but absorbed into the community and protected by them, and they in turn actually collaborate in the healing process.

In a society in a state of transformation, growing more and more distant from community ties and evolving to a state of sociocultural disintegration, continually greater regression of hysterical manifestations appear, and a deeper refinement of conflicts becomes more likely.

Though they still remain in the context of body language, today psychosomatic manifestations find release more and more in hyperexpressive outbursts as a means of expressing the individual's isolation.

The most common disturbances are headache, asthenia, and visceral problems. It is necessary to mention that even the most intensive studies rarely succeed in scratching the surfaces of the subject's defenses, so that the real causes of the deep disturbances can be found. The patient talks always about the existing somatic disturbances, personal problems are systematically avoided and relative figures remain shadowy. It is only with the greatest difficulty that any information on situations of conflict can be obtained. The reality that the sick person refuses to recognize is that the new sociocultural settings offer him dangers and conflicts while at the same time they negate the tradition in which his sickness would have been experienced for and by the community. Since it has become impossible for the community to manipulate and organize cultural meanings, it can no longer be the mediator between the sick person and his illness. Thus in many cases under the impact of new models of society, and often felt as anguish, psychic disturbances are expressed without any mediation of social conflict. While in traditional cultural models, direct expression of hysterical disorders was prevalent in the phenomenon of conversion which permitted an escape from unbearable problems and pressures and at the present time psychosomatic disturbances prevail. Opler has written "the psychosomatic patient, on the other hand, stands alone to a greater extent and wholly internalizes his difficulties with real and damaging bodily or organ misfunctioning. For this reason, I call the psychosomatic illness more harmful and dangerous, more serious and difficult to treat, and ultimately a later evolutionary development in which the terrible loss of relationship to others is more clearly symbolized."[13]

Particularly frequent among the young, and especially among young women, are bouffées délirants which can be classified in traditional nosology as schizophrenic forms. However the possibility of a rapid, even spontaneous diminution, is worth noting, so these states might be more exactly classified under the heading of "psychotic confusional states."[3]

We are concerned here with psychogenic reactions that are comprehensible in the way that Jasper spoke of them—reactions to an objectionable environmental situation that has made the possibility of defense for the subject impossible, and as such are qualitatively and quantitatively abnormal responses to the experienced event. These forms of reaction are clearly different from those schizophrenic reactions that can be observed in urban settings. The latter, being more complex, are refractory to any form of therapy and cause much greater and longer-lasying psychological damage. An example of this occurrence with one of our patients seems particularly significant.

Luciana, aged 23, is the youngest of eight children. The father is an illiterate fisherman, the mother attends to the household and children. The family is described as being united, with good relations between the parents. Luciana, who completed the fifth grade in school, worked as a domestic for a family in Northern Italy while she was between the ages of 16 and 21. This period of living in an extremely different emotional environment considerably changed her existing I-World relationship. She came to learn different concepts of reality and relationships with others. Her mother's illness forced her to suddenly return home. Because she was the oldest daughter, the responsibility of running the house and caring for the younger children became hers. When she returned to her village, she was greeted with a cold, almost hostile environment. She was closely observed, almost spied upon, to see "whether she had become a bad girl up North" during her long absence. Her comings and goings from the house were strictly controlled by her father, and she was only allowed to have female friends (and these were selected by her father). Any friendships with boys created violent family discussion, and sometimes maltreatment.

A year after her return, Luciana became engaged to a boy her own age, although she was only allowed to see him in the presence of a member of her family. Bit by bit, she began to feel so spied upon and controlled that she closed herself like a mute, sometimes suspicious, sometimes indifferent.

Her breaking point came 2 or 3 days before her admission to the hospital. Her father met her on the main street of the town while she was arm in arm with her fiancé. Her father took her home, took away her clothes, and locked her in the house, accusing her of being a "whore." Luciana reacted to being locked up by trying to run away from home half-undressed; her father and brothers then tied her to the bed and kept her there for 2 days. She was brought to the hospital because of grave delusional symptoms and psychomotor agitation. Upon entering the hospital she was clutched by marked agitation. Terrified by everyone and everything she shouted continually that they were spying on her with television sets and that they wanted to kill her. She tried to find support by grabbing the doctors' arms. She tried to undress and run away from the hospital; she repeated continually "they all say I'm a whore; they spy on me; they want to hurt me. . . ."

After many days of therapy with psychopharmaceuticals, the symptoms declined and a good psychotherapeutic relationship became possible. The disturbances were completely gone after a few months.

As has been said before apropos to hysterical and psychic disturbances, we can currently see the coexistance of two pathologies. One is more similar to the traditional forms, and the other is perfectly applicable to those that have been observed in urban and industrial environments, with a slow but definite progression toward the latter.

Our observations are applicable to those made in African environments, where, as in our studies, there was a convergence of all of the factors introduced by social and racial changes. Such changes facilitated schizophrenic disturbances from both a genetic, dynamic, and structural point of view.

In his research Collomb[4] has noted that the percentage of schizophrenia is raised in proportion to the outlay of bouffées délirants which as much as affirms that there can no longer be any ethnopsychiatry with homogenization of culture.

SITUATION OF THE YOUNG

Particularly in families of schizophrenics, the parent-child relationship becomes quite disrupted. Filled with problems, anguish, and anxiety, it can cause a rupture of in-family communications and can lead to an intersection of recognized pathological difficulties.

Zempleni[22] has noted in Africa that the general line of the process of cultural transition and transformation can lead to a series of conflicting situations with a difficult gestation period, owing to the following.

1. The problem of illiterate parents (or those who have become illiterate again) who place all of their ambitions for social promotion on the education of a child, without being able to handle the resulting personal necessities and psychological evolution.

2. The anxiety of such a child, who sees in himself the investment of his entire family, but does not receive adequate emotional support from them. It is important to remember that in a family on such a low economic and social level, only one of the children will be able to get an education and all the rest will have to work to support his studies. It then becomes the "duty" of the chosen one to succeed professionally and to support his family with his new skills.

3. The conflict that arises between the new values learned at school and the traditional family structure. Added to this is the anxiety over whether an eventual success could become the object of persecution with magic by the rest of group (envy or the "evil eye").

Adolescence and young adulthood are characterized by an even more conflicting situation on personal or familial levels.

In a society like the Sardinian, a parent's word is law, and community law is based on the patriarchal family. Even today the elders of the village decide and sanction justice and punishment together, which is followed far more than the laws of the state (these being systematically ignored).

In a cultural climate based on respect for, and obedience to, the village elders, who are all tied to traditional values and ways of thinking, the life of a young person is subject to certain limitations and coercions. These are in radical contrast to that which the young observe in their contact with the "foreigners" on the island, and this is particularly true for the young women.

Although we would be justified in doing so, we are not maintaining that such forms of pathological manifestations of psychoses and antisocial behavior, which are so frequent among young women, are the result of any particular liability or disposition. They should instead be seen in relationship to a continual accumulation of opposing restrictions and coercions which finally becomes intolerable.

These young women are not merely faced with having to readjust their morals which the Catholic church has so strongly influenced in the past and still affects today, but must completely redefine their role as women in society, moving more and more toward the liberated ideals that the mass media has given them. Problems concerning the right to an education and the choosing of an autonomous career are very much the order of the day in talks between doctor and patient.

It has been traditional that in large families the older daughters would leave school, often before they had finished the third grade, to help their mothers raise the younger children and run the home. This custom resulted in the creation of a class of adult women who were completely dependent on their family clan and totally unprepared for autonomous choices. Today this past role is systematically opposed, and this produces conflicts of a violence that is hard to imagine. Until fairly recently, in areas of Southern Italy and on the Italian islands (and in the 1960s in central Italy as well), an ancient patriarchal culture, which was undoubtably far more permissive with the male children than with the female, was in force. The male children had to tolerate paternal authority that demanded unquestioned obedience, but the females were subject to an authority that was much more severe. It was not just a submission to the authority of parents and elders, but also a severe curtailment of the freedom of movement, with limits placed both on the amount of time out of the house and at the very places they were allowed to go. Even the most inattentive of travelers through these towns noticed that these are "towns without women," in that one meets only those women on the streets who are too old to be considered sexually attractive. However, a more progressive political movement will come to these towns, too, and movements for the emancipation of women, divorce, abortion, and emancipation from familial authority will be everyday things. It is easy to imagine the conditions of tension that this will generate, and the battle for supremacy between two cultural codes that will ensue, and consequently favor an insurgence of reciprocal persecution projections (Canestrari). In this, more than in any other time, the young come to see their elders as obstacles that must be overcome if they are to pursue the possibility of personal expression. The adult, in his turn, comes to see in the young a threat, not just to his prestige and authority, but also to his internal equilibrium— an equilibrium that is already being tested by the same joining of cultures that is agitating the young, and which when amplified by family struggles, threatens to destroy all of his systems of reference.

To such adults there remains no other alternative than to embrace violently all the ancient patriarchal and authoritative systems and to become ruthless enemies of "new" tendencies as the only possible means of defense against the anguish that threatens them. The mobilization of aggression, as F. Fornari has noted,[6] accompanies the demands and arbitrariness of the vicissitudes of life under a certain cultural code, either in autoaggressive form (guilt feelings) or in the form of heteroaggression.

An increase in the number of suicide attempts among adolescents is an indication of the increase of the incidence of depression when they are faced with the arbitrariness of a cultural code and without the comfort of group consensus for what to believe in. This is aggravated by the guilt created by breaking traditions. It has been recorded in Cagliari, the regional capital of Sardinia, that in the 3 years between 1970 and 1973 there were 239 attempted suicides by women. This is in comparison to 49 that were recorded between 1960 and 1963, and 13 between 1950 and 1953. These facts have been reported in various publications and indicate the unease of young adults. While the statistics from other parts of Italy and foreign countries indicate that sentimental problems are the prevailing motive for attempted suicide, in our causality, 80% of the attempted suicides were the result of family conflicts. These familiar conflicts, emerging from interviews with patients and their families, could always be traced to cultural conflicts—but there is no dialogue between cultures.

As we have already had occasion to say, the kind of tradition that existed in Sardinia was built upon the rigid authority of the elders, and on the necessary order and consensus of the group to make it function. This was possible only if transgressions were acknowledged; in the families that we observed, those who strayed from the cultural code were at least ostracized and exiled when they were not treated as outright enemies. A conflicting situation like this could only offer a young person the dubious comfort of being in the right according to the new and modern mores, and could not possibly be experienced without tremendous anguish and feelings of persecution. In addition, the sense of estrangement and the loss of real ties of affection with family and clan would also be felt as a form of persecution.

This kind of situation, which is conditioned so strongly by rapid and violent social change, is caused by the industrialization that was purposely designed to change the traditional economy of the region because it had seemed paradigmatic and instructive to do so.

In a general sphere, one can see that economic problems cannot be resolved around a table while cultural traditions are ignored and forgotten. The path of progress must respect the existing social organization and economic structure of a people. Psychic disorders, the spread of antisocial behavior, the oil-spot-like spreading of insecurity and anxiety, and drug abuse and alcoholism do not necessarily have to go hand in hand with the conservation and innovations to which man owes his survival. A different kind of planning, elaborated in concurrence with the interests of the population, could permit paths of progress, that were less disruptive to them and generally more harmonious.

REFERENCES

1. Adler, G.: Introduzione al Sesto Congresso di Psicologia Analitica (1974), *Riv. Psicol. Anal.* **6**(1):5 (1975).

2. Ammar, S. and Ledyri, H.: Les conditions familiales de développement de la schizophrenie. *Rapport de Psychiatrie au LXX Congrés de Psychiatrie et de Neurologie de langue francaise, Tunis, 1972*, Masson, Paris, 1973.

3. Carothers, J. C.: A study of mental derangement in Africans. *Psychiatry* **2**:47, 1948.

4. Collomb, H.: Psychiatrie et cultures. Quelques considerations génerales. *Psychopath. Afr.* **2**:2, 1966 (citato da Ammar S., Ledyri H., 1972).

5. Gallini, C.: *I rituali dell'Argia*, Cedam, Padova, 1967.

6. Fornari, F.: Ideale dell'Io e codice culturale. *Tempi Mod.* **15**:13, 39, 1973.

7. Freud, S.: *Das Unbehagen in der Kultur*, Wien, 1929.

8. Lambo, T. A.: Schizophrenic and borderline states. In *Transcultural Psychiatry*, CIBA Foundation Symposium, Little, Brown, Boston, 1965.

9. Le Guerinel, N.: Le langage du corp chez l'africain. *Psychopath. Afr.* **12**(1):13, 1971.

10. Guntern, G.: Changement social et consommation d'alcool dans un village de montagne. *Schweirer Archiv Neurol., Psichiat. Neurocir.* **116**:2, 353, 1975.

11. Leighton, A. H.: Social disintegration and mental disorder. In *American Handbook of Psychiatry*, S. Arieti (Ed.), Vol. II, 2nd ed., Basic Books, New York, 1974.

12. Opler, M. K.: Sociocultural patterns and types of schizophrenias. *Psychopath. Afr.*, **7**(3):443, 1971.

13. Opler, M. K.: The evolution of behavioral disorders according to culture patterns. *Psychopath. Afr.* **13**(1):91, 1972.

14. Simone, F. and Felici, F.: Note preliminari sui rapporti fra ambiente, famiglia, "malattia mentale" nel contesto socio-culturale Sardo. *Osp. Psichiat.*, 209, April–September, 1971.

15. Simone, F. and Felici, F.: Nosografia e linguistica. *Osp. Psichiat.*, 247, April–September, 1971.

16. Simone, F., Felici, F., and Congia, S.: Il tentativo di suicidio in una società in transformazione. *Osp. Psichiat.* **4**:455, 1972.

17. Simone, F.: Scuola, ambiente e famiglia e disadattamento giovanile. Comunicazione tenuta al: Convegno: "Università, Enti locali e Scuola nella programmazione educativa e nell'intervento pedagogico." *Cagliari*, November 1971; 20–23, *Scuola e città*, 3–4, 1973.

18. Simone, F. and Felici, F.: L'occhio e lo sguardo: approccio fenomenologico. Collana P. B. N., diretta da Vizioli R., Il Pensiero Scientifico Editore, Roma, 1973.

19. Simone, F., Felici, F., Marrosu, M., and Marrosu, F.: Il tentativo di suicidio e gli adolescenti. *Rass. Med. Sarda* **77**, 87, 1974.

20. Simone, F. and Felici, F.: The attempts of suicide and the teenagers: Revision of Casuistry of three years in Cagliari (1970–73). Comunicazione presentata al VII Internationale Congress on Suicide Prevention, Amsterdam, 1973.

21. Simone, F., Felici, F., and Valerio, P.: Industrie a tecnologia avanzata in aree sottosviluppate: rapporto con la migrazione interna ed il disadattamento. Comunicazione al Convegno su "Psicodinamica e sociodinamica della migrazione interna," Varese, 1974.

22. Zempleni, A.: Milieu africain et development. *Psychopath. Afr.* **8**(2):233, 1972.

CHAPTER FIVE

PSYCHOTHERAPY
FOR THE ILLITERATE

ERNA M. HOCH, M.D.

W estern methods of psychotherapy seem to take it for granted that the patients who are to benefit by them are educated and have minds trained to think, not only about things in general, but also introspectively and self-reflectively about themselves, that they are interested in further developing this self-awareness and in finding rational explanations in the past for the way they are experiencing the present. It is also assumed that psychotherapy is a lengthy process that has to be stimulated and guided by an expert, either in a close relationship of one-to-one or within a group of similarly disposed fellow patients.

Even in the West, however, when psychotherapy became popular and attempts were made to widen its scope, it was found that the prevailing theories and practices do not all lend themselves easily for use at any and every level of social emancipation, but that there are, in every population, "underprivileged" strata, who are excluded from such methods of treatment, not only for economic reasons, but also because these methods are beyond the level of their understanding and do not correspond to their felt needs and aspirations.

If this is the case even in highly developed Western countries, then what about the regions of the "Third World," where formal education, even at the level of mere literacy, has only just started to be available to the broad masses? Is there any form of psychotherapy, apart from the practices of the indigenous healers, that is applicable at their level?

During almost 20 years of psychiatric work in India, and in particular during the last 6 years, which were devoted to building up psychiatric services and teaching in Kashmir, the northern-most part of India, secluded between high mountains and with a still largely illiterate population, I have had ample opportunity to explore how far, under what conditions, and in what form a psychotherapeutic approach is possible in a setting of this kind.

Some aspects of this situation have already been presented in two papers. As far back as 1970, during the Eighth International Congress of Psychotherapy at Milan, when "transcultural psychiatry" hardly attracted attention as yet, I tried to formulate how far psychotherapy in the Western sense could make a contribution to any program of "aid for development."[3] Three years later, during the Ninth International Congress of Psychotherapy at Oslo, interest in the problems of the Third World was very much in the foreground. I had an opportunity to speak about my experiences not only in a panel discussion on "Psychotherapy in Different Cultures," but also during a symposium on "Shamanism and Psychotherapy." My contribution to the latter was subsequently formulated in writing and published in *The Human Context*.[4]

An invitation to take part in a symposium on "Problems Imposed on Psychotherapeutic Intervention in Traditional Milieux," held during the Fifth International Congress of Social Psychiatry at Athens in 1974, stimulated me to reflect in greater detail on some of the difficulties encountered in my attempts at introducing a psychotherapeutic approach in dealing with illiterate patients and in particular into examining how far one is justified in speaking about a "traditional milieu." Every society, after all, has its "traditions" of more or less venerable age. The West, however, appears to be labeling as "traditional" societies or social strata in which values, beliefs, customs, and institutions still conform to old indigenous patterns, handed on from generation to generation over hundreds or even thousands of years, without having undergone contamination and transformation by Western influences of industrialization, urbanization, and rationalization.

As, unfortunately, I finally could not attend the Congress, the material compiled in preparation for it is presented in this chapter.

TRADITIONAL OR TRANSITIONAL?

In every society that one can characterize as "traditional" according to the criteria suggested above, but which is sufficiently open to admit at least an observer from a more developed or differently developed area, one has to distinguish three sectors: first, the one that is traditional in the strictest sense, in which old values and customs persist undisturbed. At the other extreme, one will find groups and individuals who have already emancipated themselves and who no longer conform to the old pattern. In between these two, one can perceive a transitional sector, so-to-speak the growing edge, in which emergence is only just starting and values are mixed or often confused. If we wish to talk about psychotherapy "in traditional milieux," we have to be clear which of these three sectors is to be considered.

On the basis of my experience I would say that, in the most emancipated sector—in India for instance in the upper and middle strata of the big cities and even here in Kashmir among college students and adults with an academic background—psychotherapy often can follow more or less the Western patterns. Of course one may have to introduce certain modifications that take account of the relative lack of information and sophistication and the persistence of infantile tendencies, partly connected with methods of early upbringing, which is still mostly in the hands of traditionally oriented mothers. Supportive and re-educative elements and usually a somewhat authoritarian approach are often indicated far more than with similar patients in the West (see also Ref. 1).

In the sector that is still completely "traditional" in the strictest sense, one will find a perfect "fit" between popular theories and beliefs about origin and nature of mental illness, the prevailing symptomatology of emotional disorders, and the indigenous methods for their treatment. Any "intervention" of a therapist with a Western training and outlook would in itself break up this close congruence and consequently the traditional character of the milieu, thus bringing the situation to the level at which values and practices are mixed. It is this middle sector and the psychotherapeutic possibilities existing within it that should form the object of investigation. Correspondingly, one should not talk about "psychotherapy in traditional milieux," but rather "in transitional milieux" or, preferably, "against a traditional background."

SOME OF THE PROBLEMS ENCOUNTERED IN THE "TRANSITIONAL SECTOR"

In what I have just characterized as the "transitional sector," one of the most decisive changes which the people passing through it have to face is the need to emerge into individual responsibility, self-awareness, and self-reflection from a previous condition of being sheltered in collective securities, within which consciousness only had to illuminate a very limited "here and now." This transformation, which often does not come about as the result of a natural process of maturation but is forced on a person by the pressure of social change, implies quite a few hazards for mental health, and one would readily assume that psychotherapeutic guidance should be very welcome and beneficial. In the paper already mentioned[3] I discussed in detail what obstacles stand in the way of applying psychotherapy as "aid for development" in this situation. In the present context, I only want to pick out a few of these problems.

In my present field of work in Kashmir, psychiatry has had quite a boom during the last 6 years. Initially, most patients were referred to our newly organized out-patient service from the other departments of the general hospital attached to Government Medical College. They soon learned that these new "mental doctors" do not deal with "mad" patients only, but that they give effective treatment for such troubles as headaches, palpitations, giddiness, vague aches, and pains; that is, the very complaints that other doctors designate as being "nothing wrong" and yet that they do not succeed in curing. The skillful use of tranquilizers and antidepressants which, though also at the disposition of the general practitioners, are often applied rather indiscriminately by them of course established quite a good reputation for us. People, however, also realized that what we give is more than drugs. They call it "hamdardi," which means fairly literally "sympathy" or "compassion," in other words, an attitude of human concern, of readiness to listen to the patient's problems, which up to now they had not found anywhere else. At the same time, however, very few of these people are ready to embark on prolonged psychotherapy. Some 20 to 30% of newly registered patients never come back after a first visit. This seemed very disappointing to us at first, until we realized that even these patients occasionally become "sources of referral" for further customers, a plain indication that they "got something out" of the one contact they had with us. Rather than regretting the lack of sophistication and individual awareness of our illiterate patients, we therefore tried to learn with what expectations and concepts they approach a healer according to their own tradition, and how we, in our role of modern psychiatrists, can try to do justice to them by integrating some of the old patterns into our own therapeutic activities.

One of the essential features of traditional healing by the local "Pīr" and "Faqir"[4] is that the contact between the healer and the patient is usually of short duration. Furthermore, the patient expects the healer to be invested with magic or divine powers which, if he is properly approached and pleased, he will wield for the benefit of the patient. The latter remains mostly a passive recipient or even victim of the various practices performed on him. Inquiries and instructions on the part of the healer are often not directed at the patient, but at the "ghost" by whom he is supposed to be possessed. Often the relatives have to be more active than the patient in procuring various remedies, engaging in ceremonies and sacrifices at holy shrines, and paying "penalty" in the form of donations or feasts for the poor and sick. By his extraordinary powers, either the healer can produce an immediate, miraculous change during a first consultation, or he will be considered as ineffective, and the journey then hopefully continues to a next celebrity.

This obviously means that the therapist with a Western orientation who tries to treat patients from a traditional background, unless he is prepared to lose the majority of his patients and, along with them, also his reputation, also must try to "score a goal" of some kind or other in the first encounter with the patient and/or his relatives, be it in the form of a spectacular symptomatic "cure," or at least an establishment of sufficient confidence and respect to serve as a solid base for a more prolonged therapeutic relationship.

TECHNIQUES FOR MAKING A FIRST AND POSSIBLY ONLY CONSULTATION PSYCHOTHERAPEUTICALLY MEANINGFUL

If the techniques used during a first and perhaps only interview are to be helpful in creating a favorable impression and to convey a therapeutic message, they have to serve the following purposes:

1.   *The therapist must evaluate the patient's readiness for emerging as an individual.* Has he been coming up against obstacles, either environmental or intrapsychic, in the course of a process of emancipation for which his

capacities are basically adequate, or has he been forced into venturing out of his traditional shelter prematurely, under the pressure of unfortunate circumstances? It is hardly possible to avoid wrong judgment in all cases. Often only prolonged exploration can reveal the patient's potential. Even a short interview, however, can often give some valuable hints:

Already the way in which the patient approaches the psychiatrist may be characteristic. A patient who is brought by relatives, neighbors, or even police as a passive or struggling victim seldom is a hopeful candidate for a psychotherapeutic challenge. Even then, it may be worthwhile trying to address oneself to the patient himself. The relatives or neighbors usually are only too ready to offer their information, assuming that the patient is "out of senses" and therefore incapable of giving a relevant account of himself. They respond with surprise, perhaps annoyance if we make the patient himself the center of our concern. The patient, however, often gratefully acknowledges or at times even imperiously demands such personal concern and respect. His being given the dignity of a subject instead of being disposed of as a passive object or, worse, as an awkward impediment, often brings a first ray of hope and at the same time a chance of his getting a hearing for his real complaints.

Among the illiterate, a person usually is considered "mad" only when he starts making a public nuisance of himself. Silent suffering, in particular in a phase of depression or during the early stages of schizophrenia, but also due to neurotic conflict, is not likely to attract the attention and sympathy of the environment. It therefore seems that patients often *have* to become violent or at least disturbing if they are to be heard and to obtain help. Our being able to perceive the "real trouble" underneath a superficial layer of noisy agitation or stubborn resistance often brings about a much more reasonable and calm behavior in the patient. He may accept that he is "sick," though he protests against the allegation that he is "mad."

In dealing with children and adolescents, even in the West, a suggestion that the doctor wants to have a few words with the boy or girl alone often shows how far there is hope of establishing a direct therapeutic relationship. If both child and parents readily consent, the chances are best; it the child is eager to talk, but the parents reluctant to leave him, perhaps peeping and listening at the door, while one is trying to have a private discussion, this would show that the young patient, even if he is willing to become more independent, has to face considerable obstacles and will need an extraordinary amount of determination and perseverance if he is to free himself from the ties of the family. Finally, if both parents and child insist on remaining together for the whole interview or if the child anxiously clings to his escort, and the latter does not appear to be quite wholehearted in his encouraging the child to remain with the therapist, or even triumphantly enjoys the child's display of attachment, the prospects of psychotherapeutic work with the patient himself are of course poor. While in the West, the patterns just sketched out would apply only to children and perhaps very young adolescents, we here can observe them even when a patient is of adult age.

The ideas that patient and relatives have about the causing agent or precipitating factors responsible for the illness give some further indication of the level of emancipation. Belief in possession, magic spells, or the casting of the "evil eye," fits in much better with the techniques of the indigenous healers than with what we can offer. We have actually noted that, though gross conversion reactions and possession states are quite frequent, only few of these patients come to us for treatment. Presumably, for them the traditional practices of exorcism still are more effective than our more sober modern approach.

2. Because many of our nonpsychotic patients, who, in first line, could become candidates for a psychotherapeutic approach, present physical symptoms, one of the tasks to achieve in a first interview is to bring insight from the first level up to the second one, that is, from acknowledging sickness as such to *recognizing that this sickness is emotional.*

In illiterate and little-educated patients, we cannot take for granted any knowledge about the structure and functions of the body. Pain or some uncomfortable sensation or a disturbance in the smooth running of the various organs is often the first thing that brings the body into awareness as something that can give trouble and that has to be cared for. This often causes consternation and sets going a vicious circle of aroused emotions and vegetative responses. The helplessness or lack of concern of physically oriented doctors contributes to "escalation," undermining the patient's confidence not only in his own body, but also in those whose job it ought to be to repair it effectively. An experience of physical suffering and impairment, associated with ill-digested information through hearsay about some other person's illness and perhaps death, may, for the first time, make a person aware of the fragility of human life and the constant threat of deterioration and dissolution that hangs over physical existence.

The patient, experiencing his illness in the physical sphere and recognizing only the physical and material as "real," naturally expects physical treatment and will at first be very reluctant to accept any verdict of "emotional trouble." This, to him, is synonymous with "vehem," that is, an imaginary disease, a mere fuss about nothing, coming close to malingering. The patient wants to know why other doctors have told him "nothing is wrong" and yet have prescribed expensive drugs; he insists perhaps on further physical investigations, such as X-ray, blood tests, or even an exploratory operation.

Our first task therefore often is to give the patient some kind of "health education," to explain to him the structure and functioning of his body, in particular the close connection between emotions and vegetative nervous system. I usually do this in the form of a metaphor:

> I take the example of a horse and a cart. Suppose every time the cart starts moving, it will jolt or deviate from its course or even topple over; the first thing would be to inspect the horse—whether its hooves are tightly fitted, whether harness and bit are properly adjusted, whether the horse itself is well nourished and in fit condition. Then one would inspect the cart and make sure that every nail and bolt are in their proper places and the axle well oiled. But what, if all this has been found in order, and the vehicle still does not take a smooth course? Sometimes the patient himself will then state, or else we have to point out to him, that then it is presumably the driver who does not know how and when to use the whip and when the reins or the brake. We then explain that every organ and part of the body has two nerves: one serving as a "whip," the other one as a "brake." And who is the driver? Obviously the mind, but not only that part of the mind of which we remain aware, but also the "hidden mind," the "storeroom," in which we put away what serves no obvious purpose or what is a hindrance to the activity of the "open mind." If the mind is divided; that is, when there is too much contrast between the "hidden" and the "open" mind, and there is dilemma between wanting to go forward and some hesitation, the "whip" and the "brake" will receive conflicting orders, and the functions of the body or one of its organs will be disturbed.
>
> If the patient tends to go into hysterical fits of unconsciousness, we point out that any good doctor, if he has to inflict pain or discomfort on a patient during an investigation or operation, will apply an anaesthesia. Similarly, the mind itself, if a person has to face something which he cannot bear while in his senses, can drop the curtain of unconsciousness. We then encourage the patient that, with our help and added bearing power, he or she may perhaps dare to face what was so terrifying or disturbing.

These or similar explanations, kept in simple everyday language, are usually fairly convincing, at least for the moment. The patient has arrived at the second level of insight: "I am emotionally sick."

3. The next step then should consist of establishing insight on the third level by *relating the physical symptoms, now recognized as signs of emotional conflict, to some specific problem* of which the patient may or may not have been aware up to that moment.

An illiterate or little-educated patient's awareness even of pathogenic situations that to us appear to be very obvious again can be taken much less for granted than this is the case in more emancipated people. He is likely to live still very much in unreflected manner, in an immediate "here and now," and thus lacks understanding for the historical continuity and wholeness of existence. Even educated patients here rarely remember events of their early childhood, nor do their parents recall what may have happened to any particular one of their usually numerous children. It is characteristic that in some Indian languages the term for "yesterday," "tomorrow," and "some time later," which may perhaps be "never," is the same, so that the only clear distinction is between a definite "today" or "now" that comes into clear focus, and all else hidden in a uniform mist of "not yet" or "no longer." Spontaneous confession of already known conflicts and useful cooperation in uncovering forgotten events or "unconscious" complexes is therefore minimal and seldom fruitful.

The search for precipitating factors or causal conflicts would thus be almost hopeless, unless an other peculiarity characteristic of our illiterate and little educated patients, came to our aid.

When comparing them with their more emancipated counterparts, either in the West or in India itself, one is again and again struck by the lack of individual variations in their life histories. Situations and experiences at any particular age level are so uniform, conforming closely to institutionalized patterns, that it is relatively easy for the therapist to make a clever guess about the patient's problems according to his age, sex, and social status. Of course this presupposes that he has detailed knowledge, not only about life in the particular country in general, but very specifically about the area in which he works and, within it, again about the different religious communities and social groups.

As people at this level still spend their lives mostly within the circle of the extended family, wider contacts only reaching out to the immediate neighborhood and perhaps a place of work, the most important item of information to be collected is the family history. By combining the individual family constellation with his knowledge about traditional family patterns, and by taking into account the approximate period of onset of the illness, the therapist can often arrive at a plausible conjecture about the patient's problems. Though it may not always be advisable to confront the patient with this hypothesis and thus perhaps to conjure up resistance, the therapist's skill for putting his finger on the sore spot already during a first contact is often what invests him with the necessary prestige and what creates respect and confidence in the patient.

A few illustrative examples can show how relatively simple such "guesswork" is, provided one has adequate background knowledge:

A 14- to 15-year-old girl, daughter of a "gujar," that is, a half-nomadic cowherder, is brought to us with a hysterical abasia. I find out that the girl is engaged to be married. Knowing that in Muslim families, and in particular among the "gujars," after marriage the girl does not always go to live at the in-laws, but sometimes, together with her husband, remains in the parental home, I ask: "When you get married, will you remain at home or go to your husband's family?" The prompt answer is: "How can I go to my in-laws, if I cannot walk?"

A young girl, also engaged to be married, goes into fits of unconsciousness several times a day, but nearly always between 10.00 a.m. and 4 p.m. As this is the official working time in Government offices and also private business in Srinagar, I inquire who goes to work during that time. When I learn that it is the father, I ask what is different or lacking during father's absence. The patient and her mother then explain that the people in the neighboring houseboat resent the patient's engagement—of course arranged by the parents!—to a young man from a distant part of the city, as they had hoped that their own son would be given preference. They now frequently engage in teasing and abusing the patient and her mother, but do not dare to do so while the father is at home!

In other cases, if we survey the succession of children to whom an exhausted young woman has given birth, we immediately realize that a "family planning" problem may be involved, particularly if the symptoms have started at the time when, a few months after the last delivery, a first menstruation indicates that there is risk of a renewed conception, and the husband can be kept from intimate approach only by the wife's illness.[2]

Sometimes it is not the wife, but the husband on whom the burden of a rapidly growing family falls or whose own infantile needs are frustrated or old sibling rivalries revived by the birth of a first or second child.

The arrival of a new daughter-in-law in a hitherto well balanced family can create difficulties for the mother-in-law or one of her daughters or a previously established daughter-in-law, but of course also for the newcomer herself.

Particular problems may harass a girl who, according to Muslim custom, is married to a cousin in a close-knit joint family, where no emotional outlet is possible, as parental family and in-laws are almost identical.

A frequent pattern that we encounter in our female Muslim patients is a very close alliance between mother and daughter. At the time when, according to custom, the latter ought to get married, which still is soon after menarche, either mother or daughter develops some functional symptoms, covering up the conflict between the duty of getting the daughter married and, on the other hand, wanting to keep her at home as a female companion and helper in the household. This happens particularly if no compensation is to be expected in the form of a daughter-in-law, either because there is no son old enough to be married or because the prospective or actual wife of a son is too emancipated to accommodate herself under the rule of an old-fashioned mother-in-law.

Between a widow and her only son a similar problem may exist, and either one or the other has to pay with sickness for the unwillingness to break the close relationship.

Death or severe illness of a close relative, neighbor, or perhaps friend often sets off an anxiety reaction and, though the patient and his relatives of course remember the event as such, no one has as yet established a connection between it and the patient's palpitations or fainting fits.

A mother may have started getting depressed 2 years ago. All we find out on taking the family history is that she has five children, the youngest of whom is now 7 years old. On inquiry, according to our "hunch," we actually find that 2 years ago this last child started going to school and that since then the illiterate mother feels lonely, useless, and without purpose in life.

On the other hand, the position of a person who is the first in his family to enter school or to go in for higher education, trivial as by now this may appear, is also something that often has to be pointed out, as it can lead either to anxiety and a sense of isolation or, on the contrary, to maniform inflation.

It may be noteworthy that these common constellations, picked out at random from a whole collection of problematic situations observed in our patients and their families, would not all apply in Hindu families in this same area and not entirely to Muslims in some other parts of India. When coming to Srinagar 6 years ago, after having worked in other areas of India where Hindus are in the majority, I knew very well that the experience gained among them would not be fully applicable here. It took me some time, not only observing patients but also keeping my eyes open while wandering through the narrow lanes of the old city or hearing people talk in the street or in the bus, until I was able to unravel the possible complications of the situations and relationships in this particular setting where Muslim tradition is predominant. The culture-bound specificity of factors that make for or against mental health has to be kept in mind very clearly, whereas, as already mentioned, one can almost neglect the impact of individual variations.

Whether one wants to interpret in Freudian terms the critical situations that have thus been revealed and which mostly concern family constellations and events is probably a matter of personal taste. If one so wishes, one can certainly detect Oedipal situations, incest wishes, and guilt about forbidden libidinal strivings, behind many of the manifestations that our patients present. It may be pleasing to the therapist to be able to label and interpret according to some known Western school of psychotherapy, just as one may derive some satisfaction from being able to accommodate the diagnosis within an approved international classification. The patient, however, risks being shocked and deterred if one serves him the analysis of his conflicts in terms of erotic involvements or even incestuous tendencies. To talk of "immaturity," "need for security," as against the capacity to face individual responsibility and venturing forth into some degree of independence, usually makes more sense and has a better chance of being accepted. Even then one frequently finds that, on the occasion of the next interview, whatever had been opened up and apparently understood during a first visit has again been conveniently forgotten or repressed.

4. Already during the first interview, apart from prescribing drugs which are expected as a token of the doctor's magic power, some *constructive and supportive help for dealing with the problems that have been identified* should be given. Frequently this is already implied in satisfying the needs just mentioned under steps 2 and 3; that is, by enlightening the patient about the functions of the body and their connections with his emotions and with particular situations and experiences apt to arouse them. It is usually helpful to formulate interpretations and advice in terms of traditional concepts, drawing metaphors from everyday life, borrowing from folklore, religion, and philosophy of the patient's background. On the other hand, modern "scientific" information, which can stimulate confidence in the adaptative, restitutive, and creative potential of life, may also be acceptable, particularly to those who attach prestige to modern education.

An example of using a traditional feature of Hindu religion for creating a more hopeful outlook in neurotic or even paranoid patients is included in the paper already mentioned[3] and deserves to be quoted in this context:

> ... for Hindus, time is measured in terms of characteristically patterned epochs of astronomical dimension, which alternate with equally long phases of general dissolution, and [that] nowadays we are approaching the climax of the last stage of a series of 4 epochs, in which virtue successively loses one of its 4 feet; thus, at this time, we are standing on our last leg in a precarious manner. Falsehood, greed, ruthless aggression and iron hardness and masculine emancipation of women are some of the characteristics of this degenerated Kali Yuga, after which a new golden age is expected to arise. If one allows oneself to reflect on this theory without prejudice, one realizes that an epoch of this kind, if it is to come to fulfilment, needs not only the broad mass of people living in it for *ex*pressing itself through them, but, if its character of hardness. of ruthlessness and exploitation is to be perceived as such, it also needs a minority of human beings who are *imp*ressed or even *sup*pressed by it. It seems to me, however, that it is from amongst this very minority of the sensitive and the vulnerable, of those who cannot swim along with the stream of their time, but who also do not have sufficient strength to keep up a firm stand against it, that the majority of our patients is recruited.

To help them see their suffering, their weakness, not only as a personal misfortune, but also from a higher point of view, as a meaningful happening, would seem to be one of the psychotherapeutic possibilities for leading patients, even if they are relatively uneducated, from inner loneliness and estrangement back into a feeling of belonging to their environment.

Islam also provides various resources which one can tap for creating hope, a sense of security, and trust in an ultimate justice.

To illustrate the instant effect of a more modern interpretation, the following two examples, taken from recent experience, may serve:

A young teacher, unmarried, cherished only son of a widow, in a state of depression and utter disgust with life, was brought to us by his worried mother. He had been particularly terrified by a recent dream which conveyed to him that he had "one foot in the grave." What he made responsible for his deplorable condition was a period of unemployment after completing his studies, during which he had drifted into the habit of excessive masturbation. Though at the time he consulted us he had started working as a teacher, he was still ruminating about his past "misdeeds," obviously fearing punishment in some form or another. At the end of the first interview, during which I had tried to bring about some insight according to the methods already described, I casually remarked: "You know, what is in the grave, is that which is past. I think your constant worrying about having 'one foot in the grave,' just means that half of your mind is occupied with the past. Try to turn it to the present and the future." Of course one could have mentioned that the future obviously was blocked, as he could not grow up further without risk of either having to "desert" the widowed mother by getting married or otherwise realizing the incestuous nature of his attachment to her. Eventually, in later interviews, I was able to help him to understand this. But the effect of this parting remark on the occasion of the first interview was that, for the next consultation, he came as a changed man: alert, hopeful, smartly dressed and groomed, and ready to take up his work again after having remained on leave, moping about for a few weeks.

Another patient, a middle-aged Government employee, was carrying about with him an old X-ray report, indicating that he had "chronic duodenal ulcer." As gastric and duodenal ulcers are rather frequent here in Kashmir, often leading to dramatic complications, anyone in whom this diagnosis is even only suspected risks being very much impressed and discouraged by it. In this particular patient, it had created a severe hypochondriac reaction and, in addition, justified doubts with regard to the credibility and trustworthiness of doctors, as some of them had played down or negated the X-ray findings. I simply told him: "You know, it is true that you have had an ulcer some time in the past, and that the scar of it is still visible. But apparently it is equally true that you had the forces of resistance and the vitality to overcome it. Why not think of this positive, creative aspect a little more, instead of only remembering that your body is vulnerable?"

Though the drugs I prescribed were hardly different from what he had already been taking on the advice of general practitioners, he reported marked improvement, when he came next time.

Explaining to a patient how to get rid of swallowed and accumulated anger by engaging in "redirected action" is often very useful at this point.

It may perhaps be worth mentioning that even the prescribing of drugs can be turned into a therapeutic experience. I am often shocked and pained to find how little concern most doctors, in particular young ones, have for the needs of illiterate patients. If one looks at their prescriptions, one feels all that mattered was to demonstrate their up-to-date knowledge about the latest drugs. Whether the patient is economically in a position to buy the medicines, and whether he understands, when and how to take them, what their effects and side effects are likely to be, hardly bothers them. Most of these patients are not only economically "poor," but also poor in understanding, in fact completely helpless and puzzled, when faced with written instructions. I always make it a point in my own work and in teaching young doctors and social workers to emphasize that great care must be taken to ensure that the patient gets his due supply of free drugs and that he knows what to buy, how much approximately it will cost him, and when and how he has to take the medicines. A pictorial method of marking the doses and timings for medication can be very useful.

Most traditionally minded patients also expect to be given some instructions about diet and are disappointed if we neglect or even refuse to respond to their often anxious inquiries about "forbidden" and "recommended" food articles.

It is to a great extent our concern for these apparently trivial details that gives us the reputation of treating our patients with "hamdardi," that is, sympathy or compassion.

THE BACKGROUND OF THE THERAPIST

If intimate knowledge of the local setting and a capacity to formulate interpretations and explanations in terms familiar to the patient are so essential for dealing with patients from a traditional background, the ques-

tion arises whether a therapist who does not belong to the sociocultural setting in which he works is fit to venture into work of this type. Some authors
seem to doubt this.[5] On the basis of my long experience, I would however
dare to say that the foreign therapist, provided he is well acquainted with
the cultural setting concerned, and if he has at least some command of a
local language, has some distinct assets.

An outsider is often more likely to recognize even "normal," but to him
unfamiliar situations, as potentially pathogenic than is the indigenous
colleague, for whom they are customary and who, without questioning, takes
them for granted.

He is, or at least ought to be, free from cultural values and therefore can
reduce the patient's inhibitions and scruples against revealing tendencies
and ideas of his own that are in contrast and conflict with the traditional
background, from which he is about to emerge. The foreigner in particular
often enjoys greater confidence with regard to his respect for the medical
secret than the local doctor, who frequently is himself intensively involved
in the social network.

The foreign doctor's presence and example as "different," "other,"—and
a successful and respected "other" at that—stimulates the patient to
identify with him or, if one wants to express it in Jungian terms, into discovering and integrating his "shadow." The therapist by his knowledge of
and respect for the traditional culture, on one hand, can provide much
needed support and shelter, while, on the other hand, as the one who is
"standing out," he represents that which the patient is not yet and what
potentially he can become. This provides a creative tension in the therapeutic field. The therapist's "double-faced" situation challenges the patient
into making his choice between the possibilities of emerging into existence
as a unique individual and, on the other hand, of remaining safely embedded
in institutionalized patterns of behavior and in collective securities.[4]

A technique that I have found useful for eliciting the patient's response to
this challenge and for testing his capacity for coming up to it is the following.

As I speak fluently only Urdu, the language of the educated, but do not
understand Kashmiri well, I often have to use an interpreter (junior doctor
or social worker) for communicating with the more traditionally oriented
patients. When I want to draw the patient's attention to some possible conflict in his mind between adherence to tradition and venturing into more
individual ideas or forms of behavior, I ask the interpreter to convey my
question or remark in a way that keeps him or her, that is, the local
interpreter, at a doubting distance from my point of view or even makes
him or her appear critical or disapproving. In the case of an overburdened

mother who has broken down after the birth of her sixth child, it may for
instance be: "This foreign doctor thinks that, perhaps, after already having
so many children, you might not have been very happy to have another
baby?" If the patient needs to cling for security to her traditional beliefs and
customs, she will discover the slight note of disbelief and perhaps even
ridicule in the interpreter's words and be quick to protest: "No, no!
Mothers always want to have more children." If, however, the forces of
rebellion against the fate of a woman in her traditional setting have been
stirred and have come close to awareness, the answer may be: "Yes, of
course, she is right." Accordingly, one can then "cover up" and continue
with a purely supportive approach, or, in the second instance, help the
woman to see that her resentment is justified, that nowadays it has its legiti-
mate place even within official health and economic policies and perhaps
suggest in the end that she should bring her husband for discussing "family
planning." The technique can of course be used with appropriate variations
in other situations too.

DIFFICULTIES FACED DURING PROLONGED PSYCHOTHERAPY

What I have tried to sketch up to now are a few approaches that can help
make a first and perhaps only interview therapeutically meaningful and
effective. Some of the patients thus dealt with never come back; some of
them, not satisfied, continue their round from doctor to quack, from quack
to Faqir, and so on. Others, however, as "satisfied customers," send us
more patients, thus giving some indication that our methods are not without
success. But what if the patient "catches on" and continues therapy beyond
the first visit and ready for more than just collecting of a weekly ration of
drugs? Again, the problems one has to face are numerous, and I only want
to mention two of them.

Foreign guests, from Europe or the United States, who occasionally drop
in to observe our work, have often been impressed by one serious handicap,
which one tends to forget or to underrate, if one has worked for a long time
in a country like India. When discussing a case with us, they hopefully
make a number of suggestions about how the patient's situation could be
manipulated, what aims should be set up before him, and what creative
possibilities should be realized. They become almost speechless if we then
explain how few of these options, if any, are open to a person who, though
on the road toward individual emancipation, still remains tightly wedged in
between traditional structures. The degrees of freedom are often minimal,
not only with regard to selecting a marriage partner or engaging in other
personal relationships, but also with regard to the educational, vocational,

and professional field, not to speak of the economic restrictions, which can be quite paralyzing. For adolescents and young adults in particular, the situation often is hemmed in on all sides. Whereas the young person in the West enjoys a period of economic freedom, no longer dependent on his parents and, on the other hand, not yet responsible for a family of his own, when he is capable of earning and saving money that allows him to fulfill his heart's desires and to roam about in the world free from all obligations, the young Indian, and even more the young Kashmiri, very frequently has to move from a situation of dependence immediately into one of being "depended upon." With regard to family ties, it is in some cases hardly exaggerated if one pointedly formulates that a boy exchanges his mother's bed with the nuptial couch without any interval. Economically, as soon as he earns, he may not only have to pay back "educational loans" to the Government or to relatives, but, in addition to the routine task of providing for aging parents, beside his own wife and children, he may have to support a widowed sister and orphaned nephews and nieces or to finance the education of his younger brothers and the dowry of his sisters. Social mobility and professional opportunities for all are still more of a utopia than a reality.

Under these circumstances, therapy often has to aim at resigned acceptance or philosophical transcendence of unavoidable, cramping conditions rather than at stimulating the patient into undertaking creative ventures into independence.

This limitation of degrees of freedom, however, concerns not only the external life situation but often also the ability of the patient to let his mind roam freely. Used to thinking in terms of stereotypes and to focusing on the concrete "here and now," patients generally find it very difficult, if not impossible, to go into free association. They expect the therapist to talk, to give suggestions to "tell them what to do." Being left in silence, possibly while lying on the couch, is a situation that seldom is meaningful and often provokes panic.

Group methods, on the other hand, often come up against the Eastern lack of "time consciousness," which makes the regular and punctual assembling of a group of out-patients almost impossible.

CONCLUSIONS

One may object that most of what I have presented sounds disappointingly simple or even ridiculously trivial. This is quite true. The question, however, is whether one should, in autistic fashion, satisfy one's own needs for being "up to date" and for conforming to the latest sophisticated theories and techniques of the West, or whether, in a humble spirit of true human care and concern, one is ready to meet one's fellow human beings, and in particular one's patients, on the level that is meaningful for them.

While thus in the Western sense psychotherapy, in particular if it is to be of analytical type, is seldom feasible in the "transitional sector," a psychotherapeutic approach that respects the dignity of the individual, that sees a human being as a whole, with its past, present, and future, as emerging into individual consciousness and responsibility, while yet creatively participating in the social context, that can show the hopeful creative aspects of anxiety and suffering and encourage a sense of personal responsibility for overcoming them, is certainly something that is possible and well worth striving for.

REFERENCES

1. Hoch, E. M.: Psychotherapy in India. In *Indo-Asian Culture,* Vol. 12, No. 3, Indian Council for Cultural Relations, New Delhi, 1963.

2. Hoch, E. M.: Psychiatric symptoms as methods of family planning. *Indian J. Psychiat.* **10**(1):2–11, January 1968.

3. Hoch, E. M.: Psychotherapy as aid for development. *Psychother. Psychosom.* **20**:226–240, 1973.

4. Hoch, E. M.: Pir, faqir and psychotherapist. In *The Human Context,* Vol. VI, No. 3, UK-ISSN 0018-7151, autumn 1974, pp. 668–677.

5. Wittkower, E. D. and Warnes, H.: Cultural aspects of psychotherapy. *Proc. 9th Int. Congr. Psychother.,* Oslo 1973 Karger, 1975, pp. 111–118 ISBN 3-8055-2057-3.

CHAPTER SIX

DEPENDENCE: CROSS-CULTURAL CONSIDERATION OF DYNAMICS

J. S. NEKI, MA. FRCPsych., FAMS

M an being an altricial organism, dependence is the fate of every human
infant. Since learning in the child is by and large culture-conditioned,
a culture materially influences the direction that maturation of dependence is
going to take in the individuals subscribing to it. Feelings of dependency,
therefore, do not correspond in point-to-point fashion to the theoretical
expected "realities" of the environmental-dependency situation. As Ausubel
and Sullivan state "More proximate than these 'realities' in determining
dependency situation are the actual behaviour of parents and of child's perception of them."[1] These, in turn, are determined to a large measure by
cultural expectancies. Maturational dynamics of dependence, therefore, are
shaped predominantly by cultural determiners.

Barring very few examples, such as the work of Doi,[14] all that has been
said about dependence has emerged mainly from the setting of the Western
culture—and much of it still awaits to be divested of ethnocentricity. There
is need, therefore, for cross-cultural evaluation of dependence as a dynamic
of social and therapeutic relationships.

PEJORATORY CONNOTATION IN THE WEST

In the Western psychological and psychoanalytic literature, dependence has
received a pejorative connotation: "A common judgement is that for a
person to be dependent is less good than for him to be independent: in fact,
to call someone dependent in his personal relations is a condition to be
avoided or left behind."[8] Perhaps no terms are used more frequently than
"dependent" and "overdependent." A child who tends to be clinging, an
adolescent reluctant to leave home, a wife or husband who maintains close
contact with mother, an invalid who demands company—all these and
others are likely sooner or later to be described with one of these words. As
Bowlby states: "Always in their use there is an aura of disapproval, of dis-
paragement."[9] When discovered in patients, dependency is considered a
'defect to be exorcised'.[31]

What is the reason for this pejoration of dependency so ubiquitously seen
all over the Western world? The reasons appear in part to be linguistic in
origin and in part sociohistorical.

LINGUISTIC ROOTS

Whorf,[39] whose studies of language have played a significant role in contemporary psychology, points out that differences among European languages
are very minor. Linguistic analysis of "dependence" stands testimony to

this. Dependence is derived from Lain *dependentia,* old French *dépendance* which is equivalent to *depend(re)* + *ance,* and Lain *dependers* [OF depend(re)] has the lexicographic meaning: "to be suspended, to hang down." Pejoration can be seen embedded in the very root meaning of dependence. One who is dependent hangs down from another's neck. It is, therefore, a condition to be disparaged.

By contrast, *āṣrāyaṇa,* which is the dictionary equivalent of dependence in Hindi-Sanskrit, is derived from *ṣrī,* which according to Monier-Williams[24] means to attach oneself to, to rest on, to seek refuge in, to take shelter, protection or security, and so on. None of these root meanings has a derogatory connotation.

Another linguistic nuance worth noting is that *independent* is the linguistic antonym of *dependent* in its sociopolitical connotations, but in its developmental connotation, *dependable* will be its counterpart. However, in the psychological literature in English and related languages, "dependence–independence" has also been posed as a developmental bipolarity. The developmental counterpart of dependence, even logically, can only be "dependability," on which "dependence" can lean; "independence" can merely thwart dependence and not sustain it. The semantic confusion in considering dependence–independence as a developmental bipolarity continues to prevail inspite of scientific evidence strongly suggesting these two being distinct unitary concepts. This evidence came from the factor analytic studies of Beller[4, 5] and Wittenborn.[41] Notwithstanding this, if the bipolar view still continues to hold ground, the reasons are not merely linguistic, but, even more particularly, sociohistorical.

SOCIOHISTORICAL ROOTS

"Independence" as a political concept was bound to be cherished in the Western world—in the United States, because American War of Independence marked the founding of that nation; and in Europe, because of the building of empires through colonization and creation of "dependencies." Dependency thus became a despicable term and independence a cherished value. With these connotations these terms became cultural stereotypes. Thereafter, one leap was needed to bridge the gap between political independence and personal liberty—and Protestant Ethic[38] provided this: "The social and political freedom which modern democratic communities accord the person express the belated convictions of modern communities, gained after desperate struggle, that the community must give the person a social freedom which corresponds to the essential freedom of his nature."[30]

Encyclopedia of the Social Sciences[33] analyzes the historical reasons on account of which social dependence, which until the 15th century in Europe had an "honourable status" (hence the resurgence of the condemnation of the rich for the injustices by popular religious revivalists), came to be stigmatized thereafter: "The very recognition that widespread dependency created a grave social problem tended to reflect adversely upon the dependents." New religious ideas of the 17th & 18th centuries and the concomitant economic changes destroyed almost entirely any concept of dependency not resulting solely from the fault of the dependent: "This view of dependency persisted long after its underlying religious sanction had lost their vitality. New sanctions were found in the theory of evolution and its current interpretations as proof of 'the survival of the fittest.'" [33]

DEVELOPMENTAL IDEALS

Johnson and Medinnus[22] have pointed out that "the concern of American psychologists over dependence versus independence reflects the importance attached by society to the development of independent behaviour.' The individual who is able to operate as an independent agent is regarded as a mature adult. However, anthropologists have shown that American emphasis on early independent training is not shared by all other cultures."

It is possible, says Child,[13] "that the development of a general tendency towards independence *per se* occurs only in a few societies or a few individuals and that dependence is more characteristically replaced by several separate tendencies which compete with it, e.g. cooperative social interaction among equals or nurturance of younger or more helpless individuals." And achievement is merely one such tendency that has become particularly important in the Western society.

It may be safely assumed that parents, at least initially, are accepting of the child's total reliance on them. However, sooner or later—sooner in some cultures, and later in others—the child is expected to forego some of his dependence (culture determining how much) and strive towards developing more mature and culturally approved patterns. Patterns considered to be "mature" may be those of "independence," of "interdependence," or even of "dependability"—as determined by cultural demands and socially acceptable adjustment-equilibria.

Developmental patterns are, of necessity, consequent on the developmental goals accepted by a culture. If these goals are distinctive, so shall be the relevant developmental patterns. As an example, one may contrast developmental patterns in the West with those in India. In contradistinction to *independence* as the developmental goal accepted in Western societies, the Indian society seems to posit *dependability* as the developmental goal.

Dependability may be defined as altruistic purposiveness. It is the natural counterpart of *dependence* in the early symbiotic human relationship. It is the soil in which "basic trust"[15, 16] sprouts. Its main characteristics are: ready responsivity to need/distress (of others); ability and desire to provide (love, care, support, affection, indulgence, and such); predictability (or reliability); and stability (or constancy). It is not pleasure-oriented, but often sacrifices personal pleasure and comfort.

The bonding between dependence and dependability is what has been termed as attachment. Dependence and dependability are mutually reciprocal in every way. While dependence is characterized by helplessness, dependability, by altruistic helpfulness; the former signifies the identification of the child with the parent, the latter, a reverse identification; the former is characterized by approval and contact seeking, the latter by approval and contact providing; while the former subsumes separation anxiety in the child, the latter that in the parent.

Dependability is not antithetical to self-reliance. It subsumes self-reliance, but this self-reliance is not just for the benefit of self. Dependency is, however, semantically antithetical to independence in that while the former supports dependence, the latter has an antidependence stance. In the West, independence and self-reliance are mutually confused. The real situation, as summed up by Parens and Saul[31] is that "the social attitude towards dependence in our culture, tends to be negative. Children are often prematurely pushed toward independence, and conflicts arising from excessive frustration of dependent needs may be disregarded. Indeed, many see dependence in the infant as a problem" (p. 6).

TWO DISTINCT DEVELOPMENTAL PATTERNS

Let us now examine what happens to dependency-strivings and consequential behavior patterns in these two distinctive cultures. In the West, where personal independence is prized as a developmental ideal, parents are at pains to make their children independent as quickly as possible. The newborn baby is put in a separate crib, restored to the mother only periodically for the satisfaction of its physiological needs. The psychological "umbilical cord" is not allowed to persist. Weaning is hastened, and mothering is intermittent. The parents, who cherish and jealously preserve their own personal independence, set before their children the same model to emulate. They reinforce and reward all independent behavior in their children and encourage them to be on their own. For the Western children, even the period of biologically necessitated dependence also is made as brief as possible—so that they may be able to enjoy their *independence* for as long a period as they can. As children grow up, they quickly become independent of parents. They have their separate bedrooms, separate social groups, and separate activities. Children are banished from adult groups as much as adults are banished from children's groups. However, peer groups are by their very nature a temporary arrangement for providing a sense of belongingness. The thirst for belongingness, however, remains basically unquenched until one meets a prospective mate—and then even relatively minor infatuations, because they open avenues for belongingness, tend to assume major significance in life.

The model of personal independence, which individuals have valued asserts even within marital relationships—thus turning marriage into a relatively fragile institution.

The Western ideal of independence seems to reckon without the second phase of biological dependence—namely, that of old age—which is as valid as the first phase (i.e., childhood), but emotionally even more traumatic. According to Bolk: "Man ripens slowly, his maturity is protracted and his senilization decelerated"[6]—and decelerated senilization breeds a second phase of dependence. When adults grow old, however, they find that their children have already grown independent, and so there are none to depend on. That is the reason why the aged, in the West, are mostly seen in hostels or in hospitals.

In India, as in some other oriental cultures, though independence may be prized as a sociopolitical ideal, as a goal of individual development it is not much cherished. In fact, the Indian culture tends to foster dependence right from birth. The infant stays and sleeps in the same bed as the mother—in close physical contact with her almost all the time. Mothering is indulgent, uninterrupted, and prolonged. There is no hurry to wean children off the breast. The Indian child receives mothering not only from his biological mother, but also from several mother-surrogates in the extended family—all of whom are as indulgent as the mother, and sometimes even outdo her and supplement the mother's spoiling.[12] The mother is never in a hurry to put the child to sleep in order to be able to enjoy her personal "independence." The child is permitted to stay awake and be with the family adults as long as they are awake or until the child himself chooses to doze off. Medard Boss[7] described how a number of adults in an Indian home gather around a child telling him stories, singing him songs day after day with inexhaustible patience in an attempt to cajole him into eating. He has been struck with the "sheltering nest-warmth and constantly reassuring atmosphere of forbearance and security" of the Indian home. "This," he thinks, "may be at the root of the frequently observed tendency of the Indians to give greater priority to the personal, affective rapport with the other person than to the bare objective facts of business in hand." As the child grows up, he finds before him in the adults in the family the model of dependability rather than that of personal independence. There is no hurry in an Indian home to curb children's dependence. It automatically grows down as the child grows up and is able to meet most of his biological needs himself. While dependence is going down, the child imbibes by emulation and conditioning the model of dependability. Thus while dependence is not terminated with childhood, but is permitted to be carried even into adulthood, it is automatically tapering off due to maturation. And while it tapers, dependability is being nurtured. In fact, it begins to be nurtured from birth onward. It is not the child alone who is dependent on parents; parents also know they have to depend on him. For the woman, the child is a symbol of dignity—who as a mother becomes worshipful. For the father, the child is the passport to a place in paradise—for, "a son-less one cannot attain salvation" (*Aitreya Brahmaṇa*). This fact makes the Indian family child centered—especially male-child centered. As children grow up, the permitted *dependence* and fostered *dependability* together weave a pattern of *interdependence*. In such a culture structured interpersonal relations are essential for the self-realization of the individual. This is something quite different from the subordination of the individual to the group. This relationship is not atomistic because the group is not based on the assumption of separateness of individuals who then consider how they may get linked. Nor even is it based on related persons' considering how they may develop their individuality within the group. The social group is not a series of links, but exists as a continuum. The dependence is also not unidirectional, but symbiotic. Marital relations then come to be embedded within this matrix of the familial symbiotic interrelationship.

When aging begins, and the second phase of biological dependence sets in, children who have already imbibed the model of dependability are available to lend their young and strong shoulders for their infirm and old parents to lean upon—the aged are, thus, not abandoned, but looked after in their own homes by their own children.

So divergent are the sociocultural modes of dealing with dependency-strivings in the two cultures that an observer from one can easily be bewildered by patterns prevailing in the other.[7, 12, 35, 36] Table 1 presents in a summary fashion the fate of dependency-strivings and consequential behavior in the two cultural settings.

DEPENDENCE IN THE THERAPEUTIC SETTING

Dependence in the therapeutic situation may be a reliving inside the therapeutic situation of the style of object-relations learned by the patient dur-

TABLE 1. DEPENDENCE AND CONSEQUENTIAL BEHAVIOR IN TWO PSYCHIC SYSTEMS

	Psychic System	
	Differentiating	Affiliating
Developmental ideal	Independence.	Dependability.
Social mechanism	Individuation.	Belongingness.
Relational orientation.	Vertical—hierarchical.	Horizontal—affectionate.
Direction of motivation.	Achievement-oriented.	Approval-seeking.
Patterns of socialization		
(a) Type of attachment to parents.	Dependent and affiliative attachment permitted during childhood only—to be overcome as quickly as possible.	Strong interdependent affiliative attachments fostered and carried over into adulthood.
(b) Type of family bonds.	Strong bonds with marital family —almost to the exclusion of the extended family.	Emphasis on bonds with extended family subsuming those with the marital family.
(c) Reaction to contact by the family.	Unsought contact by the extended family considered intrusion—and hence strongly disfavoured and even resented.	Even unsought contact by the extended family considered comforting or supporting, and hence favored or at least acquiesced.
Patterns of verbalization		
(a) Verbal interaction.	*Self-oriented:* talk more, interrupt oftener, and dominate in most verbal conversations.	*Other-oriented:* listen more, accommodate differences, defer more and show greater consideration.
(b) Emotive content.	Verbal interaction mostly business-like, attending mainly to objective facts of the business.	Verbal interaction based on personal affective rapport.
(c) Degree of verbal facility.	Verbalize ideas and emotions more successfully and more directly—even aggressively.	Verbal expression of ideas and strong emotions often blocked by shyness, reticence, and even suppression unless a personal affective rapport is established.
(a) Relational anxiety.	Fear of dependence: "lest others disappoint."	Fear of independence: "lest others foresake."
(b) Consequence of psychic system rigidity.	Overdifferentiation leads to feelings of *loneliness*—remedy for which is sought by resorting to extrafamilial socialization of all kinds.	Overaffiliating leads to feelings of *social overwhelming*—remedy for which is sought by soliciting solitude.
Therapeutic relating		
(a) Reliance on therapist only as an *aid* to self-help.		Reliance on the therapist maximal; self-help only as much as directed by the therapist.
(b) Therapist abhors patient dependence—which is considered a bug-bear of therapy.		Therapist fosters and skillfully utilizes patient dependence for therapeutic purposes.

ing his early childhood. However, there is something within the therapeutic situation, especially the stresses of transference and countertransference, that enhances the release of dependence states.

Balint observed, "There are many factors in every doctor-patient relationship which push the patient into a dependent childish relationship to his doctor. This is inevitable. The only question is how much dependency is desirable."[2] Obviously, one expects wide interindividual variations, because both patients and therapists vary respectively in their needs for dependence and their ability to handle it. Obviously too, one would expect intercultural variations because different cultures prescribe different norms of expectancies and responsibilities associated with dependency behavior in the therapeutic situation.

Within the Western culture itself therapist attitudes range widely between an utter abhorrance of any kind of dependency-needs on the one hand to actual mitigation of these needs by providing real gratification on the other. Even among the psychoanalysts one is able to identify two broad categories of therapists depending on their attitudes toward dependence—the "paternalists" and the "maternalists." Although some British psychiatrists[2, 3] make a distinction between *infantile* and *mature* dependence, most Western psychotherapists hold a unitary view about it and whatever their conceptual explanation for the phenomenon of dependence, they become anxious to a varying degree if it shows up during the therapeutic process. Many of them have considered it the "bug bear" of the therapist.[42] They have, at times, shown "furious intolerance" for it.[11] It has also been considered as "the most obstinate" of the characterological resistances to psychotherapy.[43] "While hostile or affectional transference feelings seem to be more adequately resolved by counselors," observe Brammer and Shostrom,[10] "it is . . . persistent form of dependency which gives them most difficulty."

As such, most Western therapists seem to be most ill at ease when signs of dependence show up in their patients.

The patient himself is afraid to allow himself to depend on other people "lest they disappoint him."[29] In the therapeutic situation the patient becomes aware of his own helplessness and impotence and feels himself to be ""putty" in the hands of an "omniscient" therapist, and begins to feel threatened that this will cause him to lose any outline and definition."[34]

It is not difficult to see, then, that whenever dependence raises its head, disguised or undisguised, in the therapeutic situation in Western psychotherapy, the therapist as well as the patient generally feel threatened in their own respective places for their own respective reasons. Sometimes, the whole situation can even become surcharged with hostility, and aggressive transference may ensue.

To the average Western psychotherapist, "being depended upon" appears equivalent to "being exploited" and "being abused." For this reason he may misperceive that the dependent person (who, in fact, is utterly helpless) really (or, as they say, "unconsciously") desires to control the situation. On account of this desire he may seek to "shower the therapist with gifts and favors, or he may develop a sentimental attachment that assumes a sexual form."[42] It is not hard to see that through such maneuvers the patient is really trying to create for himself a climate of greater security, but the apprehensive therapist believes that the patient's real motive is to "devaluate the therapist, to enslave him, to test his convictions, or to fuse with him; in this way taking a short-cut to cure."[42] Couldn't this be the therapist's own paranoia?

It appears to me that the participants in the therapeutic encounter in the setting of the Western culture, by virtue of their uneasy notions about dependence, tend to become defensive. This they do in their own respective ways. The patient is unable to cope with the regressive dependence produced by illness now made resurgent in the therapeutic situation. He fears that this is going to subvert his self-respect. Presumably, he also feels a threat to his own personal outline and definition which he fears might suffer dissolution in the course of the therapeutic process. The therapist, on the other hand, seems to feel threatened that the patient, by leaning on him too heavily on account of his resurgent dependency-needs, is going to subvert his independence. Thus it appears that both of them engage in a struggle for defending their own personal independence in a climate that inevitably becomes surcharged with anxiety and sometimes even with hostility.

MATTER OF PROPORTION

Balint[2] points out, "the problem is that of proportion; how much maturity should be demanded and how much child-like dependence on the doctor should be tolerated?" The answer cannot be a simple one. Every culture tends to prescribe its own norms for mature behavior. It sets some kind of limits on the demands that can be made on the patients in therapy. It also prescribes the role of the therapist—which often gets fashioned to some extent after the models of traditional helpers that historically antedated him or are concurrently competing with him.

In the West, the traditional forerunner of the therapist has been the priest, and in some situations he still continues to fulfill therapeutic functions. The priest comes into contact with his clients when they turn to him for help. He enables them unburden their anxieties and feelings of guilt (as through a confessional), refurbishes their hope, and prescribes some anxiolytic activity for them (such as prayer, charity, etc.), and restores them back to their usual lives.

In India, however, the counterpart of the priest who has traditionally fulfilled the therapeutic function is the guru. His clients do not usually establish contact with him only occasionally but generally stay with him for an extended period of time—sometimes even for good—and refashion their lives after his example and precept under his personal surveillance. He vanquishes their ego and overcomes their resistances. Stripped of their resistances, his clients thirst for his words of wisdom, which they receive in their awaiting consciousness. This generates a process that can bring about illumination and transformation. The dynamics of the guru–chela relationship, and their bearing on psychotherapy have been studied and reported elsewhere.[26, 27] These, then, are the distinctive models that have influenced therapist roles and client expectations in the respective cultural settings.

However, the other very important factor that has a direct bearing on the therapeutic setting is the quantum of dependence fostered by the culture during childhood and how much of it is permitted to be carried into adult life? Once again, it is a matter of proportion; but in the average Indian population the proportion of dependence that is permitted to be carried forward is enormous.

That is why the average Indian patient brings to the therapeutic setting really strong dependence-needs which, by Western standards, may be considered "atrocious." Although the therapeutic situation even in the West has been described as one of "vigorous dependency" by some,[11] its *vigor* is anergic compared to that of the therapeutic dependence witnessed in India.

In fact, even the defenses that the Western therapists build up against the development of dependence in therapy do not hold good in the Indian situation. Take, for example, the Western psychotherapists' taboo on socializing with the patient and abhorrence of physical contact and informal relationship with him (to safeguard against seductive dependence). A formal relationship is, to quote Mahal, "distrusted by our [Indian] patients, so that workable relationship does not develop and therapy does not really get off the ground. The patient becomes increasingly dissatisfied and quits. This happens in a considerable number of cases in spite of the fact that these patients are assessed to be suitable for psychotherapy, and this continues to hold good. This happens before the patient has really worked on his problem and approached his conflicts. . . . The difficulty here is of inability on the part of the patient to orient himself to a formal relationship which leaves him dissatisfied."[23] Indian patients seek an informal personal relationship with the therapist, rather than a strictly professional formal one. "In order to achieve this, they bring letters of introduction; in their conversation, they introduce familiarity and strive to establish a friendly relationship, and look for signs of reciprocity in the therapist's behaviour and utterance. They offer gifts, extend invitations to visit their residences or to marriages and other social functions. They feel assured if they belong to the same religion, caste, linguistic group or geographical area as the therapist. This behaviour is in no way peculiar to the therapeutic situation. . . . A distrust of formal contacts and a cosy feeling of security and reassurance in informal contacts is the common characteristic of our people. Even if we are buying some goods from a shopkeeper, we either try to transact business with a known person or attempt to develop familiarity during the business.[23]

Cross-cultural variation with regard to induction of sexual feeling in the patient is even greater. In the West, young female patients generally do not feel uncomfortable being alone with the therapist in a closed room— closed for the sake of privacy, cherished so much in the West, but not necessarily so in the East.[28] An Indian young female patient would feel very uncomfortable in the kind of setting universally associated with Western psychotherapy. To allay her discomfort, she may suggest a brother–sister or father–daughter relationship with the male therapist. Such a relationship is not merely suggested, but often freely verbalized (as is customary in the general population between unrelated males and females if they communicate with each other). The therapist's response to this is carefully watched. Should he be insensitive, cold, and indifferent, and maintain silence, or alternatively try to offer interpretations of this relationship in psychodynamic terms the patient quits therapy. A verbal token reciprocation of this relationship on the part of the therapist makes for the establishment of a relationship of trust, and therapy can proceed.

In India, a patient generally comes to the therapist with the same sense of surrender and faith with which he would approach a guru seeking benevolent refuge with him. Though he may not believe that the therapist can conjure up for him a fanciful Nirvāna, yet he does believe that the therapist is going to be the *vehicle* through whom God is going to work the miracle of cure. It is not easy and perhaps not even expedient to wean such patients from their dependent attitude toward the therapist. Even if the therapist conveys that he is no omniscient, omnipotent personage, the patient considers this to be a sign of utter humility on the part of the therapist, and his faith in him further increases. If the therapist persists in his antidependency attitude, the patient only feels dejected and bereft of the munificence of his "grace," and so would consider himself an unfortunate reject.

Many a Western psychotherapist believes that dependency makes for poverty of motivation for therapy: "Dependent persons are often brought to the therapist not because they feel a need for change, but rather because parents, marital partners, or friends insist that something be done for them. Visits to the therapist, in such cases, are kept merely as a formality. The patient expects that no change will occur, and he will be resistant to any effort to get him to participate in the treatment process . . . with a defective motivation such as this, little progress can be expected."[42]

This is interesting reading from the point of view of the Indian psychiatrist and his experiences with his patients. His patients are almost invariably accompanied by relatives who bring them to the therapist and are not only willing to stay with the patient in the hospital if permitted to do so, but if not permitted, still continue to hang around, sleeping during the nights under the canopy of the sky in the lawns of the hospital unwilling to desert their sick relative. Obviously, if a therapeutic system has never reckoned with fostering of dependency of such a degree, "little progress can be expected" with it, and even "months and years of therapy may effect little alteration in the inner dynamics of the personality."[42]

DEPENDENCE—BENIGN AND MALIGNANT

What is deemed normal dependence in the context of one culture might be considered excessive in another. Anxiety in the therapeutic situation may thus be created by incongruity between the patient and therapist expectancies with regard to the dependency states.

It has to be appreciated that no patient puts forth dependency needs beyond the combined dictates of his illness (which produces protective regression), his personality make up (which, in part at least, is his own culture lived by him), and the therapeutic situation (in which the therapist himself is the co-author of resurgent dependency strivings).

This has also to be realized, then, that the emotive climate in therapy rests a greal deal on the respective stances that the patient and the therapist take with regard to these dependency needs. Emergence of dependence per se does not cause alarm. It is the parataxity of the expectancies of the patient and the therapist that generate anxiety and even paranoid hostility. Although dependence is often looked on as abnormal on account of the anxiety generated by this parataxity, the quantum of dependence per se released in the therapeutic setting is, in fact, no measure of its abnormality.

Dependence may, however, be abnormal, though, if it can be considered *age-excessive,* (as in hysterical personalities), or insufficient (as in antisocial characters) within a given cultural context.

However, some forms of dependence can be identified which would almost ubiquitously be considered pathological. From clinical experience, the following subtypes of malignant dependence can be identified:

1.   *Anxious dependence.* This can arise in a severe form out of an inescapable dependency on a tyrranical person especially when there is a constant fear of displeasing him. If this tyrranical person is also erratic and unpredictable, which can easily thwart the efforts to anticipate his wishes,

the anxiety generated can assume enormous dimensions. There is thus an obligatory dependence with a simultaneous hatred for the other person—but the hatred has to be repressed because of the obligatory dependence.

In a milder form it can also arise when the dependability of the person depended on is considered uncertain.

2. *Clinging dependence.* This often arises when need for dependence is coupled with low personal worth. The dependent person can't believe that others are interested in him. Thus he engages in a continual exercise of testing out their interest by a demanding clinging type of dependence.

3. *Guilt-laden dependence.* This arises when need for dependence is coupled with guilt about one's own "parasitism." This kind of a situation can arise when the person depended on fosters dependence by readily meeting dependency needs of the other person but at the same time makes him conscious of "how much" he is doing for him.

4. *Narcissistic dependence.* This arises when one considers oneself rightfully worthy of others' love. Mutuality in dependency relations is then forsaken and fulfilment of dependency needs is sought as a "right."

5. *Aggressive dependence.* If the excessive or abnormal dependency needs are not fulfilled, active aggression or a sulking, complaining behavior is unleashed. In the latter case, attempt is made to transfer guilt feelings to the other person for not providing sufficient care. In this he might as well be projecting his own undependability in interpersonal relations on the other person concerned.

6. *Passive dependence.* This kind of dependence emerges when there is fear of being active, and the anger is devoted not to the expression of frustrated needs but to their suppression. One such passive dependent, thus, is the *dependent masochist.*

7. *Apathetic dependence.* This variety of dependence tends to occur especially when love-hate valences so counterbalance each other that an emotional paralysis ensues and a state of apathetic dependence remains behind devoid of any affective substratum. If, instead of causing emotional paralysis, the despair leads to a social withdrawal, the emptied self also feels depersonalized.

8. *Substitutive dependence.* In this variety of dependence, the object itself is substituted. This is seen in drug addicts and alcoholics. Here dependence "on what" and "for what" is blurred. One lives on the drug for the drug. There seems to be a reactive substitution of the chemical for the object.

The exact behavioral manifestations of these subtypes will obviously vary from culture to culture, just as the behavioral expression of normal dependence varies. However, in spite of manifest differences, one should expect to be able to identify a thematic communality between the manifestation of any given subtype in different cultural settings. To be able to do so, however, one would need to have a cross-cultural vision without any ethnocentric biases.

MANAGEMENT OF DEPENDENCE IN THERAPY

Management of dependence in therapy depends on several factors—the chief among which is the syntaxity of the participants' expectancies in the matter of therapeutic relationship. These expectancies are culturally conditioned. If the patient's need for dependence and the therapist's ability to contend with it are mutually syntactic, they lead to a comfortable, harmonious therapeutic relationship; if paratactic, to a turbulant, disturbed relationship fraught with all kinds of anxieties, hostilities, and paranoid proclivities.

If dependence in a given patient is interpreted from the standpoint of a disparate culture, it would only generate further anxieties rather than relieve the existing anxieties. A therapist with a Western stance—who holds "independence" as the goal of therapy—for example, would face severe parataxity when dealing with an Indian patient who has high dependency needs. His "interpretation" of dependence in the way he is accustomed to make would at best push the patient to false independence, and this would produce new interpersonal anxieties between the patient and those he depends on. Likewise, an Indian therapist accustomed to fostering and supporting dependency needs and providing "active" rather than "passive" help would experience similar parataxity when dealing with a Western patient who cherishes personal "independence." Should he try to foster dependence even mildly by saying "I will help you," the patient would, likely, take it as an affront to his self-respect and retort, "But doctor, don't you think I have to help myself?"

It has been said that most if not entire psychotherapeutic practice is procrustean.[21] Procrustes was the innkeeper outside Athens who stretched or chopped his guests to fit his bed. Most therapists fit their patients to their therapeutic beds (here, not the physical couch but the matrix of their own concepts, beliefs and attitudes). This is amply evident from how they deal with dependency needs.

We have already identified a group of Western psychotherapists who view dependence as a source of transference distortion. They consider it a bugbear of psychotherapy and become anxious when it emerges. For them dependence spells the patient's desire "to maneuver the therapist into a position where demand for constant favours will be forthcoming." A therapist of this kind is less sure of himself when dependency needs well up in the patient during the course of therapy; and if, sensing his diffidence, the patient rejects him, he labels him as "aggressive." He is at pains to interpret dependency needs as soon as they emerge. Interpretation unfortunately cannot automatically lead to true self-reliance although in haste it can push one to false independence. Thus an illusion of having dealt with dependence can easily be created—but that is about all that is often achieved.

A second group considers dependence as the basic pathology of all psychiatric disorders. In their view the treatment approach that is necessary is to help the patient go into full clinical regression,[40] to get behind the infantile dependence,[17] and let the patient start from a "new beginning,"[2] provide him with a model of good object relations,[20] and, if necessary, gratify the patient's dependence needs by the "mothering technique."[19]

A third group who consider dependence in the therapeutic setting not only inevitable but also necessary and therapeutically serviceable actually foster and even enhance it—and then make use of it for the benefit of the patient. They differ from the group mentioned immediately above in that they do not consider dependency as a characterological problem but one of social rearrangement—from a unidirectional relationship (of dependency) to a bidirectional one (of interdependency i.e. dependence plus dependability). Therapeutic dependence can become serviceable only if it does not generate anxiety in the patient as well as the therapist, and that is possible only if "independence" has not been set as the goal of therapy. Most Indian psychotherapists, I am inclined to think, if they are not blindly applying one or another brand of Western psychotherapy, are obliged to adopt this third strategem.

Several factors seem to weigh in favor of the adoption of this technique in the Indian setting and these include: high threshold of toleration of dependence in the culture, patient expectancies of direct help from the therapist, and population characteristics (poverty, illiteracy, lack of sophistication, etc.).

It is essential to decipher whether it is merely an unusual quantum of normal dependence or is it some variety of pathological dependence one is confronted with. No amount of normal dependence, perhaps, outstrips the human capacity to endure it—for it surely cannot be greater than the "absolute dependence" of the human infant. Abnormal quantities of normal dependence are released in any illness as a result of protective regression. Its absence, in fact, might be pathological—as in patients, say, with coronary artery disease, who lightly take their illness and refuse to take bed rest because they fear a state of dependence.

It is pathological dependence that generally creates difficulty—and in such cases, dependence may not be the primary pathology. Dependence in some cases may be inextricably intertwined with some other concurrent primary psychopathology. If this primary pathology can be successfully dealt with, abnormal dependence can be expected, in most instances, to revert to the normal variety.

Normal dependence of any magnitude may have to be supported—even more so when it signifies a state of utter dependency, as in psychoses. This seems to be the real intent even of Winnicott's[40] "management" therapy and Ferenczi's[19] mothering technique—in spite of the different vocabularies they employ.

Supporting the dependency needs forges a harmonious syntaxity between patient expectancy and therapist responsiveness. The model of dependability that the therapist himself sets before the patient helps him to grow up step-by-step from dependency to dependability.

Though normal dependence may not require any "interpretation," it definitely requires proper restitution. The first step is to help the patient to greater self-confidence and self-reliance while still supporting his dependency needs.

The next essential step is to enable the patient to see and identify his own personality resources that have become clouded behind the resurgent dependency needs—thus enabling him to rediscover his own potentialities (for responsibility), which is the harbinger of dependability.

Unless paratactic anxiety has been unleashed, and therapeutic relations complicated on that account, dependency needs of the patient go on getting less and less as therapy proceeds.[32] What remains at the end is generally a reasonable quantum of dependence which the significant others in the patient's life can support and be willing to support.

It appears that even some of the most indulgent Western psychotherapists cannot permit a dependency relationship to hang on to them. So they are at pains either to "cure" this dependence (through interpretation), curb it (through coercive or punitive measures), refer the patient to some worthier colleague, or discharge him. But "any discharge in psychotherapy," observes Murphy,[25] "should be treated more as an 'au revoir' than a good-bye. This assists the patient to tolerate the 'loss' of a key figure in his life *until he has found someone to take his place* [italics mine]." However, the sting of the situation lies in that the Western patient is generally "alone," and the therapist hardly finds anyone else (apart from another therapist) on whom he can transfer his client's dependency yearnings. In India, on the other hand, a variety of significant "others" are almost always available in a patient's life who are intimately interested in his welfare and who are generally ready to lend their shoulders to his dependency leanings. What the therapist needs to do is to plan in time the mode of the eventual restitution of the residual dependency needs of the patient. The therapist will not have to say: "If I were to act like the traditional authority, it would eventually infantilize you; you would have to keep me around as a leaning post the rest of your life," because the patient is likely to have several more willing and more dependable leaning posts in his real life.

CONCLUSION

Fairbairn mentioned Gitelson as holding four factors on which psychoanalytic cure rests: insight, recall of infantile memories, catharsis, and relationship with the analyst. He himself, however, considered that "the really decisive factor is the relationship of the patient to the analyst" (p. 379).[18] He considered interpretation in itself as insufficient. In my view interpretation of dependency needs is a necessity dictated by the culture that holds "independence" as an ideal of personal development. It must be realized further, that the nature of transference phenomenon is mostly an echo in the therapeutic situation of the culturally prescribed norms of dependence. Guntrip[20] seems to realize this, for he says, "when the forces of our culture have for his lifetime driven the patient to believe that 'salvation' for him lies in strength, independence, a somewhat aggressive self-reliance, opposition to interference, contempt for and resentment at dependent ties, it is extremely humiliating to have to face the need for what Balint calls a 'new beginning' of personality growth from the starting place of a passive dependence on a therapist" (p. 442).

It can be easily seen that most of the conceptual formulations about therapeutic relationship, and the methodological strategies employed in therapy derive from how a culture prescribes the norms relating to dependency behavior. Any psychotherapeutic system, then, cannot neglect cross-cultural echoes and build on ethnocentric assumptions if it aims to claim universal validity of its concepts and relevance of its techniques across cultures.

REFERENCES

1. Ausubel, D. P. and Sullivan, L. V.: *Theory and Problems of Child Development,* Grune & Stratton New York, 1970.

2. Balint, M.: *Primary Love and Psychoanalytic Technique,* Pitman Medical Publishing Co., 1952, p. 248.

3. Beller, E. K.: Dependency and independence in young children. *J. Genet. Psychol.* **87**:23–25, 1955.

4. Beller, E. K.: Dependency and autonomous achievement striving related to orality in early childhood. *Child Develop.* **28**:287–315, 1957.

5. Beller, E. K.: and Turner, J. Le B.: 1962, quoted by Watson (1967).[37]

6. Bolk, L.: *Das Problem der Menschwerdung,* Fischer, Jena, 1926.

7. Boss, M.: *A Psychiatrist Discovers India,* Oswald Wolff, London, 1965.

8. Bowlby, J.: *Attachment and Loss,* Vol. I, *Attachment,* Hogarth Press, London, 1969.

9. Bowlby, J.: *Attachment and Loss,* Vol. II, *Separation,* Hogarth Press, London, 1973.

10. Brammer, L. M., and Shostrom, E. L.: *Therapeutic Psychology,* Prentice-Hall, Englewood Cliffs, N.J., 1968.

11. Burton, A.: *Interpersonal Psychotherapy,* Prentice-Hall, Englewood Cliffs, N.J., 1972.

12. Carstairs, G. M.: *The Twice Born,* Indiana University Press, Bloomington, 1961.

13. Child, I. L.: Socializing. In *Handbook of Social Psychology,* Vol. II, Gardner Lindzey (Ed.) Addison-Wesley, Massachusetts, 1959.

14. Doi. T.: *The Anatomy of Dependence,* Kodansha International, New York, 1973.

15. Erikson, E. H.: *Childhood and Society,* 2nd ed, Norton, New York, 1963.

16. Erikson, E. H.: *Identity and the Life Cycle* (Psychological Issues Monograph I.), International Universities Press, New York, 1959.

17. Fairbairn, W. R. D.: *Psychoanalytic Studies of the Personality,* Tavistock Publication, London; Basic Books, New York, 1952.

18. Fairbairn, S.: On the nature and aims of psychoanalytical treatment. *Int. J. Psycho-Anal.* **29:**374–85, 1958.

19. Ferenczi, S.: *Further Contribution to the Theory and Technique of Psychoanalysis,* Transl. J. I. Suttle, Basic Books, New York, 1952.

20. Guntrip, H.: *Personality Structure and Human Interaction,* Hogarth Press, London, 1961.

21. Hornick, E. J.: My Failures: Some of them and how they grew. In *Success and Failure in Psychoanalysis and Psychotherapy,* Benjamin B. Wolman (Ed.), Macmillan, New York, 1972.

22. Johnson, R. L., and Medinnus, G. R.: *Child Psychology: Behavior and Development,* Wiley, New York, 1969.

23. Mahal, A. S.: Problems of Psychotherapy with Indian Patients. In *Personality Development and Personal Illness,* J. S. Neki and G. G. Prabhu (Eds.), All-India Institute of Medical Sciences, New Delhi, (Mental Health Monographs No. 2), 1974.

24. Monier-William, W.: *Sanskrit-English Dichinary,* Oxford University Press, 1950.

25. Murphy, W. F.: *The Tactics of Psychotherapy,* International Universities Press, New York, 1965.

26. Neki, J. S.: Guru-Chela relationship: The possibility of a therapeutic paradigm. *Amer. J. Orthopsychiat.* **43:**755, 766, 1973.

27. Neki, J. S.: A re-examination of the Guru-Chela relationship as a therapeutic paradigm. *Int. Ment. Health Res. Newslett.* **16:**2–7, 1974.

28. Neki, J. S., and Ironside, W.: Privacy, secrecy and confidentiality (manuscript), 1974.

29. Nemiah, J. C.: *Foundations of Psychopathology,* Oxford University Press, New York, 1961.

30. Niebuhr, R.: Freedom. In *A Handbook of Christian Theology* M. Halverson and A. Cohen (Eds.), Collins (Fontana Books), London, 1964.

31. Parens, H., and Saul, L. J.: *Dependence in Man: A Psychoanalytic Study,* International Universities Press, New York, 1971.

32. Schuldt, J. W.: Psychotherapists' approach-avoidance responses and the client's expression of dependency. *J. Couns. Psychol.* **13**:78–83, 1964.
33. Seligman, and Johnson: *Encyclopaedia of Social Sciences,* Macmillan, New York, 1962.
34. Singer, E.: *Key Concepts in Psychotherapy,* Basic Books, New York, 1965.
35. Slater, C.: *The Dravidian Element in Indian Culture,* Longmans, London, 1924.
36. Spratt, P.: *Hindu Culture and Personality,* Manaktalas, Bombay, 1956.
37. Watson, R. I.: *Psychology of the Child,* John Wiley, New York, 1967.
38. Weber, M.: *Protestant Ethic and the Spirit of Capitalism,* Transl., T. Parsons, Allen and Unwin, London, 1930.
39. Whorf, B. L.: *Language, Thought and Reality,* Technology Press, Cambridge, Mass., 1956.
40. Winnicott, O.: *Collected Papers: Through Paediatrics to Psychoanalysis.* Tavistock Publication, London; Basic Books, New York, 1958.
41. Wittenborn, J. R. et al.: 1956, quoted by Watson (1967).
42. Wolberg, L. R.: *The Technique of Psychotherapy,* Grune & Stratton, New York, 1954.
43. Wolstein, B.: *Transference,* Grune & Stratton, New York, 1964.

CHAPTER SEVEN

PSYCHIATRY AND THE PSYCHIATRIST
IN MODERN INDUSTRIALIZED NORWAY

CHRISTIAN FANGEL, M.D.

The resident in psychiatry took a close look at me and said: "Do you really think it will be of any use whatsoever to give my patient psychotherapy? I know for sure that when he returns home there will be no job for him that he will be able to do. Within a few weeks he will become anxious and depressed again, and most likely return to the hospital for a new admission. I think it is a waste to offer this man any intensive treatment. Within less than 2 years he will have his disability pension anyhow. You know just as well as I do that he is a victim of our modern capitalistic society. It can not use men of middle age with impaired working ability like this man. His painful back will always prevent him from doing the strenuous job he previously did in the fishing industry."

My young colleague was an outspoken Marxist-Leninist, which is not uncommon among Norwegian students and young professionals within the psychiatric field today. And surely he brought into focus once again: will psychiatry be able at all to meet the challenge of the modern industrialized society? And if so, how? What to do when society itself seems to foster new clients much faster than any psychiatric service can take care of? No wonder that many psychiatrists feel that they are in a serious identity crisis.

INTRODUCTION

Having listened to and talked with colleagues from abroad during the last years, I have often got the impression that quite a few think that a stable social democratic development, like the one we have had in Norway, may lead up to a society of equality, justice, and welfare. At the Eighth International Congress of Psychotherapy, Milano, 1970, I felt these viewpoints were underlying many of the statements given by different participants. In his epilogue to the congress, Boss[1] summarizes his impressions of the congress, thereby also giving his opinions on some of the major problems underlying the professional situation of psychiatrists and psychotherapists today.

In this paper I put forward some ideas on the present state of psychiatry within the Norwegian society, and on the relationship between social development and mental health in this country.

Norway is a small country with a small population. For good reasons most foreigners do not know very much about this country.

Accordingly I first give some brief information on the development of the Norwegian society during the last generation. Then I give some data on our society today, with special emphasis on the borderline between mental health, politics, and psychiatric service. Eventually I forward some personal points of view concerning the relationship between psychiatry and modern society in the years to come.

References will be given in the language of the original papers or reports, mostly Norwegian. Titles in English, given in parenthesis, are my translations, as are quotations in English of Norwegian papers or reports.

SOME GENERAL INFORMATION

Norway is the country in the northwest corner of the European continent. Mostly it is a country of islands, coast, and mountains, the southernmost point being at about 58′ northern latitude, the northernmost point being at about 71′ northern latitude. In comparison I mention that the southernmost point of Greenland is about 2′ north of the southernmost point of Norway. North of 63′ northern latitude the country is very long and narrow.

Most tourists find the climate cold and wet, and so do many Norwegians. A large part of the southern, and some part of the northeastern Norway is characterized by inland climate, however, with reasonably warm summers and pretty cold winters. The rest of the country has a typical coastal climate, with fairly cold summers and comparatively mild winters.

Land area fit for forestry or farming is about 25% of the total, agriculture utilizing only 3%. In the old days the country offered its inhabitants rich supplies of fish and game, large and productive forests in the southern part of the country, but fairly poor conditions for farming.

The natural resources that were the original qualifications for the development of a modern industrialized society were the rich supplies of fish all along the long coast, the forest, minerals, and first of all our waterfalls giving energy for cheap and abundant electrical power.

Due to Norway's geographic location, the rich fisheries, numerous good harbors, and the fact that most of our coast is free of ice during the winter, Norwegians have been familiar with sea and sailing from very old days.

Norway is one of the few constitutional monarchies left. The King has no real political power, however. Parliamentarism was gradually introduced from the end of last century.

The Norwegian Labor Party, which on the whole has been the most powerful political factor in the country since 1935, was founded in 1887. For a period in the beginning of this century, the Labor Party had a revolutionary profile, closely connected to Russian communism. The Moskow theses (1920) were the reason for the Labor Party's breach with Comintern. From 1927 the party has generally had a clear social democratic political profile.

The fact that there always has been a very close connection between The Labor Party and The Trade Unions in Norway has been of great importance for the political stability in the country during the last 40 years, as has the Main Agreement between The Trade Unions and The Norwegian Employers Association that was attained in 1935.

The first Labor Party government was formed in 1928. The period 1935 to 1961 was characterized by Labor Party governments and great political stability. World War II was of course a great strain on people and society. The resistance to the Nazi regime was very strong, however, and the legal Norwegian government was active from London during the whole war.

It is said about the period 1949 to 1965:

> The welfare state was developed in Norway during this time. That is not to say that a problemless society was created—of course not. But a form of society was developed that contained all the elements we consider characteristics of what we call 'the welfare state.' We had the planned economy based on society's total responsibility for the economic development. We had the implements of the planned economy: the national budget, the long-term budget, national planning, direct governmental participation in the economy, the extensive common expenditure. And we had the new social policy with a comprehensive Social and Health Insurance system as its keystone.[2]

I think this is only partly true. The social and health insurance was not the ultimate keystone, and our society is far from without problems. One of my main objects with this article is to illustrate this. But let me tell a little more about the political background: Obviously the long and stable social democratic period previously mentioned was one important element in the growth of the welfare state. Since World War II there has been a gradual liberalization of the nonsocialist political parties in Norway, at least until recently. The last 15 years have brought new interesting characteristics into the picture: additional small political parties have been formed, among them two socialist parties besides the old Norwegian Communist Party. One of the new ones is a revolutionary communist party (Marxist-Leninist), and one may be called a revolutionary social democratic party. The political discussion in the nation gradually seems to become more vivid, and to me it seems that Norwegians gradually are becoming more politically conscious. This was quite clearly demonstrated in 1972 by the intense political activity before the referendum concerning Norwegian membership in the European Common Market. The result was that we did not apply for membership. The political involvement in 1972 was much more active than the one prior to Norway's entrance in NATO in 1949.

THE POPULATION

We know that the country was inhabited some 8000 years ago. The first official population census, of 1769, showed some 720,000 inhabitants. At the end of 1950 there were 3.28 million inhabitants, at the end of 1973 almost 3.98 million. Today the population has passed 4 million, and is estimated to be about 4.6 million in 1990.

From a somatic point of view, the health situation today must be regarded as very good. Figure 1, 2, and 3 illustrate this. Figure 1 shows life expectancy, by sex and age. From the period 1901 to 1910, compared to the period 1966 to 1970, life expectancy increased about 16 years for newborn boys, and about 19 years for newborn girls. It is interesting to note that the life expectancy for newborn boys gradually increased till the period 1956 to 1960. Later there has been a slight decrease in life expectancy for newborn boys. This means that the increase in death rate for males above 40 years of age more than compensates for the still ongoing decrease in death rate of newborn and small boys. Figure 2 shows death rate of infants, 0–1 year, in Norway for the period 1915 to 1967. Figure 3 shows the height of Norwegian men at time of common, compulsory military service, age about 20 years, from the beginning of this century till 1973. Figure 4 shows population by age and sex, in 1950, 1960, and 1970. I here point out the gradually increasing number of elderly people, which is of interest in connection with psychogeriatric problems. Also I will mention that until the end of 1972 Norwegians retired at 70 years of age. Since the beginning of 1973 the retirement age has been 67 years. During the last years there has also been a gradual increase in the proportion of young people in education.

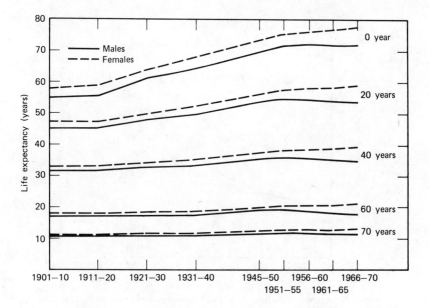

Figure 1.   From Ref. 3. Life expectancy, by sex and age.

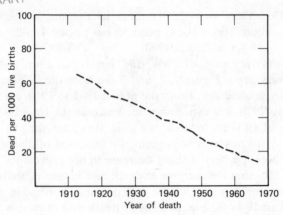

Figure 2.   From Ref. 4. Death rate of infants 1915 to 1967.

Accordingly, an everdecreasing part of the total population has to carry the economic burden of the welfare state. On the other hand, an everincreasing part of the total population is economically unproductive. These people do not experience in their daily life the good feeling of doing a job to the benefit of both themselves and the community.

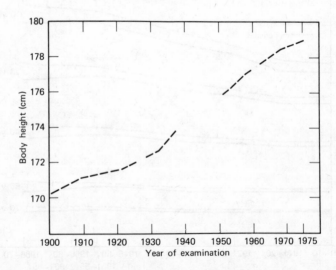

Figure 3.   From Ref. 5. Body height of Norwegian men about 20 years of age.

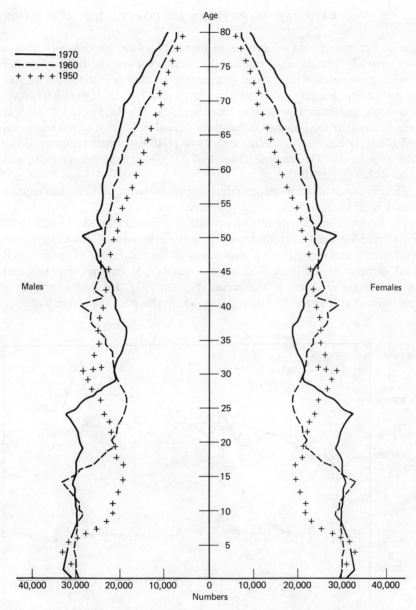

Figure 4.   From Ref. 6. Population by age and sex in 1950, 1960, and 1970.

GEOGRAPHIC PATTERN OF POPULATION AND WORK

Due to her nature and conditions of living, Norway has generally always been sparsely populated. Traditionally most Norwegians lived in rather small communities, with a close relationship to their neighbors. Many also lived in quite desolate areas with no or just a few other families within reasonable distance. Towns were small and few. On the whole I think it is right to say that the population has been typical rural, that urban traditions and life-style has been familiar only to a relatively small segment of the total population. The capital, Oslo, had 340,000 inhabitants in 1930, and about 487,000 in 1970.

The development of modern, industrialized Norway certainly has made a considerable change in the social structure.

The keyword in this connection is centralization. During the last 20 to 30 years there has been a strong pressure on the urban areas, great changes in rural areas, and depopulation and threat of disintegration of many small rural communities. Figure 5 shows the number of internal migrants and internal single migrants in the period 1950 to 1972. Internal migration is here defined as leaving the municipality where you until then have had your

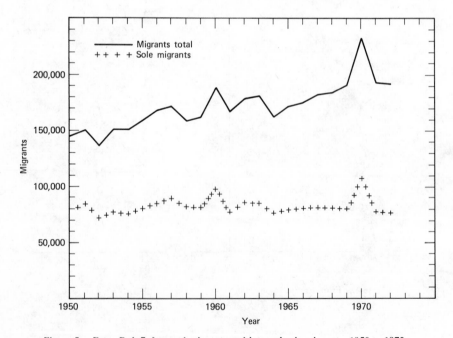

Figure 5.   From Ref. 7. Internal migrants and internal sole migrants, 1950 to 1972.

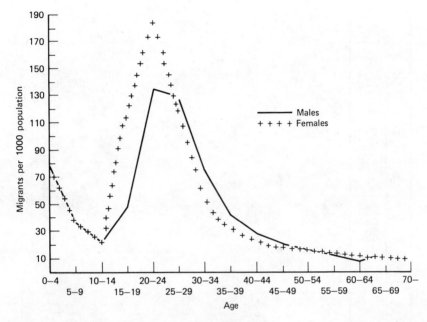

Figure 6. From Ref. 8. Migrants per 1000 population by sex and age, average numbers per year or the period 1966 to 1970.

permanent address to live in another municipality. The number of single migrants is fairly stable, but the number of people migrating with their families is gradually increasing. In 1950 single migrants were 54.1% of the total, while in 1971 single migrants were 39.5% of the total. (The peak in 1960 and 1970 is due to migrants previously unknown, registered at population census in 1960 and 1970.) Figure 6 shows migrants per 1000 population by age and sex, average number per year for the period 1966 to 1970. To me it clearly illustrates that the majority of migrants are young adults, many of them leaving their place of birth and childhood, leaving the old generation behind. Hence the old ones will have no children or young relatives to take care of them, and to carry on their work.

In 1960 57% of the total population was living in densely populated areas; in 1970 the percentage was 66. A densely populated area in this connection is defined as an area of 200 inhabitants or more, with a distance between houses no longer than 50 meters.[9] I think this definition also says something about the original rural character of Norwegian society.

Table 1 shows the distribution of the economically productive part of the population, in 1950, 1960, and 1970. (For females the percentage is given of the total economically active population for the given industry at the given

TABLE 1

Industry	1950 Economically Active Population (%)	1950 Of Which Females (%)	1960 Economically Active Population (%)	1960 Of Which Females (%)	1970 Economically Active Population (%)	1970 Of Which Females (%)
Agriculture	18.1	10.5	13.4	6.5	7.7	8.2
Forestry, etc.	2.9	0.9	2.2	0.8	0.8	1.8
Fishing, etc., and whaling	5.0	0.4	3.9	0.3	1.9	0.7
Mining and quarrying	0.7	2.8	0.6	2.3	0.6	4.6
Manufacturing	25.8	23.0	25.5	18.9	27.3	18.0
Construction	9.3	1.6	9.5	1.7	8.9	2.4
Electricity, gas, water, sanitary services	0.8	7.4	0.9	8.1	1.1	8.4
Wholesale and retail trade	9.5	40.8	11.6	39.5	13.4	40.1
Financial institution and real estate	1.2	35.2	1.7	·39.8	2.3	45.3
Water transport	4.7	4.8	6.0	6.8	4.7	9.9
Transport and communications other than water transport	5.4	17.5	5.9	17.4	6.3	19.6
Government services	2.9	23.4	3.8	22.5	6.1	20.0
Community and business service	6.9	54.3	9.3	52.6	14.8	53.1
Personal services	6.4	87.1	5.3	83.5	3.9	73.6
Activities not adequately described	0.5	10.2	0.4	5.2	0.3	27.7

From Ref. 10.

time.) We recognize typical trends of other societies during periods of rapid industrialization and great social changes. The percentage of the economically productive population in agriculture has dropped from 18.1 to 7.7 in this 20-year period. At the same time governmental services increased its part from 2.9% to 6.1%, while community and business services increased from 6.9% to 14.8%. The percentage employed in manufacturing industries does not change very much during this period, from 25.8% to 27.3%. This may seem surprising, considering that the total productivity of manufacturing industries increased very much from 1950 to 1970. I think, from our point of view, it says something about rationalization and a strong demand for efficiency in modern manufacturing industries.

Table 1 also gives some informative data on the distribution of females within the economically productive population, demonstrating well-known attitudes to sex roles and suitable jobs. For instance, female taxi drivers, bus drivers, and police officers were practically unknown until a few years ago.

YOUTH AND EDUCATION

In accordance with the differentiation and specialization within a modern society, the Norwegian society has invested abundant human and economical resources in the educational systems during the last generation. The high social and economic status achieved by highly educated people has also been a strong motivating factor for young people to seek further education.

Up until 1969 primary school was 7 years, since 1969, 9 years. Except for some very few private primary schools, all primary schools are free. In general a higher number of adolescents have sought further education than the educational system has been able to receive. By now we have four universities in the whole country. Over the last years more and more university faculties have not had the capacity to admit all students applying for admission. These students then have had either to give up their plans for an academic education, or have entered a study that was not included in their original plans.

Students, and most adolescents having passed primary school, are given governmental grants and loans on favorable terms while taking further education, terms sufficient to keep a normal living standard and complete their education, provided they progress at a reasonable level. Figure 7 shows the percentage of the age groups 15, 17, 19 and 24 years in educational systems during the period 1962 to 1971. In 1950 about 13.5% of the total population was in educational systems; in 1971 the percentage was about

20. Figure 8 shows number of students at universities and colleges. In 1963 the number of students in their first year of study was about 4700, some 26% of them females. In 1972 first-year students were about 8700, some 40% of them females.

The humanities and social sciences are the fields of study that more than any of the others have had an increasing number of students. In the period 1961 to 1971 students of the humanities increased from about 3000 to about 10,000, and students of social sciences from about 700 to about 7000. There are probably several reasons for this. I think one main reason is that the capacity for admitting new students has been greater for faculties in humanistic and social sciences in this period than for other faculties. As for social sciences I also think that the rapid increase in number of students is due to an increasing interest in this field among young Norwegians. As for the humanities I think that many female students, having no other field of special interest, feel that humanities is a suitable field for them. Many of these students leave university before they have graduated.

The number of students in medical faculties has been fairly stable for the

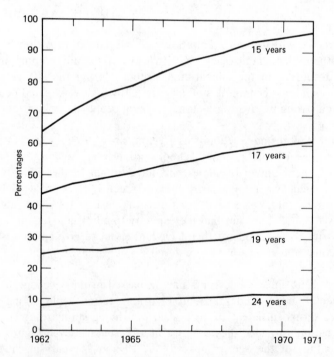

Figure 7.   From Ref. 11. Age groups 15, 17, 19 and 24 years old in educational systems 1962 to 1971.

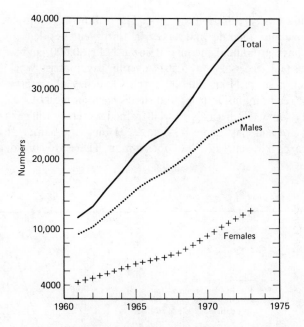

Figure 8.   From Ref. 12. Number of students at universities and colleges 1961 to 1973.

period 1961 to 1971 with about 8.5% of the total number of students. Since World War II the capacity for admitting students to our medical faculties has been far below the number of students wanting to study medicine. Roughly 30% of Norwegian medical students studied at universities abroad during this period.

ECONOMY

The material living standard has increased considerably during the last 10 to 15 years for most Norwegians. Norway has become a very rich nation and is supposed to become even more so as the oil production in the Norwegian part of the North Sea increases in the years to come. *The Economist*[13] assumes that Norway will become the most wealthy nation in the world.

A great number of Norwegians today feel that their private economy is quite satisfying and are a bit sceptical as to the advantage of a further increase in material living standard. But there are still great social differences, and many people do have a real need for a better personal economy. Taxation is hard, and progressively harder the more you earn. The system for calculation of taxes is very complicated, taking into consideration many different factors. The following examples may give some ideas about income and taxes: a third-year resident in psychiatry today will have an annual income of some N.kr 80.000, and will pay some 40% in taxes (1 U.S.$ ≈ N.Kr. 5.50). A senior psychiatrist, working at a hospital, will earn some N.kr 120.000 a year, and pay about 50% in taxes. A trained worker in manufacturing industries earns some N.kr 65.000 a year, and will pay some 35% in taxes. A well-trained secretary will earn about N.kr 45.000 a year and pay some 40% taxes. Doing the same job, a woman generally earns a lower wage than does a man. There are considerable varia-

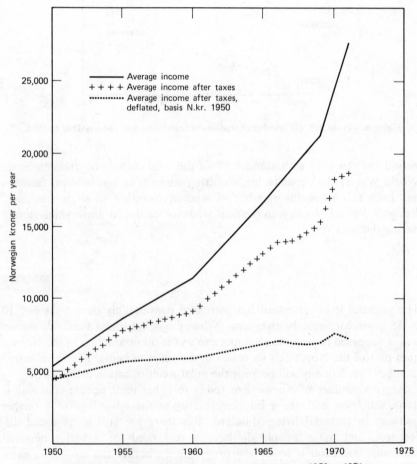

Figure 9.   From Ref. 14. Average income per taxpayer, 1950 to 1971.

TABLE 2

Private Consumption, Percentages of Total, 1946–1973	1946 (%)	1950 (%)	1970 (%)	1973 (%)
Food	32.0	30.0	24.0	22.8
Beverages and tobacco	10.8	8.9	7.7	7.7
Housing	10.0	8.3	13.8	13.8
Furniture and houseware	6.9	8.4	7.9	7.8
Clothing and shoes	13.5	16.6	10.5	9.3
Health service and personal hygiene	4.7	4.5	7.0	8.5
Travel and transport	5.8	5.8	11.1	12.1
Leisure and education	5.4	4.9	7.2	7.1
Other consumption	10.9	12.6	10.0	10.9

From Ref. 15.

tions; in manufacturing industries women get roughly 75% of what a man makes.

The inflation has been pronounced during the last years, wages and prices rising quite rapidly. Figure 9 shows the average income per taxpayer in 1950 to 1971. The rapid increase in average income is clearly demonstrated. The figure also gives information on the inflation, comparing average income after taxes to average income after taxes deflated to 1953 value of the N.kr. The tendency shown in the figure has continued after 1971.

Table 2 gives some information on how Norwegians use their money, showing the development in private consumption 1946 until 1973. There is a marked increase in percentage of consumption of health services and personal hygiene, travel and transport, and also leisure and education. (Money spent on holidays and recreation is part of leisure expenses.)

CRIMINALITY

Norwegian society is a blend of a capitalistic and a socialdemocratic society, gradually developed on a socialdemocratic basis. It tries to combine individualism and collectivism, which is not easy. Daily life for Norwegians is controlled by numerous rules, regulations, and laws. To give some examples: moonshining is prohibited; the production of wine and spirits is under firm governmental control; and all sale of wine and spirits, which are very expensive, only take place in special shops run and owned by the state. Advertising for the sale of tobacco has recently been prohibited. You are obliged to use a

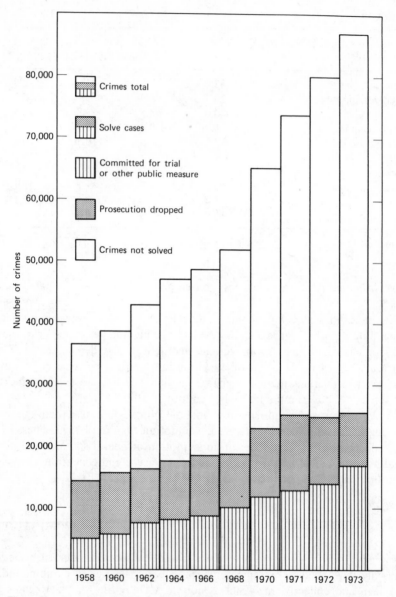

Figure 10. From Ref. 16. Crimes investigated by the police in the period 1958 to 1973.

safety belt when driving a car. There are strict speed limits for driving on all roads and streets. You are not allowed, by law, to drive a car if you have more than 0.5 alcohol pro mille in the blood. You are liable to punishment if you do not give correct information about your income for the local authorities to calculate the tax you are going to pay. It is prohibited to possess, sell, or use cannabis.

On the whole, it is almost impossible not to break some law or regulation now and again. One may wonder what this does to our sense of justice?

However, apart from all the minor crimes most people commit from time to time consciously or unconsciously, the number of more serious crimes also have increased rapidly. Figure 10 shows crimes investigated by the police in the period 1958 to 1973. I try not to give more detailed data here, just mention some trends: the number of crimes increased more rapidly in urban than in rural areas. Boys and young men, aged 10 to 25 years, were responsible for more crimes than was any other part of the population. The percentage of second offenders is gradually increasing. In the period 1960 to 1971 the number of reported sexual offenses did not increase, whereas offenses against property and offenses of violence steadily increased. Figure 10 also clearly demonstrates, looking at unsolved crimes, that the Norwegian police does not have adequate capacity to meet the continuing increase in criminality.

MAJORITY AND MINORITIES

I think that up until quite recently most Norwegians would deny that we have any serious problems in accepting minority groups. There has existed some peculiar ideas among many Norwegians that we are more tolerant and accepting than most nations. There has been quite a widespread feeling of disapproval of racial and minority discrimination in other countries. However, during the last years the original Norwegian minority, the Laps, has made it quite clear that our tolerance of minorities is an illusion. Also, foreigners coming to work in Norway have experienced that we are just as intolerant and discriminating as most other people.

In 1955 there were about 15,500 economically productive foreigners in Norway, in 1973 just over 21,000. The majority are men and have citizenship in other Scandinavian countries.

HEALTH AND SOCIETY

I think that the urgent problems within psychiatry today are closely linked to the present development of modern industrialized society. Also, I strongly feel that a welfare state like the Norwegian one by no means has solved the multiple problems of fundamental nature that a rapidly changing society presents to people.

The general information on Norway and the Norwegian society has been given for three main reasons: first, to give the reader the necessary background for the understanding of the rest of this paper; secondly, to give the reader the possibility to make comparisons between the Norwegian society and societies he may be familiar with; third, because I think that many of the daily main problems for most Norwegians, including mental problems, are closely connected to the development that the given background information illustrates.

In this part of the chapter I give a brief survey of the situation within the field of psychiatry in Norway today, the problems that are presented to us, and how we try to meet them.

HEALTH INSURANCE AND SOCIAL ASSISTANCE

One of the fundamental ideas about the Welfare State is that any inhabitant, regardless of social, economic, or religious background, regardless of sex, age, and marital status, and so on, shall have the same right to the necessary assistance, treatment, or financial support when illness, death, injury, or any other mishappening occurs that make him/her or his/her family unable to take care of themselves.

The history of the Norwegian health insurance system and social security systems is a long history, going back more than a hundred years. The Poverty Act of 1845 was the first step of many leading up to our present social assistance systems. The Insanity Act of 1848 gave the first regulations for the care and treatment of the mentally ill. The Public Health Act of 1860 formed the basis for a public health system. The Occupational Injury Act of 1894 was our first law on health insurance.

From these first steps the creation of our health insurance and social assistance system has gradually taken place; in some periods most emphasis has been on the improvement of the social assistance system, in other periods on the improvement of the health insurance system. Obviously the national economy has always had a major influence on the implications and the extent of each new step. For a very long time numerous private organizations working from religious, humanistic, and idealistic motivations have given social support and aid. Many of these are still active; some have considerable importance. However, the recognition of public responsibility for social aid and support has gradually become more outspoken.

A few more very important laws should be mentioned. The Old Age Pension Act of 1936 established a system of old age pension at 70 years for the whole population. In 1956 Health Insurance was made compulsary and general. From 1909 till 1956 Health Insurance existed, but membership was voluntary for great parts of the population. Health Insurance covers all expenses for treatment in hospital, nearly all expenses related to outpatient examination and treatment, and all drug expenses related to chronic or serious illness.

In 1966 the National Insurance Scheme was passed by the Parliament. This comprises sickness benefits, old age pension, benefits for rehabilitation, disability pension, death grants, benefits to surviving spouse, benefits for children and unmarried mothers, plus aid and support in some more special cases. The expenses related to the National Insurance Scheme are enormous, and are covered by membership duty, duty from all employers, and considerable contributions from the State and all municipalities.

From a psychiatric point of view, the Mental Health Act of 1961, was of special importance. This clearly formulates the responsibility of the combined county–municipality administration to organize comprehensive psychiatric services in each county, including the necessary institutions for psychiatric treatment and care for children, adolescents, and adults. It also stresses the responsibility for organizing precare and postcare in connection with hospitalization, and formulates when and to what extent a person may be under psychiatric care and treatment against his own will.

Taking a broad look at all the different laws, regulations, and directives that have been given on health insurance and social support in Norway during this century, and how they have been administered, I think some interesting trends may be seen. The importance of the national economy has been mentioned. It is an interesting fact that the intentions of each new step in the development have been quite good, but that the public economy often was insufficient to fullfill the good intentions. Also, in many cases, the information given to the common man about the consequences of new steps has been inadequate. Accordingly, quite often, great parts of the population have not been aware of aid and support they were entitled to. Another interesting trend is that there has often been a dilemma whether the new laws should be locally or centrally administrated. Often the solution for this dilemma has been a combined local and central governmental administration, which often has given a bureaucratic taste to the field. Furthermore, most new steps both within health insurance and social support have been aiming at special groups within the population which at the given time have been clearly suffering or underprivileged in some respect. In this respect I think the development of our health insurance and social support systems has been defensive, trying to make it easier and safer for people to live within the changing society. Generally I think it is right to say that during the last years new laws, propositions to the Parliament, official analyses, and so on, of social and health problems have gradually become more offensive by also being directed to the underlying causes of the problems they are dealing with. I also think it is right to say that as Norway gradually became a wealthy nation, there has been obvious trends of competition between some of the political parties as to which one of them dared to promise the most rapid development of the Welfare State.

The reader particularly interested in Norwegian systems of health insurance and social assistance is recommended to read *Social Insurance in Norway.*[17]

A brief formulation of the aim of social politics was given in 1972 by a committee appointed by the Norwegian Government: "The Committee feels that the aim for all social policy must be to make it possible for each individual to fulfill himself and function as a responsible human being in what is a meaningful context for the individual."[18]

So simple to say and so difficult to achieve.

NORWEGIAN HEALTH SERVICES

Expectancy of life and mortality rate of newborn and small children are often regarded as valid indicators of the physical health of a population. Figure 1 and 2 may thus indicate that the physical health of the Norwegian population is very good. I think this is true, at least in comparison to the population of most other countries.

The morbidity and the panorama of illnesses are generally the same as those found in other industrialized Western European countries—malignant neoplasms and cardiovascular diseases, including heart infarction, being the most common causes of death both for men and women.

The central administration of our Health Services is the responsibility of the Department of Health, one of the departments underlying the Ministry of Social Affairs. There is a direct administrative link from the Department of Health to the primary health services in the municipalities, through Public Health Officers at different levels. Also, our hospitals are under the control and supervision of the Department of Health.

I have previously stated that the Welfare State of Norway is characterized by a mixture of individualism and collectivism. This is also shown in our Health Services. Most of our hospitals are owned and run by the public, some by the state, some by the counties, and some by the municipalities. But there are quite a few hospitals run by private organizations as well. The National Insurance Scheme covers 75% of total expences for all hospitals, public or private. For the public hospitals the rest, 25%, is covered by the hospital owner. For the private hospitals this 25% is partly covered by the patients and partly by public contributions.

A fairly marked differentiation between general practice and hospital services is characteristic of our health services. Hospital treatment generally means that the patient is "handed over" from the primary health service/ general practitioner to the hospital and its specialized services, and is meant to be "handed back" when hospital treatment is no longer required. In many cases the aftercare is also provided by the hospitals' outpatient service. Generally this system works satisfactorily for the treatment of the physical illness as such. But it often proves inadequate for establishing a continuity in the treatment of the patient, and also it often proves very difficult to establish close cooperation between the specialist in the hospital and the general practitioner in the primary health service. Most Norwegian hospitals are quite up-to-date, well equipped and rather efficient. However, most of them are also quite up-to-date on the feeling of alienation many patients experience during an inpatient stay. Figure 11 shows population per physician, dentist, and nurse during 1950 to 1972. Today there are about 600 inhabitants per physician. There are, however, marked differences throughout the country. In 1971 there were 264 inhabitants in Oslo per physician, and 1115 inhabitants per physician in the County of Finnmark, the northernmost County of Norway. Today there seems to be an increasing tendency for the young physicians to find a job within the primary health service. There are more than one explanation for this. One is that it is gradually becoming harder to get a job as a resident in general hospitals, especially in the larger ones. Another is that both the social and professional prestige of the general practitioner seems to be increasing. Furthermore, the increasing interest in social sciences and political problems that has been quite marked among Norwegian students for some years also applies to the medical students, making the importance of general practice a challenge for many of them.

General practitioners in Norway mainly get their income directly from the health insurance system, covered by the National Insurance Scheme, the payment they get directly from the patient being quite minimal. We have a complicated system of payment from the National Insurance Scheme, nominating a fixed price for each of all the different examinations and treatment services the doctor gives his patient. However, the system does not specify the amount of time the doctor is supposed to use in his dealing with each type of patient.

There are two obvious and serious drawbacks in this system. One is that the doctor will earn more money the faster he works, which of course may become a threat to the quality of his work. Another is that this system favors treatment and is unfavourable to preventive medicine. And the need

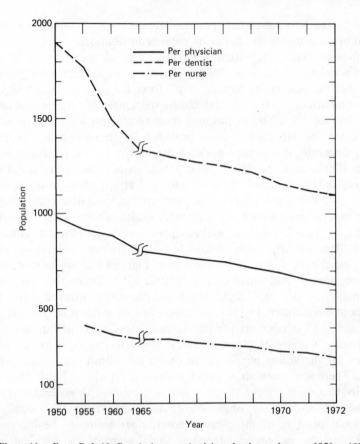

Figure 11.   From Ref. 19. Population per physician, dentist, and nurse, 1950 to 1972.

of prevention is the most urgent problem of our health service today. Public Health Officers are supposed to practice preventive medicine, and also do so. But most of them are supposed to run a general practice as well. Medical doctors working in hospitals or institutions are generally paid a fixed salary, but also regularly have some extra income by private practice, often organized in connection with the hospital's outpatient clinic.

Another peculiar characteristic should be mentioned. The expenses covered by the National Insurance Scheme for running a hospital is a fixed price per inpatient per day. The price differs for the different types of hospitals. This of course may favor that a doctor identifying with the hospital's economy may recommend inpatient treatment even when outpatient treatment would be preferable from a strict medical or psychiatric evaluation of the case. The staff representing the hospital administration, or the board of the hospital representing the owners, may feel obliged to consider the economy of the hospital most important, whereas the treatment staff may consider strict medical or psychiatric evaluation the most important. Especially in psychiatric hospitals this may lead to conflicts between the treatment staff and the hospital administration.

Ultimately I shall just mention that the lack of nurses is today probably the most important problem for Norwegian hospitals, especially so for the general hospitals. During the last years hospital wards have far too often been closed for shorter or longer periods, because of a lack of nurses.

MENTAL MORBIDITY IN THE POPULATION

In Norway we have a long tradition of social-psychiatric and psychiatric-epidemiologic research. I think my Norwegian colleagues will agree when I mention Prof. Ørnulv Ødegård as the Norwegian Nestor in this connection. The Norwegian Central Register of Psychoses was established before World War II, at Gaustad Mental Hospital; the files of the Central Register give information on admissions of psychotic patients in Norwegian Mental Hospital, back to 1916.

I shall here just briefly mention a few investigations from abroad and from Norway. They all tell the same thing: there is a widespread and large mental morbidity in modern societies.

In his study carried out in 1944, Bremer[20] studied both the physical and mental health of the population of Berlevaag, in the county of Finnmark in Norway. He found that 20% of the population suffered from a psychiatric disease. (A preliminary report on a follow-up of the Berlevaag study was published in 1975 by Bjarnar et al.[21].) In a comprehensive study in Sweden, Hagnell[22] studied the psychiatric morbidity in 1957, finding a point prevalence of 22%. In his studies at Samsø in Denmark, Strømgren[23] found a prevalence of 27%.

Essen-Møller[24], in his investigation of a rural population in a small area in southern Sweden, found 1.5% psychotics, 1% oligophrenics, and 1% "organic defective." Neuroses were found in about 4% of males and 8% of females, and about 10% suffered from neurasthenia or psychopathia.

In his retrospective cohort investigation in Iceland, Helgason[25] found 28.6% of the cohort had a mental disorder.

The figures from these investigations correlate well with the results from other well-known investigations (e.g., the Midtown Manhattan Study and the Stirling County Studies).

However, many investigations have also given interesting information on the distribution of different mental disorders within the population compared to social class, economic situation, physical illness, and such. There seems to be no doubt that mental illness is more common in lower social classes. The Midtown Manhattan Study[26] clearly points out that low social status gives a markedly higher prevalence of psychiatric morbidity than high social status does. There is, in this respect, a marked correlation both for the father's social status and the patient's own social status. Ødegård[27] points out that those parts of the population that are characterized by the lowest educational level, with the poorest occupational training and the lowest income, show the highest prevalence of psychoses. He also points out that the course of the psychoses is most serious in these parts of the population.

Commuting is a characteristic phenomenon in many Norwegian areas with a rapid urban growth. In a pilot study on commuting and psychiatric illness, Sørensen[28] studied the commuting frequency among patients admitted to the University Psychiatric Clinic in Oslo. He found that among the male patients there were more commuters than would be expected from the commuting frequency in the residential municipalities of the patients. He also showed that the risk of becoming a psychiatric patient increased with the distance between the commuter's residential municipality and Oslo. The author believes that the explanation for his findings is probably the strain to which the commuter is exposed, partly by his long travel from home to work, by his minimal leisure time, and by the commuter's role conflict by having a rural residence and an urban employment.

In his study on migration and functional psychoses in Oslo, Dalgard[29] points out that internal migration is correlated with increased rate of psychoses only in the case where migration implies social mobility, upward or downward. The author also discusses the difficult question of selection of personality types versus the importance of stress factors in relation to migration, and states: "The concept of psycho-social disequilibrance probably gives the most adequate description of the situation in which migration, or other social acts, is linked to mental illness."([29] page 158.)

Ultimately the results from some investigations from general practice in Norway shall be mentioned. A pilot study was carried out in March through May 1971, registering 1803 patients from 10 different general practices. Øgar[30] found that in 31% of the patients who consulted the doctor or were examined in their homes, the main problem was of mental origin. Of these 19% had a mixed mental and somatic problem, while 12% had a purely mental problem. More women than men suffered from mental problems, 32.8% versus 29.3%, respectively. Neuroses were most common, 10.7% in men and 18% in women. For psychoses the numbers were 0.7% for men and 1.1% for women.

In his study from a fishing community in Northern Norway, Fugelli[31] preliminarily reports 31% of his patients having a mental disorder. Neuroses make up 57% of all mental disorders. Psychiatric disorders are most common in age groups 40 to 70 years, but it is also important to note that he finds 25% of his patients in age group 0 to 9 years having a mental disorder, and 24% in age group 10 to 19 years.

Andersen[32] in a preliminary report on a comparative study of physical and mental illness in a Lapp and a Norwegian population figures life prevalence of psychoses to be 4.3% in female Lapps and 2.1% in female Norwegians, 6.6% in male Lapps and 2.7% in male Norwegians. As for neuroses, he reports 10.1% in female Lapps and 23% in female Norwegians, whereas the percentage was 6.7% in male Lapps and 10.1% in male Norwegians.

In his comprehensive study from a general practice, Bentsen[33] reports that out of 1261 registered patients, 21.7% were registered with mental disorders.

To summarize: studies both from Norway and abroad shows that 20 to 30% of the population suffers from mental disorders, and that there is a significant correlation between mental morbidity and social class, the lower social classes showing a distinctly higher prevalence of mental morbidity than do the higher classes. Females show a higher prevalence than do males.

CARE OF THE MENTALLY ILL

Up till 1940 Norwegian psychiatry was dominantly influenced by European continental psychiatric tradition. After 1945 it gradually became more influenced from England and the United States. Psychoanalysis gained considerable interest from the 1920s, especially among psychologists and certain groups of intellectuals, but did not have any important influence on clinical psychiatry in general. Ever since Wilhelm Reich lived in Norway, 1934 to 1939, there has been some interest in character analysis. This interest, especially in character-analytic vegetotherapy, has been increasing during the last years. During the last 10 years clinical psychiatry in Norway has become more and more psychodynamically oriented; psychotherapy is today generally accepted as an important and valuable therapeutic measure among most Norwegian psychiatrists. Today all residents in psychiatry shall have at least 1 year of qualified individual supervision in psychotherapy as part of their training. Behavioral therapy has gained some interest during the last years, but has not up until today become of any clinical importance on a larger scale. In Norway, as elsewhere, the introduction of the neuroleptic drugs about 20 years ago was of outstanding importance.

The Psychoanalytic Institute and the Institute of Psychotherapy, both in Oslo, have played important roles as training institutes during the last 10 years. Generally there has been very good relations between the two institutes. In 1975 the Norwegian Child Psychiatric Association had about 80 members, the Norwegian Psychiatric Association about 460 members, and the Norwegian Psychologist Association about 400 members.

Generally one may say that the care of the mentally ill is the responsibility of the primary health service, the social agencies, and the specialized services. Both Øgar[30] and Bentsen[33] found that about 85% of the mentally ill seen by the general practitioners are taken care of by the general practitioners themselves. Øgar gives these additional data: 21% got no treatment. From 10% to 40% got tranquilizers. In 50% of the cases the doctor discussed the problems with the patient. (The character of this treatment probably varies considerably, from short-term psychotherapy to "plain talk.") Antidepressives are used fairly often; no figures were given however. Of the mentally ill patients seen by the general practitioner, 2.5% are sent to psychiatrist for ambulatory treatment, 6.5% to other specialists. (Psychosomatic states are quite common.) Of the women 4.7% and 2.9% of the men were admitted to hospital due to their mental illness; not all of them were admitted to a mental hospital however.

The General Social Act of 1965 states that social support generally shall be given to people who need this "to overcome a difficult life-situation," or who "are not able to take care of themselves." It is well known that a considerable part of the clients taken care of by the social agencies do suffer from mental illness or belong to high-risk groups. (Reliable data are, however, hard to give.) It is also known that many of them suffer from physical illness, or belong to high-risk groups also in this respect. Many of our maladjusted alcoholics as well as adolescents using cannabis receive social support for long periods. The social agencies are also quite familiar with the "multiproblem families," often characterized by poor economy and housing, alcohol abuse, psychosomatic states, depressions, emotionally deprived children with various mental sufferings, shortcoming at school, enuresis, and so on. Especially in poor municipalities the economic capacity often is insufficient to meet the needs for help. Accordingly, to get access to financial support from the National Insurance Scheme, the social agency staff often feel that they have to take part in the medical "diagnostic culture," thus converting the clients of the social agency into medical patients. Surely enough, social clients quite often are physically or mentally ill. But a medical frame of reference often will represent a distortion and undue oversimplification of a complex situation characterized by multiple functional failures and social maladjustment.

An overview of the specialized psychiatric services will show a broad variety of different types of institutions: mental hospitals, psychiatric clinics, child guidance clinics, treatment homes for children and adolescents, family guidance clinics, psychiatric nursing homes, rehabilitation centers, institutions and homes for mentally retarded, educational-psychologic district centers, clinics for alcoholics, and such. (To describe them all is beyond the scope of this chapter.)

The inspiring results achieved by psychopharmacology, and also the great inspiration mediated by the theories of psychodynamic psychotherapy, brought much enthusiasm and optimism to people working within the specialized psychiatric services. During the last 10 to 20 years I think we have been very quick and willing to adopt new therapeutic methods. A broad variety of therapeutic measures are generally used within our mental hospitals and psychiatric clinics today: the therapeutic community, group psychotherapy, individual psychotherapy, family therapy, neuroleptic drugs, occupational therapy, physiotherapy, rehabilitation training, ECT, and so on. I think that the general enthusiasm has brought many results of considerable value. However, I also feel that professionals within the field have attained some competence in the use of many therapeutic measures, but too many of us do not master any measure with full competence.

The staffing of our psychiatric institutions has generally improved considerably during the last 10 years. In accordance with a general public and political acceptance of the importance of the psychiatric service within a modern society, investments in psychiatric service systems have been considerable. Nevertheless, most people working within psychiatric institutions seem to work rather hard. The need for psychiatric service seems to be without limits. Also, to keep up with the generally accepted importance of inservice and postgraduate training represents an additional burden to many. I feel that the enthusiasm and optimism that were characteristic during many years are gradually vanishing. A doubt as to the efficiency of our therapeutic measures is gradually emerging. Also, I think, there is a gradually oncoming feeling that our work may be more or less in vain, as the society seems to create new patients much faster than we are able to treat them.

Some additional information on our mental hospitals shall be given. Traditionally mental hospitals admitted primarily psychotic patients, whereas neurotic patients primarily were treated in psychiatric clinics. This differentiation has gradually disappeared during the last years. Mental hospitals in Norway usually have beds for some 400 inpatients. Table 3 illustrates changes in admission patterns and patient "turnover" in Norwegian mental hospitals. There is a gradual decrease in average covering of approved beds. One reason for this is that the number of beds has increased; another is that the capacity for outpatient treatment has improved. About 1950 the needs for beds in mental hospitals and psychiatric nursing homes was estimated to be 40 per 10,000 inhabitants; in 1973 the estimation was 18

TABLE 3

Year	Average Covering in % of Approved Beds	Admissions and Dismissions in % of Average Covering	Percentage Distributions of Admissions	
			First Admissions	Readmissions
1950	125.2	67.6	55.6	44.4
1955	124.7	69.4	50.0	50.0
1960	115.4	109.2	46.1	53.9
1965	104.4	149.0	43.2	56.8
1970	95.7	176.5	40.0	60.0
1971	95.4	203.4	42.4	57.6
1972	93.8	212.5	40.1	59.9
1973	91.0	227.3	38.8	61.2

From Ref. 34.

to 20 beds per 10,000 inhabitants. On a country scale this is now attained.[35] Numerous reports on outpatient treatment of psychotic patients have been published. In a follow-up study from Oslo,[36] the results of outpatient treatment appeared to be approximately the same as for hospital treatment. Table 3 also illustrates the increasing turnover of patients in mental hospitals, characterized by numbers of admissions and dismissions, and also by the increasing number of readmissions.

Table 4 illustrates first admissions by age, 1960 to 1970 to 1973. There is a marked increase in numbers of young patients. This probably illustrates an increasing tendency to hospitalize cannabis/drug-abusing adolescents

TABLE 4

Age	Percentages of total		
	1960	1970	1973
Under 20 years	4.3	8.4	8.9
20–24 years	6.0	9.1	10.7
25–29 years	6.9	6.4	8.8
30–39 years	21.7	13.8	12.3
40–49 years	18.6	16.2	13.9
50–59 years	17.5	15.6	15.7
60 years and over	25.0	30.5	29.7

From Ref. 37.

and young adults, and probably also deviant and maladjusted young people generally. There is, however, also an increase in first admissions of old patients, illustrating the increasing need for psychogeriatric services.

The primary health service will, also in the future, take care of the majority of the mentally ill patients. To strengthen the primary health service is in Norway regarded as one of the major tasks in the years to come. An integration of the primary health and social services is part of the fulfilment of these plans. Integrated health and social centers have been in operation a few places during the last 2 to 3 years. Mellbye[38] describes the plans for Oslo. Here the plans are to establish 150 units, each unit comprising a general practitioner, a public health nurse, and a generally trained social worker, and each unit in average serving 3,000 inhabitants. Two to four such units will be closely connected to each other in a center, where physiotherapist and home nurses shall also have their offices. The consultation services of the different specialized health and social services, including the psychiatric, also shall take place in the center.

The plans for the further development of the specialized psychiatric services may be characterized by: regionalization, continuity, and flexibility. The Mental Health Act of 1961 divided the country into 15 regions of Mental Health Service. The standard model for the psychiatric service within a region is a mental hospital cooperating with nursing homes, private care, homes for aftercare, integrated outpatient service, a psychiatric clinic preferably integrated in a general hospital, and an outpatient clinic for children and adolescents in cooperation with treatment homes.

According to Steenfeldt-Foss, "The main problem today is not primarily lack of psychiatric institutions, but rather lack of better qualified personnel within the psychiatric services, a more even distribution of this personnel throughout the country, and greater flexibility in the use of existing resources."[35] Steenfeldt-Foss also states: "Only by having a comprehensive knowledge in, and understanding of sociodynamic and psychodynamic processes, the professional within the Mental health service will be able to encounter the individual or the group with a differenciated therapeutic offer, characterized by realism and quality."

Many years will go before the existing plans for the development of our psychiatric services have been fulfilled throughout the country. As for prevention of mental illness, the future seems uncertain. By the Mother and Child Guidance-Center Act of 1971, the principle is stated that the National Insurance Scheme also shall contribute financially to a service primarily of preventive nature. This is new and important. An interesting and stimulating report[39] on the possible role and function of the Mother and Child Guidance-Center within preventive psychiatry has gained considerable attention.

Leighton[40] describes how the disintegrating process in a small community could be reversed, and how the prevalence of mental disorders decreased as the general situation in the community improved. Richter[41] gives an interesting report on the psychoanalyst's role in cooperation with action groups actively interfering in a slum population to induce social changes.

In my opinion studies like these two are very important, but it remains an open question as to whether they indicate a field of work for the psychiatrist in the future.

THE OTHER SIDE OF THE COIN

Norwegians generally have a rather high material living standard, and the Welfare State also gives much safety to people by the comprehensive systems of health insurance and social support, based on the principles of equal rights and opportunities to all inhabitants. For instance, psychotherapy, at least up to 200 treatment hours, is fully covered for any Norwegian by the National Insurance Scheme. In practice there are of course numerous social and psychological mechanisms in operation, resulting in a marked discrepancy between ideals and realities.

In the population there still is ambivalence both as for the philosophy and the practice of the Welfare State, although the majority of Norwegians undoubtedly are for it. The opponents are especially concerned about the public expences and what they suspect to be insurance- and support-abuse. Figure 12, based on official reports and public budgets, shows the State's expenses to the National Insurance Scheme, 1971 to 1974. In this period total expenses increased from N.kr 10.25 billion to N.kr 16.25 billion. This is a considerable increase, also taking the ongoing inflation into consideration. The tendencies shown have continued. In 1976 the State budget for health services was 22.5 billion and 4.5 billion for social support systems. In 1961 the total public expenses, the State and the municipalities together, was about N.kr 3 billion for the social support and health service systems altogether. During the last 2 to 3 years the political authorities have gradually paid more interest to the question of how all this money is spent, the concept of cost-benefit analysis becoming gradually more important.

I think that public expenses to sickness benefits, disability pensions, and social support are especially provoking to many people. It seems provoking to know that a considerable proportion of the population, apparently quite healthy, live on money they receive from the National Insurance Scheme, achieved by a heavy taxation that also hits yourself. Figure 13 shows disability pensioners per 100 population, by sex and age, 1966 and 1972. The increase in percentage of disability pensioners is clearly demonstrated.

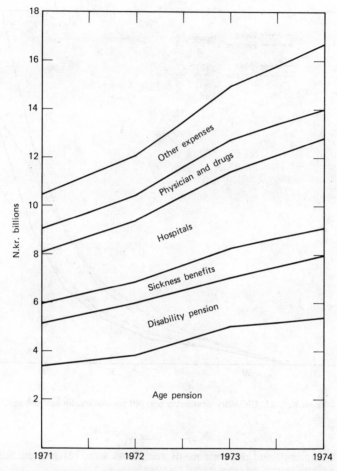

Figure 12. From Ref. 42. Norwegian state's expenses to the National Insurance Scheme, 1971 to 1974.

It is remarkable that in 1972 about 10% of Norwegians at age 55 were disability pensioners. It is also important to note that about 30% of all disability pensioners have a psychiatric diagnosis.

Figure 14 shows recipients of social support by age, percentages of total, 1966 to 1968 to 1971. Most remarkable is the proportional increase in age group under 30 years, from 14.4% in 1966 to 26.7% in 1971. I think it is natural to associate these data with data on migration rates and what has been reported about the "suburb-poverty." A few total numbers on persons receiving social support shall be given[45]: in 1966, 32,010; 1970, 37,160; 1971,

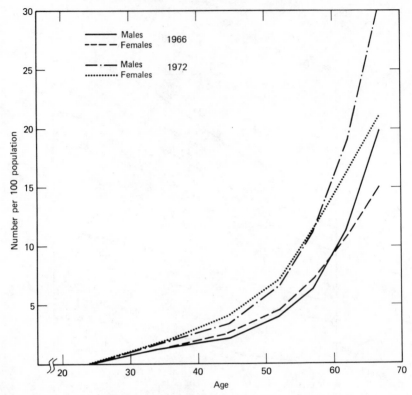

Figure 13. From Ref. 43. Disability pensioners per 100 population, by sex and age, 1966 and 1972.

37,506. Recipients and dependents of recipients were (estimated numbers): in 1966, 65,170; 1970, 74,300; 1971, 75,500.

In their book, *The Use of Tranquilizers in Norway,* Bakka, Johnsen, et al[46] give numerous interesting information. Their data refer to patients who got tranquilizers prescribed at public expenses.

During the 10-year period, 1962 to 1972, the sales of psychopharmaca from the Norwegian Drug and Pharmacy Depot to local pharmacies increased very much, measured in price value from N.kr 9.2 million to N.kr 38.4 million, in percentages of total sales of drugs from 10.7% to 13.2%. (The Norwegian Drug and Pharmacy Depot has a monopoly on wholesale of all drugs in Norway that are obtainable only on a doctor's prescription.) In the period 1965 to 1970 there was a rapid increase in the sales of tranquilizers, and this came on top of already existing considerable use of hypnotics. In the material the following groups showed an overrepresentation among those using tranquilizers: women, and especially younger ones, married people in contrast to unmarried, both men and women at age 45 to 69 years as compared to those age groups adjacent to them, and patients with chronic physical illness. A total use that gave a fair reason to suspect abuse was found in 10% of the users in Oslo. It is to be noted that the total use of tranquilizers did not decrease when the National Insurance Scheme did not cover the expenses any more.

The data refer to a certain period in 1970. It seems obvious that the life situation of many Norwegians, at least at that time, was of such a character that the use of tranquilizers seemed to be an important help to them.

In his book *InsuranceNorway,* Kolberg[47] presents his studies on the use of health insurance and social support in Norway. As a sociologist he is using a social frame of reference. His studies clearly demonstrate obvious connections between certain social conditions and the use of certain types of health insurance and social support.

The frequency of disability pensioners is positively higher in rural than in urban municipalities, and especially so in stagnating rural municipalities economically primarily based on farming and fishing. The use of unemployment insurance is the most frequent in rural fishing municipalities, the least frequent in municipalities based on manufacturing industries. The same was found as to support to unmarried mothers.

On the other hand, the use of medical doctor's services is marked more frequent in urban areas, and especially so in wealthy and expanding municipalities. This also goes for inpatient hospital treatment, although differences here are less outstanding. The use of sickness benefits shows the same pat-

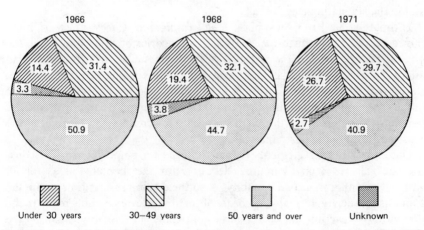

Figure 14.   From Ref. 44. Recipients of social support by age, percentages of total, 1966, 1968 and 1971.

tern. The frequency of social support is highest in the economically best situated municipalities.

Generally, slowly expanding rural municipalities, with an economy based on farming and industry, seem to show what might be called the most "balanced and natural" consumption of health insurance and social support.

The underlying explanations of Kolberg's findings are not readily accessible. The political, physical, social, and psychological factors governing our lives are multiple, many of them are not well known, and they interact in complicated manners. Nevertheless, his findings confirm obviously the close relations between physical and social conditions and health. The data revealed by his study also are hard to combine with any theory of insurance-abuse based on individual moral traits. Most likely, geographical differences and uneven distribution of health services throughout our country are part of the explanation for some of his findings, for example, the use of doctor's services. But undoubtedly also characteristic trends in the development of our society are revealed by his study.

The rehabilitation of disabled persons is difficult. In stagnating, or nonexpanding rural areas, a new job is hard to get. In Norway too many adults have had to choose between disability pension and migration to rural, expanding communities. From the data given on disability pension it seems that adults of age about 50 years represent a new social "drop-out" group. The data seem to justify the statement that there is a considerable degree of hidden unemployment in Norway, covered by the disability pension.

It seems that the development in a rapidly changing society represents a considerable burden to people, both in the rapidly expanding urban areas and in the stagnating rural areas.

Ultimately K. Ericsson's book *The Ambiguous Care*[42] must be mentioned. Based on the historical-materialistic theories of Marx and Lenin she gives a historical overview of the care of the mentally ill in Norway, also analyzing present-day psychiatric care within this frame of reference. She states that the society's attitude to deviants and mentally ill has been influenced mainly by two important forces: the economic capitalism and the humanistic tradition. Of those, the capitalistic force has by large been the most powerful in the past, and still is.

One of her main statements is that the need for employees in the industries has always been of major relevance, for the mentally ill as for all employees with a marginal capacity. Also the economic situation within the capitalistic society has always been of major relevance. She regards the present-day reaction among many politicians in Norway against the enormous public expenses in social and health service systems as a reflec-

tion of today's need for enormous investments in building up our new oil
industries.

THE PSYCHIATRIST IN THE SOCIETY

The background information given earlier illustrates characteristic trends in
the development of the Norwegian society. Provided these trends continue
in the years to come, psychiatry and psychiatrist are probably going to face
even greater problems than today.

Further improvement of general hygiene, more efficient preventive
medicine, and further advances in medical treatment may prolong life
expectancy even more. Old people will then proportionally be an even
greater part of the total population. At that time the pathogenetic factors of
organically based mental illness may be under control, but today we know
that the incidence of mental illness, primarily on an organic basis, rapidly
increases with increasing age. Even today psychogeriatric problems
represent a great challenge to Norwegian psychiatry. Provided our society
can afford it, which probably will be the case, the common pension age is
likely to become lower than the present 67 years, and the proportion of pensioners in the population will increase accordingly. We know today that the
step from an economically productive life to retired life represents a
considerable mental burden to people feeling that they are still capable of
doing a job.

A further increase in internal migration rate is likely to occur in Norway.
Further industrialization, especially based on crude oil from the North Sea,
will demand further centralization in new industrial areas, with a continuation or even increase in the internal migration rate. I think Dalgard's[29] concept of psychosocial disequilibrance points to a major problem. It should be
noted that he examined the relation between psychoses and internal migration. We know that internal migration represents a heavy mental burden to
many people, not necessarily resulting in a psychotic decompensation.
Family links and social networks are too often torn to pieces, for the
migrants and for the people left behind as well. From the depopulation pattern of many small rural communities in Norway we know that the elder
part of the population usually are the last ones to move out. The bigger
Norwegian towns have grown rapidly during the last generation. Accordingly, most of the inhabitants have loose and unstable urban traditions.
From numerous new suburbs we know that for most people it takes many
years to establish new social networks. Many migrants suffer from
considerable mental stress during long-time, vague, and unspecific mental

symptoms, depressions and psychosomatic disorders being quite common. For the adolescents the step to start drinking, sniffing, or using cannabis is often much too easy. The economic burden is also considerable for migrating families, in spite of the fact that better paying jobs in the urban areas regularly are the main reason for migration. Living costs are regularly considerably higher in the urban than in the rural areas, and housing is expensive. The "suburb-poverty" is well known to the social agencies. (Three years ago it was reported that about 40% of the families in a new suburb in Oslo got financial support from the local social agency.)

The equal right for all adolescents to get the education they want is one of the ideals of the Welfare State. Youth in education gets grants and loans from the State, so that social class or the private economy of the parents should not be a factor of importance for the adolescent's choice of education. However, there is a marked discrepancy between ideal and reality here. Many factors other than desire influence the choice of education, and our educational systems do not have the necessary capacity. Nevertheless, the gradually increasing proportion of adolescents and young adults in educational systems, like the gradually increasing proportion of pensioners, place the economic burden of the Welfare State on a gradually decreasing proportion of the total population.

The rapidly increasing rate of crimes is also a characteristic trend. It seems that within a modern and rapidly changing society the individual's behavior is regulated by laws and rules to such an extent that it is hard not to commit a crime now and then. Stealing is very common. It is calculated that Norwegians steal in stores and shops for a value of about N.kr 1 million every day. It seems to me that the present development of our society gradually change our attitudes to minor crimes, and probably also gradually our concepts of justice.

The true psychiatric morbidity in the Norwegian population is not known. The main reason for this is that we do not know the borderline between mental illness on the one hand, and the reduced feeling of well-being, the impaired social, and the impaired interhuman functioning on the other hand. The role and responsibility of the psychiatrist, today and in the future, is unclear and has been widely discussed. The literature on the problem is abundant; a few examples shall be mentioned. To me psychiatry is a medical profession, and the analysis and viewpoints forwarded by Illich[48] have a pertinent relevance for psychiatry as well as for the rest of our Health Services.

The political implications of the psychiatrist's role and function have been widely debated. The viewpoint that we serve as a preserving agent within an unhealthy capitalistic society is not rare. In his book *New*

Perspectives on Psychiatry, Haugsgjerd[49] states: "We shall have to function as commisars for well-being and health and engage in political work that will not always be popular with the official agencies and the dominating classes." Nyhus[50] is very sceptical to any professional imperialism and to the professionalization of fundamental questions regarding the individual's feeling of happiness and well-being. Magnussen[51] is of the opinion that, in addition to care and treatment of the psychotics, the professional responsibility of the psychiatrist is primarily in those cases where the problems are in "the inner space," "inside" the patient. As for the abundant sufferings and human disharmony in "the outer space," in interhuman relations, psychiatry may have something to offer. But other ways of handling this may often prove to be better and more relevant than psychiatric treatment.

Many authors forward the viewpoint that the psychotherapeutically trained psychiatrist, or rather the psychotherapist, will give the model for the future psychiatrist. Bettelheim[52] states: "But contrary to what the greatest need of man now is, education has not only concentrated more than ever before on the battle already won, on the mastery over nature, and has ever more come to disregard what are now the pressing problems—mastery over the unconscious and emotional sources conditioning life, culture, and society which prevent man to order things rationally." Ziferstein[53] is of the opinion that the psychotherapist preferably should engage in social issues, and that such involvement actually may broaden his perspective. He also quotes a statement given by a Committee of the American Psychoanalytic Association: "Active participation by the analyst in social issues reveals only data of a superficial nature." Ugelstad[54] forwards the viewpoint that social-psychiatry and psychotherapy must establish close cooperation, and that those two branches in psychiatry together should become important ingredients in the psychiatric work in the years to come. Sutherland[55] puts it this way: "I therefore suggest that the crucial matter is the creation of a 'socio-therapeutic system' amongst the helping professions in which the psychotherapeutic center has to play a fundamental part."

I think the situation of the psychiatrist of today may be summarized like this: he is a medical doctor, educated and trained in accordance to a medical tradition based on the triad examination, diagnosis, treatment, primarily assigned to cure individuals. He is part of a population of which at least 20 to 30%, according to present definition, do need his help. He does not really know the difference between disease and normality. In doing his job he is using a variety of therapeutic measures, the effects of which to a large extent are uncertain. And he is living and working in a society that seems to foster new patients much faster than he is at all able to cure. He is skeptical to the nature of this society, or openly antagonistic to it, but he knows that both his patients and he himself do have to live and function within it. This, I think, is the confusing situation of the psychiatrist. To me, however, there is even more to it.

QUO VADIS?

When Adam and Eve had to leave Paradise, after having eaten from the fruit of the Tree of Knowledge, they left with their souls marked by the human anxiety. Outside Paradise they met a frightening physical world that was threatening to their lives every day. Since then mankind has fought continuously to conquer the physical world, to gain control over all forces that are a threat to his life.

In modern industrialized nations man has to a large extent achieved this control over nature. Today other humans are probably representing the major physical threat to us, and we to them. The military budgets indicate this.

To me it seems that belief in God has gradually vanished as man achieved control over the physical world, leaving too many of us with no other feeling of a meaning of life than what our work, our children, and the here-and-now gratifications may give us. It is hard for the parent-generation to present to their children any ideals when they miss ideals themselves.

By conquering the threatening nature we also have lost a natural relationship to death, well known from the discussions on what the medical criteria of death shall be, and also from recent court cases where parents fight for their children's right to die. Generally there seems to be a tendency by the common man to push this problem onto the medical professions, and by the medical professions to push it onto the common man. The fact that modern medicine seems, when all possibilities are used, to be able to interfere with how and when life shall terminate, seems to be too provoking to all of us. To remind you of Erikson's words[56]: "And it seems possible to further paraphrase the relation of adult integrity and infantile trust by saying that healthy children will not fear life if their elders have integrity enough not to fear death."

On our way to the postindustrial society the value and meaning of work also are threatened. For many years we have known too well the feeling of alienation so often experienced by employees in modern industries. In the postindustrial society there will be even less need for our working capacity. This we are not at all mentally prepared to meet. Unemployment is today an increasing problem. We have seen how disability pension today is the Norwegian Welfare States' offer to so many adults, living in places where there is no job for them, or having a working capacity that is inadequate within our hard-working industries. It is a paradox that young people gradually spend more and more time in educational systems, when we know that within some years there will perhaps be no jobs for them.

The Norwegian Welfare State has been formed on the basis of good economy, a stable social democratic policy, and a humanistic tradition. On our way I think we have mixed up two important concepts: deviation and illness. There are strong demands on conformity within a modern society, and a misconceived humanistic tradition will easily lead into a situation where deviant behavior or social maladjustment is looked upon as symptoms of underlying illness. Accordingly the Welfare State will readily feel obliged to treat deviants. Personally I feel that this has been one of the underlying mechanisms in formation of what has been called the Norwegian "treatment-society."

Provided that the development of the Norwegian society continues along the same lines that it has followed during the recent 15 to 20 years, the demand for psychiatric services in the years to come will exceed all limits. I feel that we are still caught in some sort of "psychiatric imperialism;" our present plans for the development of our psychiatric services formulate how we shall achieve more and better psychiatric service for more and more people. I do believe in a decentralized comprehensive psychiatric service, based on a psychotherapeutic approach, in a qualified way also using our other therapeutic measures, and working within a social-psychiatric frame of reference.

Nevertheless, to me it is obvious that prevention is the only way out of our urgent problems. And prevention in this respect means changes in society. And changes in society are political matters. I do not believe in a society run by specialists. I feel sure that neither psychiatrists, nor any other professional group have, or shall try to achieve competence as society-planners, society engineers, or society-saviors. The concept—psychiatric illness—has rather to be narrowed than to become widened. I think that the psychiatric professions should be extremely aware of any tendency in society trying to use our professional competence to hide negative effects of society's development. And I think we shall have to be very honest and out-spoken on the limits of our professional competence. Neither a psychiatric service like the one we have in Norway today, nor the one we plan for the future, is an adequate answer to the unease, anxiety, loneliness, and life problems that so many people experience today.

Surely I do not know the answers to all the human problems within a modern society. But I feel that a vital democracy, active in the local communities, is a qualification to find the answer. The psychiatrist, like many other professionals, has a responsibility to report to the public when becoming aware of destructive trends in society's development. He shall do as best as he can the job he is educated and paid for, and he shall preferably take an active part in the political life on a common basis with his fellow citizens.

REFERENCES

1. Boss, M.: Sturmzeichen in der psychologie und psychotherapie. *Psychotherap. Psychosom.* **20**:92–106, 1972.

2. *Arbeiderbevegelsens Håndbok*, Tiden Norsk Forlag, 1975. (*Handbook of Norwegian Labor Movement*, Tiden Norwegian Press, 1975.)

3. Norwegian Central Bureau of Statistics, *Social Survey*, 1974, p. 38.

4. Forsdahl, A.: Momenter til belysning av den høye dødelighet i Finnmark Fýlke. *T. n. Laegeforen.* **93**:661–667, 1973. (F.A.: Some factors to enlighten the high death rate in Finnmark County. *J. Norw. Med. Ass.* **93**:661–667, 1973.)

5. Forsdahl, A. and Waaler, H. Th.: University of Tromsø, 1975, p.c.

6. Norwegian Central Bureau of Statistics, *Society Survey*, 1974, p. 5.

7. *Ibid.*, p. 23.

8. *Ibid.*, p. 23.

9. *Ibid.*, p. 7.

10. *Ibid.*, p. 116.

11. *Ibid.*, p. 72.

12. *Ibid.*, p. 84.

13. *The Economist*, Norway Survey, November 15, 1975.

14. Norwegian Central Bureau of Statistics, *Social Survey*, 1974, p. 140.

15. *Arbeiderbevegelsens Håndbok*, Tiden Norsk Forlag, 1975. (*Handbook of Norwegian Labor Movement*, Tiden Norwegian Press, 1975.

16. Norwegian Central Bureau of Statistics, *Social Survey*, 1974, p. 207.

17. *Social Insurance in Norway*, The National Insurance Institution, Oslo, 1973.

18. *Norges Offentlige Utredning, 30. Universitetsforlaget, 1972 p. 31. (Norwegian Official Analysis, 30* University Press, 1972.)

19. Norwegian Central Bureau of Statistics, *Social Survey*, 1974, p. 58.

20. Bremer, J.: A social psychiatric investigation of a small community in Northern Norway. *Acta Psychiat. Scand.*, Suppl. 62, 1951.

21. Bjarnar, E., Melsom, R., et al.: A social psychiatric investigation of a rural district in Northern Norway. *Acta Psychiat. Scand.* **51**:19–27, 1975.

22. Hagnell, O.: *A Prospective Study of the Incidence of Mental Disorder.* Bonniers, Lund, Sweden, 1966.

23. Strømgren, E.: Contributions to psychiatric epidemiology and genetics. *Acta Jutlandica Med. Ser.* **40**:1–86, 1968.

24. Essen-Møller, E.: Individual traits and morbidity in a Swedish rural population. *Acta Psychiat. Scand.*, Suppl. 100, 1956.

25. Helgason, T.: Epidemiology of mental disorders in Iceland. *Acta Psychiat. Scand.,* Suppl. 173, 1964.

26. Srole, L., Langer, T. S., et al.: *Mental Health in the Metropolis,* Vol. I, McGraw-Hill, New York, 1962.

27. Ødegård, Ø.: Psykosenes epidemiologi. *Nord. Psykiat. Tidsskr.* **24**:15–27, 1970. (Ø.Ø.: The epidemiology of the psychoses. *Nordic J. Psychiat.* **24**:15–27, 1970.)

28. Sørensen, T.: Pendling og psykiske lidelser. *T. n. Laegeforen.* **92**:157–161, 1972. (S.T.: Commuting and psychiatric illness. *J. Norw. Med. Ass.* **92**:157–161, 1972.)

29. Dalgard, O. S.: *Migrating and Functional Psychoses in Oslo.* University Press, Oslo, 1967.

30. Øgar, B.: Psykiatri i almenpraksis. *T. n. Laegeforen.* **92**:905–912, 1972. (Ø.B.: Psychiatry in general practice. *J. Norw. Med. Ass.* **92**:905–912, 1972.)

31. Fugelli, P.: Mental health and living conditions in a fishing community in Northern Norway. *Acta Psychiat. Scand.,* Suppl. 263, 1975.

32. Andersen, T.: Physical and mental illness in a Lapp and a Norwegian Population. *Acta Psychiat. Scand.,* Suppl. 263, 1975.

33. Bentsen, B. G.: *Illness and General Practice.* University Press, Oslo-Bergen-Tromsø, 1970.

34. Midré, M.: Psykiatriens målsetting og virkemidler i lokalsamfunnet. Institutt for samf. vitenskap, Univ. i Tromsø, 1975, stensil, p. 22. (M. M.: Goals and functions of the psychiatric service in the local community. Institute of Social Sciences, Univ. of Tromsø, 1975, stencil, p. 22.)

35. Steenfeldt-Foss, O. W.: Planlegging og organisering av psykisk helsevern i Norge. *Nord. Psykiat. Tidsskr.* **27**:225–241, 1973. (S.-F.,O.W.: Planning and organization of mental health service in Norway. *Nordic. J. Psychiat.* **27**:225–241, 1973.)

36. Bratfos, O., Hirsch, J., et al.: Out-patient treatment of psychoses. *Acta Psychiat. Scand.* **48**:30–42, 1972.

37. Midré, M.: ref. 34, p. 25.

38. Mellbye, F.: Helse- og sosialsentra som basis for den primaere helsetjeneste i byer *T. n. Laegeforen.* **94**:1501–1506, 1974. (M.F.: Integrated health and social centers as a fundament for the primary health service in towns. *J. Norw. Med. Ass.* **94**:1501–1506, 1974.)

39. Bogen, B., Sundby, H., et al.: *Helsestasjonen i støpeskjeen,* Universitetsforlaget, Oslo, 1972. (B. B., S. H., et al.: The Mother and Child Guidance Center in Reformation, University Press, Oslo, 1972.)

40. Leighton, A. H.: Poverty and social changes. *Sci. Amer.* **212**:1965.

41. Richter, H.-E.: Community development und Psychotherapie in Randschichtgettos. *Psychotherap. Psychosom.* **24**:269–280, 1974.

42. Ericsson, K.: Den tvetydige omsorgen, Universitetsforlaget, Oslo-Bergen-Tromsø, 1974, p. 167. (E. K.: *The Ambiguous Care,* University Press, Oslo-Bergen-Tromsø, 1974, p. 167.)

43. Norwegian Official Statistics, *Social Survey,* 1974, p. 187.

44. *Ibid.,* p. 196.

45. *Ibid.,* p. 195.

46. Bakka, A., Johnsen, A., et al.: *Bruk av beroligende midler i Norge,* Universitetsforlaget, Oslo-Bergen-Tromsø, 1974. (B. A., J. A., et al.: *The Use of Tranquilizers in Norway,* University Press, Oslo-Bergen-Tromsø, 1974.)

47. Kolberg, J. E.: *TrygdeNorge,* Gyldendal Norsk Forlag, Oslo, 1974. (K. J. E.: *Insurance Norway,* Gyldendal Norwegian Press, Oslo, 1974.)

48. Illich, I.: *Medical Nemesis,* Calder and Boyars Ltd., London, 1974.

49. Haugsgjerd, S.: *Nytt perspektiv på psykiatrien,* Pax Forlag, Oslo, 1971. (H. S.: *New Perspectives on Psychiatry,* Pax Press, Oslo, 1971.)

50. Nyhus, P.: Mot profesjokratiets diktatur? *T. n. Laegeforen.* **95**:1133–1138, 1975. (N. P.: Towards the dictatorship of the professionals? *J. Norw. Med. Ass.* **95**:1133–1138, 1975.)

51. Magnussen, F.: Sosialpsykiatri og psykoterapi. i: *Visjon og vilje,* Fabritius Forlag, Oslo, 1975. (M. F.: Social psychiatry and psychotherapy. In *Vision and Will,* Fabritius Press, Oslo, 1975.)

52. Bettelheim, B.: Psychotherapy and psychopedagogy. *Psychotherap. Psychosom.* **20**:92–106, 1972.

53. Ziferstein, I.: The role of the psychotherapist in a changing society. *Psychotherap. Psychosom.* **25**:283–286, 1975.

54. Ugelstad, E.: Psykoterapi i sosialt perspektiv. I: *Psykiatrien på skilleveien,* J. W. Cappelens Forlag Oslo, 1971. (U. E.: Psychotherapy in a social perspective. In *Psychiatry at the Crossroads,* J. W. Cappelens Press, Oslo, 1971)

55. Sutherland, J. D.: The consultant psychotherapist in the National Health Service: His role and training. *Brit. J. Psychiat.* **114**:509–515, 1968.

56. Erikson, E. H.: *Childhood and Society,* Penguin Books, Hogarth Press, 1965, p. 261.

CHAPTER EIGHT

THE IMPACT OF LATIN CULTURE
UPON THE WORK OF A WOMAN ANALYST

MARINA PRADO DE MOLINA, A.S.

Five years ago, I participated in a seminar, held at the School of Sociology of the University of Madrid, dealing with the problems women were facing at that given moment. Last year, in Zurich, I collaborated in the Fifth International Forum of Psychoanalytic Societies' workshop on the impact of the feminist movement on the practice of the woman analyst. In this chapter I deal with the same subject because I am able to see that what we consider feminine or masculine in a given society continues to be colored with stereotypes that cause both women and men to fall into positions that are reactionary and unjust and, in addition, dangerous to the good psychic functioning, both of the individuals and of the couples, a problem from which we psychoanalysts are not excluded. It was curious, for example, that in the previously mentioned workshop, which was filled with women, only two men appeared, one of them the husband of the coordinator.

During the last 5 years here in Spain, a high percentage of women have returned to studies once long forgotten, or begun studies as adults, a phenomenon also occurring in other countries. It is also common for a middle-class woman to begin to work after several years of marriage and even after bringing up children and grandchildren. What do these women seek in their studies or their work? It would be easy to simplify the answer, as do some men in our society—perhaps even their own husbands—by considering it a kind of pastime or by translating it into economic terms.

On the other hand, when 2 years ago I undertook a survey of the opinions of sociology students about the instinctive side of life, I had these answers to the following question: "When a woman has had sexual relations, ought she to pretend that she has not had them?"

At first, 72% felt that, yes, the woman should withhold such information. However, on analyzing further, the study showed that 80% of the women and 60% of the men did *not* wish to withhold or have withheld such information, although 40% of the men still chose to be deceived.

I would recognize in these different facts, often not seen as related to one another, an awakening to oneself, to a clearer concept of one's identity, to the necessity of greater independence of judgment, to a personal maturity and to the realization of what each woman wants as her social role, a role not imposed on her but one worked out on an individual basis.

Frequently many theories are no more than the rationalization of a deeper problem that one has tried to set apart, a display that justifies deeper emotional attitudes. It is clear, therefore, that my rational and emotional attitudes are going to be reflected in this chapter and, for this reason, the

I wish to express my appreciation to my American cousin Barbara Broome Carballal for her work in translation.

conclusions at which I may arrive will be colored by my individual experience, both as a human being and as a woman. If it were true that in the nineteenth century when one studied the paths of the stars through a telescope there were subjective errors in the measurements, it is clear that in this field in which I am an interested party, the same problem will exist. Even if the feminists of the eighteenth century were partially correct in affirming that "everything men have written about women is not to be trusted because men are both the judges and part of the judgement," one cannot, for the same reason, fall into the gross error of believing that only women are capable of dealing with the subject in which they too are interested parties.

My dilemma as a human being arises from the possibility of being treated as an object or as a subject. The system of values of a society becomes a reality when one group ascribes a determined role to another. The role requires that one behave with certain patterns. In social groups a series of pressures are produced which causes persons to act in a determined way. When this pattern is not in agreement with the internal makeup of the subjects, confusion is produced. The dissociation reflects a seriously divided social field that interrelates intimately with the individual.

To study the influence of Latin culture on the work of a woman analyst, one must do so with regard to what Viola Klein refers to as the present cultural patterns in a society in a state of transition where one finds a real situation, somewhat modified externally, but coexisting with traditional attitudes and ideologies.

In a patriarchal society, women, relatively speaking, form a group apart. As occurs in the case of other groups in similar positions, preconceived opinions, more or less oversimplified, are applied to that class in its totality without sufficiently considering individual differences. This patriarchal system has been identical, except for multiple variations, in almost all the civilizations of the earth since the beginning of written history. All of these similarities in the feminine role have their origins in the first civilizations on the Mesopotamian peninsula. Later, both the Jewish culture as well as the civilization born on the banks of the Ganges had similar development, as both Leviticus and the Laws of Manú show. In the Semitic syndiasmatic family, the chief lived in fully polygamous circumstances with the incorporation of slaves and life-and-death power over them. In the monogamous family, one finds greater solidity in the conjugal bond, the dissolution of which is no longer optional. Among the Greeks one finds this new form of the family in all its strength, although among the Spartans married women possessed still greater freedom which leads one to deduce that matrilineal influences existed.

Among the Romans, woman was freer and received more considerations.

The Roman who held life or death rights over his wife felt that her fidelity was, therefore, guaranteed, although in reality that was not true. Here too, the woman could break the matrimonial bond at will as could her husband.

At the beginning of written history in the ancient Nordic communities one finds that the transition from maternal to paternal law is still occurring, although many vestiges of the syndiasmatic family still remain. The four Scandinavian countries formed a cultural block which extended as far as Russia. They also had a great affinity toward the Germanic tribes that occupied all of the northern part of the continent as far as the Rhine where the Roman Empire began. Among these civilizations, the mother was considered the good spirit of the home even though the father held the title of *lord*. According to Plutarch, women were accustomed to the difficulties of war and assisted their husbands in this field. Plutarch tells that in the camps of the Randicos, the Germanic tribes returned to find their wives, dressed in black, killing off the deserters—even if they were husbands, fathers, or relatives. Tacitus too speaks of bands of women warriors where not only the young girls went to war but also the elderly priestesses, dressed in white linen. The Germanic girls taken prisoners by the Romans preferred suicide to losing their virginity.

With the influence of Christianity and absorption of the barbarian tribes into Western Civilization, a new era began where monogamy gave supremacy to the man but also a position of greater prestige to woman.

Within medieval Christianity the partisans of asceticism began violent attacks against the sins of the flesh and rated marriage as lustful as any illicit union. The church began its battle in favor of priestly celibacy. From the time of Gregory VII celibacy became a reality in the West, and the dangerous nature of women was underlined still more severely. This meant that if woman had attained a certain triumph through the Christian religion, she then paid for it by suppressing a part of herself, her sexual nature.

In the Middle Ages the justification of the position of women—be it real or hoped for—was sought in the realms of physiology and biology. For the last 2000 years one sector of public opinion, represented at first by the philosophers of the Enlightenment, has sustained the belief that sex is an unimportant accident of nature and that the apparent psychosexual differences are, in great part, mere differences in upbringing, easily susceptible to change. Another faction, among the Romantics, has sustained the belief (upon which the demands with respect to feminine rights are founded) that woman is different, this difference becoming converted emotionally into a slight inferiority with regard to man.

In my opinion many of the efforts made by women to rise above a situation of alienation are no more than a mirror reflection of male behavior. The acquisition of a crude vocabulary by young women is, in most cases, no more than an example of the necessity to identify with purely male patterns and the exhibition of poorly assimilated liberty. Let us emphasize the mistaken nature of this kind of identification as showing up the hidden castration from which the person suffers.

It is certainly true, in my opinion, that there exists a more balanced position, precisely that which many women would attempt without being sure of being able to carry it out. From this position, she would try to see what exists within herself, what active tendencies she possesses, what inhibited or repressed sadistic inclinations she may have, so that conscious of her self-persecution she can reduce it and, as a result, not project it externally. In short, she should try to see what men and women have in common. In my judgment, one needs to know if what Freud called masochism and what seemed to pertain specifically to women in Western culture was not due more to the sociological supremacy of the penis than to the biological fact.

Clinically, what one sees in the pathology of this generation and what one can foresee in the near future with relation to the development of Western society is a series of processes of depersonalization, of identity crisis, of the use of drugs, of suicide, and so on, in short, an escape from oneself and the outside world. In an age where one aspires to the possibility of choice, one finds paradoxically a dazzling escape from such choice. One must ask the reason for this escape, the reason for this crisis. The aspirations of women, together with the reactionary positions of both sexes, are but one of the many facets of this crisis. In my understanding, there exist notable differences between what we have been taught and what we have to practice, between what is thought and what is said, between what is said and what is felt, between parental teaching that formed an ego ideal based on love and the aggressive spirit, an all-out struggle for survival in a power-oriented society.

Now that the right to orgasm and the use of contraceptives are a sociological fact in many countries, the woman may enjoy and, in fact, does enjoy external freedom similar to the man's in sexual matters. This leads one to ask what the psychological consequences of this will be for both sexes. One cannot forget that both sexes are necessary for the continuation of the species and that mutual satisfaction is much more than merely the number of copulations. In the same sense, neither can one forget that to obtain this satisfaction, the man needs to demonstrate his sexual capacity within a general potency while the woman does not need this demonstration but does need man to show his to obtain her own satisfaction.

One of the consequences seen in other countries and, at certain social levels in my own, is that when faced with the woman's activist position, the man becomes inhibited and unconsciously takes a childlike posture similar to that he held with relation to his mother. He no longer dominates; he is dependent. Thus instead of the Eros becoming richer, the relationship is impoverished as the wife becomes the phallic mother of his early years. This way the woman defeats her own purposes if she strengthens these fantasies with her internal reality.

All of these questions are ones which one may ask when comparing the situation of women in other countries with that of those in Spain's patriarchal society where economic, social, and political circumstances have prevented such a rapid evolution in this sense but where all of these concerns previously referred to are beginning to appear.

THE POSITION OF THE WOMAN IN SPANISH SOCIETY

To study the position woman occupies in Spanish society one must study:

1. The legal status of women.
2. The division of work.
3. The ideological and moral aspects.

The Spanish legal code is clearly influenced by Roman laws and by the Napoleonic Code derived from them. Under Roman law only the man is subject to legislation as the woman is treated as an object, subject, in turn, to the head of the family. As of May 5, 1975, certain Spanish laws have been changed because of the profound transformations occurring within Spanish society, changes that have made a revision of family law both convenient and desirable. One must note here, too, that these changes correspond to pressures in Spanish society, pressures reflecting the general feeling of inequality in the legal status of men and women. Viewing the law as the crystalization of customs and social events, one can thus see the evolution which woman's role has undergone and the change in her status.

Among the most important illustrations of this inequality between men and women one might point out the changes the law of May 5th shows are as follows:

1. Marriage is now not enough in itself to transmit nationality. Previously, the Spanish nationality of the husband was automatically given to the wife and children, while this did not occur in the marriage of a Spanish woman to a foreigner.

2. The Code in which marital permission was necessary for the woman's contracts has been reformed.

3. The discriminatory terms of "obedience" as the woman's obligation and "protection" as the man's have been suppressed and replaced by terms of mutual protection.

4.   The representation that a husband held over his wife with regard to legal matters can now only be given with her permission.

5.   The clauses that prevented a married woman from being a guardian have been modified.

6.   The married woman may now accept inheritances without her husband's permission, an act not possible previously.

7.   In contracts, the clauses that compared women to the physically or psychically retarded have been suppressed.

8.   The place of residence must be decided by mutual agreement and no longer solely by the father as was previously done.

9.   While the husband continues to be the administrator of the family goods, each partner may govern the property he has acquired and the wife no longer needs her husband's permission to dispose of her property.

10.   At age 21 both sexes come of age, although the law still requires the woman to live at home till age 23 unless she leaves to marry or to enter a convent.

11.   In the Penal Code, however, a woman is still punished for adultery while the man is punished only if he brings a lover into the house or if he is flagrantly unfaithful.

With regard to the division of work, the upper-class Spanish wife attends to her social obligations, her home, and her children, although in most cases these children are in the hands of servants. Only a small minority of the women in this class have intellectual concerns and university studies. In the middle class, the woman dedicates herself, almost exclusively, to her home, especially now that she has only part-time help. In this group there are more women with academic degrees, although they continue to be in the minority. To give a personal example, of the 28 girls who finished the Spanish high school together, only 2 of us have continued with advanced studies and, at the present time, I am the only one who practices in her field. In the lower classes, the married woman works almost exclusively at home or at part-time jobs which are no more than a prolongation of her housework. For the men of this class, it is a matter of pride that their wives *not* work, a proof of their economic potency.

With regard to the woman who works, one finds that:

1.   The woman forms part of a reserve army maintained by capitalist economy and, in the case of the Spanish woman, a reserve needed for part-time jobs and for jobs a man does not wish to undertake.

2.   The woman wishing to start to work collides with competitors who have preference—men, because of their sex, even though their talents have not been tested.

3.   The shortage of jobs and the preference of men for those jobs which

do exist obliges the woman to accept lower salaries, often 70% lower, to agree to unjust situations, or, to the contrary, to take part in movements to regain their rights.

4. The work normally done by woman is that which is usually an extension of her work at home.

5. Woman's work at home and in similar fields, typical of precapitalist society, is not in relation to the real development of Spanish society today.

6. As the children grow older, women tend to fill their free hours with new projects related to the home because they are not prepared to undertake others. While a slight but increasing minority attempts to return to an active professional life, these women face enormous difficulties due to insufficient or outdated preparation, lack of practice, or age.

7. Among the 21-year-olds one finds the greatest number of women working outside the home (47.5%). As age increases, this percentage decreases progressively in such a way that one finds only 19% working at age 34—this due either to the needs of her children or the influence of her husband. From age 35 on, women again work outside the home with 23.9% working at age 55. Only when a woman renounces her role in the family because she remains single (voluntarily sometimes, more often not), or assumes the role as head of the family or pays someone to substitute her or must work to augment her husband's limited income, does she find herself in a position to select what Spanish society terms the "male pattern." But even in these cases, the marked differences in the role of each sex oblige the single woman, the widow, the childless, the woman who enjoys domestic help, as well as the worker's wife, to fulfill her obligations upon returning home, thus doubling her working hours.

8. With regard to academic studies, the number of girls entering primary school is similar to that of boys. Progressively, the girls abandon their studies on the high school level. Already at this level one finds a great difference in the size of male and female groups with regard to the preparatory degrees which allow one to continue professional studies. A marked contrast is found only in those fields that Spanish society has set apart as feminine: child care, nursing, social work, and such.

9. At the level of advanced learning, the percentage of women is much smaller than that of men and again centered in certain fields: liberal arts, fine arts, and pharmacy.

Customs, sexual ideology, all that previously have been considered moral, are undergoing great changes. In many families, gaps are occurring between parents and children, although not as great as those found in foreign countries. Youth refuses to accept the lies of present-day society, rising in rebellion against whatever might represent hypocrisy, external pressure, or social injustice. Nevertheless, many lack sufficient inner strength to assume the responsibilities that go with the position they have taken which makes this appear merely a passing phase, analogous to reactionary behavior of the time and to the identity crisis. This does not deny the existence of a minority whose behavior is consistent with its political ideas, with its social postures, or with its aspirations.

The sixth commandment concerning adultery, of such importance 25 years ago in Spain, has practically disappeared and seems no longer relevant, according to students of sociology. Instead emphasis is given to loving one's neighbor and to not stealing, and when an open question is asked, a primary position is given to social justice. This, in my judgment, would imply an important change and point to new values, perhaps long-needed ones.

Within this section one must also include as an important point the lack of agreement that exists between the source of sexual education the aforementioned students would have *liked* to have had—their parents—and that source they did have. Eighty-seven percent obtained this information from books, school, or classmates, while 97% would have preferred to have received this information from their parents.

In the study undertaken by the Molina-Nuñez Institute (previously Peña-Retama) last year, the "normal Spanish family," understanding by this the family where no one has ever had to visit a psychiatrist, consisted of a unit where the family relations were logical and where children, within general terms, agreed with their parents and with their own upbringing.

The result of investigation leads one to think that there exists a neurotic family matrix from which individual neurotic developments emerge which will take on clinically detectable symptoms in the sons or daughters most innately appropriate to relieve the family of its conflicting situation. The father figure tends to excessive control, urgent demands with regard to studies and behavior in general, and coldness and emotional distance (also extended among the children). The significant tendencies in the mother figure are sexual repression, splitting in the currents of tenderness and sexuality and those of aggressiveness and affection, feelings of dissatisfaction, and a failure to recognize her own worth. These characteristics are those of the emotionally immature personality with a certain predominance of passive dependent characteristics which one might diagnose as a hysterical personality. The father might be diagnosed as an obsessive character.

From the union of these partners, a dynamic situation arises from which the father is affectively distant although he makes his wife and children internalize these demands. Such paternal influences are, to an extent, intercepted and modified by the mother who, with her passive resistance and her hidden criticism—the fruit of her ambivalent posture with regard to the father—produces a nonconforming attitude in the offspring with regard to the father figure and his commands.

THE WORK OF A WOMAN PSYCHOANALYST
WITHIN SPANISH SOCIETY

In this section, I speak of the impact that Spanish society, as described previously, has on the work of a woman psychoanalyst together with the different influences that one's countertransference suffers due to these psychosociological conditions.

When beginning to analyze the sources through which patients are referred to someone, it is necessary to consider the place that psychoanalysis holds in Spanish society. Twenty years ago in Spain, this was a therapeutic procedure viewed with serious misgivings both by official or classic psychiatry and by the Church. If one were to crystallize the position held by many of the university professors, it would be sufficient to mention Professor López-Ibor's *The Agony of Psychoanalysis* published in 1951.[15]

On the part of the Church, psychoanalysis was considered an object of anathema because of its pansexualist tendencies. Following the advice of said institution, a priest had to request permission to undergo psychoanalysis with an analyst of Freudian orientation, since it was supposed that a psychoanalyst with a healthy religious attitude could not possibly exist. On the other hand, it is also necessary to mention the reactionary attitude of some of the neophytes of psychoanalysis who, seeing themselves as bearers of absolute truths, felt persecuted by God. Under such circumstances, it was difficult for a scientific method which possesses, as does any other, indications and counterindications to make progress. Thanks to the personal tenacity and human and scientific strength of Dr. Molina-Núñez, this was able to be done within 7 years.[16-18] In 1962 the first and only sanitorium for neurotics and psychotics using the method of analytic psychotherapy was opened in Spain.

In the last few years the panorama has changed greatly, although even today some extreme judgments are heard at the universities, proclaiming on one hand that psychoanalysis is of no use, or, on the other, that it cures everything. The latter opinion is maintained by people who have adequate theoretical knowledge but who lack a complete psychoanalytic preparation, by which I mean a didactic analysis carried out by competent persons, theoretical formation, analysis of control, and such. At the same time, phantom institutes have proliferated promising formation in a month or a year or where just one therapist carries out the analysis of the candidates, the analysis of control, and the didactic preparation. That is to say that although there exists a genuine interest among the young people who are discontent with the psychiatric formation or university studies in psychology, the panorama is so confused, the rush to undergo analysis or to demonstrate the worth or failure of a particular method are of more importance than the need that a certain person carry out the analysis, and that this psychoanalyst be of one sex or the other is of secondary importance. For this reason, I receive some patients sent by classical psychiatrists whose principal aim is to demonstrate that dynamic psychiatry or analytic psychotherapy, often confused one with the other, have no reason for being. This then becomes a prime reason in the transference of many patients, the sex of the psychotherapist being only a secondary variable. In addition, I often receive patients sent by doctors and psychiatrists with dynamic orientation for whom the preparation is more important than the sex of the analyst.

Another source of patients is that represented by former patients for whom it is extremely important that the same person who carried out their previous treatment undertake the new therapy. Many of these patients, in spite of the fact that they have had their transference analyzed, continue to have a too idealized concept of the therapist, either because they have not completely finished with their transference or because surrounding circumstances have pushed them from one medicine to another before they came to us and were able to receive consistent treatment. When a man comes to me seeking help, he may usually be assigned to one of the following constellations:

1.   He is trying to resolve, on an unconscious level, a state of great dependency with relation to his mother-substitute, represented at that moment by me. This is the case of certain homosexuals with an ego that is sufficiently strong to allow them to form a therapeutic alliance. For this reason, they are able to begin treatment with a woman analyst because they have the necessary capacity to avoid anxiety and are able to achieve bisexuality in a relatively short period of time. In this group I would also class those homosexuals—although with a less favorable prognosis—whose degree of sickness or anxiety toward the maternal image is so extreme that one must request the collaboration of a male therapist.

2.   Another type of patient is he who has a high level of aggressivity toward women and whose partial motivation in approaching us is to defeat us. Such patients have such strong sadistic fantasies that they try to convert the sessions into a battlefield. When they find an active interpretive attitude on the part of the analyst, their urge for struggle and their fear of castration, which corresponds to their projected desires, are stimulated. When

faced with a more passive interpretive attitude, they experience their fantasies or wishes such as death or physical harm with regard to the analyst with the corresponding guilt feelings. In these cases, I prefer to transfer them to a male analyst, not because a woman is incapable because of her sex to treat them, but because I believe that treatment with a male analyst would less arouse their defense mechanisms and thus be shortened in length.

Women patients who come to us may be grouped in the following way:

1.   Those who because of their oedipal guilt feelings from which they wish to be protected seek analysis with a woman.

2.   Women in highly competitive situations with men because of which they cannot bear a male analyst and thus seek out another woman as an ally stronger than themselves or as a strong penis (which they imagine the analyst has) which they wish to use for their own pathological ends.

3.   Women in search of their own identity for whom the patterns their mothers have given them do not suffice and who hope to find in me an *imago* to introject in a massive way—which shows how tied they are to oral levels, although they can show partial facets of their personality on higher levels.

When a patient comes to me, I consider first his diagnosis and prognosis in order to weigh the possibility of analysis in the case, and when these are favorable, I weigh the facts in view of the treatment—whether a male or female analyst would be preferable for the patient's internal constellation, trying to keep such treatment as short as possible. The sex of the analyst should correspond to the sex of the less-feared parent. In my opinion, a male homosexual or a man who is impotent should begin treatment with a male analyst, and later, when sufficiently prepared to face the more dangerous figure, he may, or perhaps, should, change to an analyst of the opposite sex.

One must not ignore, however, the fact that the person undergoing analysis will, depending on his fantasies, parental roles, and phases of analysis, project feelings with relation to his paternal or maternal *imago* without regard to the analyst's sex, but I feel that the emotional and corrective experience will take place more adequately and rapidly if the patient achieves the integration of his feelings within the context of reality of what is the analyst's true sex. This way, too, the period of resistance toward the feelings related to the most feared images is shortened with the presentation, in the proper moment, of the stimulus that represents the external image that is going to put such fantasies into motion and the elaboration of which will be guided by the first therapist who has been able to establish a sufficiently solid therapeutic alliance.

Now I wish to explain that I understand as cotherapy the realization of treatment by two analysts of different sexes, simultaneously or successively, in the spirit of consciously complementing each other's work, because I have worked in this manner since 1959 in collaboration principally with Dr. Molina in individual therapy. In addition, we have done cotherapy in group psychotherapy with other therapists.

In regard to individual psychotherapy, we have worked with two forms:

1.   Successive cotherapy, consisting of a change of therapist in a given moment with the idea of mobilizing concrete transferential content, easing in that way the process of identification with the parental image of the same sex.

2.   Simultaneous cotherapy in which two therapists treat the patient simultaneously in separate sessions with the idea of correcting the fantasies of destruction and separation of the married couple or the working out of conflicting situations with one of the parental images through the double action of ego strengthening by one therapist and the mobilization of transferential content by the other.

In both the individual cotherapy, as well as group cotherapy with two therapists of the opposite sex, one observes as *sine qua non* conditions:

1.   The equality of status in the therapists, each with different but inter-changeable functions, which avoids the rigid patterns of domination or sub-mission leading to the mutual resentment seen in today's society.

2.   The equality of status of the therapists with regard to the patient with the objective that each is able to stimulate the fantasies of pairing off.

3.   A similarity in theoretical orientation, since, in my judgment, therapists with totally antagonistic methodologies and orientation cannot work together.

4.   A basic mutual acceptance, a factor more important, in my under-standing, than a certain disparity in orientation and methodology.

5.   The capacity of each analyst to recognize and accept his own abilities and limitations.

6.   The capacity of each therapist to accept his partner's success in a given moment.

In the evaluation we made of our work in the year 1969 which was based on 32 cases, we noted four fundamental factors with which we believe we may justify the use of this method.

1.   The normal analytic relationship, with only one therapist, must rely on the possibilities that the patient has to project upon himself the deteriorated internal objects and the introjections later reconstructed, even

though it be only partial. In fact, this type of relationship functions as a setting that favors splitting, since the patient tends to identify with the doctor and live the negative part within himself. When the patient is seriously afflicted and his opinion of himself is very low, this situation of splitting created by the setting itself may make it impossible to overcome or extend in some clear way the working through. In the cotherapy situation, and, above all, when simultaneous, which is what I will refer to here due to the importance of countertransferential phenomena, the patient has the option from the very beginning of projecting his internal division, since it is no longer lived between the therapist and him but rather between the two therapists. If between these two, one finds the basic principle for all cotherapy technique—mutual acceptance—in the moment of the introjections, the setting of the therapeutic situation is in itself structure giving.

2.   Cotherapy makes possible the easing of the mechanisms of identification with the therapists on a less idealized base. The continual working through of the splitting projected on the therapists, contrasting it with the real and personal relationship which the two share with regard to the patient, obliges the patient to abandon his idealized fantasies about them as he begins to establish an identification more in agreement with reality.

3.   This facilitates the "being able to become" experience which I consider as having a basic value in the crisis of acceptance of the therapist, and with it, in moving on to a relationship of partial objects to total ones. In psychoanalysis certain key experiences exist that create an important and brusk mobilization of the emotional contents. At this moment, the patient recognizes the therapist's acceptance of his feared identity. The presence of an analyst of the same sex aids in the passive and homosexual identification, while at the same time the second therapist's presence supports the patient's ego faced with the fantasies of castration and of internal harm put into motion by the rivalry with the parental image of the same sex.

4.   As a final point, let us consider that cotherapy with the interplay of action of two analysts offers the best conditions for working through very dramatic situations in the sense that upon presenting them to one of the two therapists, the second analyst serves as an auxiliary ego that supports the process of differentiating between the projected material and that which corresponds to reality. That is to say, cotherapy permits a less traumatic working through of the problems in the sense that it allows the liberation of unconscious fantasies reinforcing the presence of reality and creating the optimum conditions, so that within the dynamics of the ego, the defensive structure yields when faced with conflict, and the development of another, less pathological, structure becomes possible. The moment for initiating cotherapy is that in which, having deeply worked out the projected identification with regard to the less traumatic parental image, the patient has

experienced a sufficiently dependent relationship toward that image. If one waits too long in establishing cotherapy and one lets the exact moment pass, the patient may tend toward a less productive intellectual analysis; if one establishes it too soon, the chaotic situation of W. Reich may occur.

ANALYSIS OF THE COUNTERTRANSFERENCE

Using the simplified method of Kemper[10] with a few corrections one may say that there exist in all human relationships:

1. A subject, with his constitutional data, his prior experiences, and his orientation toward the world in which he lives.

2. An object, something animate or inanimate which the subject is facing, perhaps, too, with a determined constellation which will affect in a positive or negative sense the subject on the condition that he presents certain specific characteristics.

The reactions of the so-called object depend on the subject and the object's own constellations that he perceives in accord with his own internal makeup also depend on the radiations that he receives from the subject.

The analytic situation is a specifically dual situation with characteristics that differ from any other type of human interaction. But here, too, there exists the specific constellation of the therapist, however much it may have been analyzed, with its scotomas and its own transference neurosis. On the other hand, the analyst, in trying to understand the subject, experiences a partial regression. That is to say, his ego splits into a regressed ego that identifies with the patient becoming as it were a sounding board for the patient's unconscious, and a second ego that perceives, ties together, translates, and unites in a conscious manner all that which he felt in his unconscious.

Many authors such as Flournoy[4] think that since 1950 we are living in the third age, that of countertransference, which is considered the best instrument that analysis has. This is also my opinion because I have seen in the clinic that when something goes wrong in the analysis, this signifies that something is wrong in the countertransference.

P. Heimann[9] sees the countertransference as an instrument for understanding the patient under analysis although the emotional response of the therapist is often nearer the psychological reality of the patient than his analysts' conscious judgement about the same situation.

M. Little[14] is concerned with countertransference as a hindrance in the comprehension and interpretation together with the influence of the same on the analyst's behavior. This author reemphasizes the tendency of the analyst to repeat certain aspects of the parents' behavior, thus satisfying some of his own internal needs (rather than those of the patient).

As is well known, one must always distinguish within the countertransference: (1) the transference of the analyst through which mechanisms the analyst recognizes the patient's conflicts or what Racker calls concordant identification, (2) the neurosis of countertransference which corresponds to the neurotic response of the analyst to the patient's transference, which is to say, the activation by the patient of the therapist's blind spots, or Grinberg's projective counteridentification. It is certainly true that the psychoanalytic formation of the analyst, if adequate, ought prepare him for access to the unconscious, allowing him to understand the interrelation of his own internal images with those of the patient. However, sometimes it occurs that the reactivation of his scotomas is so strong that he rejects these scotomas because he fears them as some complementary identification. (3) The normal reactions of the analyst to the patient's whole being also exist in a conscious and realistic form, which correspond to the total emotional reaction of the therapist toward the patient as a subject and as a person.

The analyst's therapeutic capacity would be in proportion to his sublimated positive transference while if he feels primarily a neurosis of countertransference with its aggressive or erotic overtones, this will cause resistence and disturbances in the psychoanalytic work.

One would have to ask at this point what kind of countertransferential reactions one would have in this society and how the sociological is going to relate to the psychological reinforcing or weakening of one's internal constellation.

In the analytic situation as in the parent-child situation, the capacity with which the analysts recognize and accept their own scotomas, their own neurotic countertransferences is highly important, since that way they will not transfer their interpretations to the patient on a conscious level nor will they transfer their own conflict filled situation in their unconscious communication. At the same time they will help the patient, having recognized their own limitations, to work through his capacity for enjoying life, for taking pleasure in the company of others, and for forming a scheme of interpersonal relationships in which the "I" and "thou" are involved and with which the patient is going to form some less persecuted introjections when they are available to him. Here, too, it is important to have analyzed one's narcissism and to recognize the satisfaction to be found in the "analyst role."

It is very probable that with the homosexual patients who correspond to a group of subjects seen frequently, the woman analyst will experience her own feelings of castration and that she will see them as babies who make no sexual demands on her, and since they do not represent a danger, the analyst may not want them to grow.

With an aggressive male, one may experience one's father or brothers in a position of superiority producing thus the logical envy and desire for hostile revenge.

With feminine patients who have a dependence on the mother *imago* one may feel a desire to protect them in the same way she herself would like to be protected by her mother with regard to her oedipal constellation, and in that way wish to obstruct their growth and individualization on an unconscious level.

With the group of women whose psychological constellation responds to competitive situations with men, the analyst's neurotic countertransference may be revived in such a way that she allows herself to be placed at the service of the pathological use that these women wish to make of her supposed phallus as she responds with regard to her sociological castration.

When faced with young women in the 20-year-old bracket, with a youth markedly different from that which analysts my age knew, young people who enjoy so much more liberty than we did, there may arise a feeling of envy coupled with competition reinforced by the social medium in which we live and in which "possessing" a man may become just one more material item as Leah Davidson notes.[3]

If one tries to differentiate with regard to countertransference in the male group or the female group, one is able to observe a greater satisfaction with the analyses of males done by female analysts. Let me emphasize here the double sociological and psychological influence that favor man over woman. The mother-son relationship which is so satisfactory for the former because she finds these erotic overtones more or less repressed or sublimated begins to have an important role here. When the analyst has had a positive relationship with her father, the son (here the patient) may represent the father of her childhood, thus repeating the oedipus fantasies. One must point out here the importance of one's incestuous fantasies towards one's sons, the fantasies most seriously forbidden in our society perhaps because they represent a deeper regression into the evolutionary period on a psychological level thus producing more anxiety. On the sociological level this would represent the desire to substitute a patriarchal society for matriarchal because the former would accept the incestuous solutions of father with daughter more in agreement with existing patterns in society.

It is curious to observe that in psychoanalytic literature there do not exist investigations about sexual acting out of feminine analysts while, yes, one finds some in regard to male therapists. What has happened? Is it that women analysts do not have scotomas? Are we not able to feel sexually attracted to a patient? Since I am not able to accept either explanation, I must suppose that those which have occured have been more repressed than those of the male analysts, although even the latter have not been sufficiently studied.

With women, one's envy of one's mother and the fear of a homosexual bond with regard to her may impede any similar approach or enjoyment of the analyst-patient relationship which one may have with the male group.

In all of the books about psychoanalytic technique the necessity of neutrality on the analyst's part is mentioned, emphasizing it as a condition for good progress in analysis. Personally, although theoretically I agree with this ideal, I find in practice the ease with which I fall and with which I see other analysts fall into positions which would cause us to doubt the subjectivity of our objectivity. My aspirations in this respect must be limited to recognizing the problem. This means that when faced with an erotic countertransference toward a patient, for example, what one ought to demand of oneself is the capacity to recognize it, dealing with it without denying it ourselves, allowing our ego to direct our Eros in such a way that it reaches and helps to create an Eros no longer feared by the patient. This objective may be achieved in agreement with the analyst's emotional growth in such a way that she feels and expresses verbally with her ego instead of with her id.

One may not forget that in normal development parents of both sexes respond to the love of their children in a more intense way than one likes to admit and that the growing out of this phase is a necessary step so that the sons and daughters may seek mates without feeling rejected as human beings. Only an ego sufficiently loved and for that reason sufficiently strong is able to accept the fact that its oedipal desires cannot be realized. I agree with Searles[24] that the unconscious mechanism of negation through which the parents do not recognize their child's importance leads more to damage of the ego than to its growth and autonomy, since the parents, and, in this case the analyst, put into motion or reinforce patterns of identification in which the ego is capable of facing his internal wishes and the external pressures represented by society. One may say, then, that good psychic functioning would be in relation to the balance achieved by the ego between the ego ideal and the superego on one side and the id on the other.

In psychopathology when faced with certain patients with insufficiently strong egos, the superego is that which takes the role of controlling the id for which reason in the psychoanalytic treatment the analyst will have to serve as an auxillary ego so that the patient may recognize reality, separating it from his unconscious fantasies. The working through of the schizoparanoid position with its partial objects to the depressive phase with total objects is an important moment in the analytic situation. For this to happen, the ego ideal and the superego have had to work out the first stages of development; that is to say, the patient must have accepted his dependence with relation to the object in the treatment with the analyst. In the same way the analyst also has to accept his feelings internally so that he does not project his partial objects on the patient.

The analyst, for his part, has to accept the feared identity of his patient on an emotional level, since the interpretations are often not more than the vehicle that makes the patient feel the capacity of the therapist's love. I find that many patients, only when they have realized this opening toward the therapist's world, are able to realize less persecuted and more realistic introjections.

One must not forget that in transference as well as in countertransference one finds the normal reactions of the patient to the analyst and of the analyst to the patient as whole beings, as subjects and persons. In the same way that a neurotic part, although quantitatively different, exists in both patient and therapist, there also exists a healthy or relatively healthy part of the patient which is capable of recognizing the internal reactions and attitudes of the analyst in a realistic way, precisely those parts not in relation to the patient's blind spots.

It is also true that some patients as they continue advancing and improving may become highly attractive persons, awakening feelings in relation to one's normal response to the opposite sex, which are unpleasant to recognize. These feelings may originate guilt feelings, anxiety, and so on. I have observed that in agreement with my own development I have been able not only to admit the feelings but also to verbalize them, often in agreement with the patient's need. For this reason, I must conclude that that which at the beginning of my analytic practice was a painful content for me, I find that with more experience I am able not only to solve but also to use in relation to the object which stimulated it independent of my own needs. The difference lies in the capacity of my ego to distinguish clearly what could be my desires, the id, and the reality and responsibility with which I, an analyst, must come face to face.

Already in 1952, Max Gitelson pointed out: "An analysis can come to an impasse because the analyst does not realize, or misunderstands, or avoids the issue of a patient's discovery of him as a person."[7]

Maurice Bouvet in 1958, following this flexible orientation, emphasized "the deliberate variations required with different types of patients in different phases of their analysis in order to maintain an optimal distance."[2]

Sacha Nacht[19] in the same panel thought all rules concerning neutrality and anonymity, if taken too strictly, could lead to a sado masochistic "analytic couple" and florid ritualism. He suggested that an analyst should be able to abandon the rigid neutrality and allow his presence to be felt.

It is in this spirit and the understanding that this presence is going to be felt, distorted partially and worked through, that we advise cotherapy for the diagnoses previously cited, emphasizing at the same time that the transference that the analysts are going to have toward the patient as well as that which they will have between themselves is going to have different characteristics than that which presents itself in an analysis done by a single therapist.

Once the adequate moment for cotherapy is established, the patient will try to situate the first analyst in the good object position and will consider the second as a bad object. When faced with this mechanism, the therapist who initiated the treatment ought to respond by analyzing the projections that the patient makes of his split world as well as the persecution object that he places on the second analyst. The reason for this technique is simple: the patient will accept more easily the interpretations that come from the good-object analyst, while if they come from the other therapist he will systematically reject them as a defense maneuver to avoid the possibility of being destroyed by what he himself has projected because he felt unable to tolerate it. In this phase, the second bad-object analyst will have to bear massive doses of aggressivity without feeling internally damaged by the patient or his cotherapist.

For this reason, basic trust between the therapists is considered essential, since the patient, upon mobilizing his internal fantasies, is going to try to project them on the two people who form the therapeutic setting. If this basic trust does not exist between the two analysts, he who receives the projections may counteridentify with them and place himself in a situation of envy or rivalry with the analyst who carries the positive part. In the same way that parents lend each other mutual support in their children's upbringing and that this support is essential in moments of difficulty, the therapists have to know how to take these feelings from the patient and return them to him in such a way that they are easy for the patient to assimilate through the interpretations of the first therapist, the second therapist receiving the projection without identifying with it.

For this reason one may say that the second analyst supplies the "corrective emotional experience" to which Alexander[1] refers or the symbolic realization of Sechehaye[25] while the therapist who began the treatment has the work of analyzing the unconscious material. In this way the patient is going to contribute new material to be analyzed.

In the cotherapy the patient relives the first matching situation of his parents in which he was the third person, excluded on an oral level. The results of this situation are more beneficial on the dynamic level but also more painful. For this reason, the patient is going to try to unite with one of the two therapists, trying to exclude the other, as a defensive maneuver, since the situation of being the third person, the excluded one, feels like a dangerous one for him.

Sometimes the patient will try to play one therapist against the other, trying to produce a power struggle so that the therapist with the more feared *imago* remains on the sidelines, separated from the network of social communication. If it is the male analyst who bears the feared *imago* and the female therapist who in the first phase takes charge of the interpretive activity, the former may resent the situation and live his passivity as castration, a situation which, if not cleared up, will produce mutual resentment. On her part, the female analyst may feel desires for retaliation against her partner if she has felt belittled with regard to the male.

The patient may also manipulate both therapists, trying to change himself into a person desirable to each of them, something like the crown of laurel given to the winner, which can cause internal resentment on the therapists' part.

In the cotherapy the true matching must be that of the therapists for which reason this attempt to exclude one must be analyzed in its deepest content. If there do not exist internal necessities of a pathological nature in the analysts, the patient will try to repeat the matching in the opposite direction, namely with the second therapist. In both cases there may arise and often do arise difficulties on an oral or incestuous level with the corresponding feelings of envy and jealousy respectively. The position of both therapists here will be that of verbalizing and working out between themselves these possible feelings so as not to transfer them to the patient (who would at first be most satisfied but who in the long run would not be helped in resolving his problems).

The matchings that the patient will try to work out correspond to both homosexual and heterosexual levels because both constellations may be put into motion in the therapists. The presence of a cotherapist of the opposite sex in a joint action tests the capacity of the analyst to abandon his fantasies in relation to his homosexual side and his own feelings of omnipotence. Both analysts should have sufficient flexibility and capacity to agree and disagree among themselves without it being in any way a dangerous situation as well as being able to approach and move away emotionally from the patient depending on the stage through which he is crossing. The more worked out the analysts have their homosexual and heterosexual positions the easier it will be for them to recognize the mobilization of those constellations within themselves as well as the reactions they mutually experience in relation to the projected matchings. The therapists ought to and can be able to feel love and hate among themselves without the latter destroying the former. The unconscious transmission of this situation will help the patient who passes through and experiences similar, though much sharper emotions, and will also give him the hope of overcoming this phase, achieving a security of object.

One must not forget that together with the attempt at separating the pair of therapists there also exists the opposite desire, that of keeping them together, and any false step in this sense on the therapists' part will be lived as a danger for the patient's infantile world and will fill him with guilt feelings which add to those of his own childhood.

From all of this which has been presented, one may deduce that one can never call cotherapy those cases worked through as defenses of the therapists, those in which one tries to compensate for a case that has gone badly. In such cases, it would become a badly worked out treatment by two analysts, serving only to augment the confusion and internal splitting of the patient. Neither can one call cotherapy that treatment in which there is a difference in status in the therapists, useful perhaps for didactic ends, but which neither corresponds to the already cited dynamics nor helps to shorten the length of treatment.

In both cases I believe that the corrections that have to be established in the analysts' transference so that their internal constellations do not trespass upon the social field are not going to justify the use of the technique previously referred to, whose end is primarily the shortening of the treatment through the analysis of the conflictive unconscious and the presentation of the correct social field. The realization of the man-woman cotherapy brings to the forefront the question of the therapists' own identity difficulties, of the yielding of their cultural attributes corresponding to the opposite sex, together with their underlying unconscious fantasies.

REFERENCES

1. Alexander, F.: *Fundamentals of Psychoanalysis,* Norton, New York, 1948.
2. Bouvet, M.: Technical variation and the concept of distance. *Int. J. Psychoanal. Vol.* **39**:1958.
3. Davidson, L.: De mujer a mujer, feminismo, transferencia y contratransferencia. *5th Forum Int. Psicoanal.,* Zurich, 1974.
4. Flournoy, O.: Du symptome au discours. Rapport presente au XXVIII Congres des Psychoanalystes de Langues Romanes, 1967.
5. Freud, A.: *Normality and Pathology in Childhood,* Hogarth Press, London, 1966.
6. Freud, S.: Sobre la psicogenesis de un caso de homosexualidad femenina. *Obras Completas,* Vol. 1, 1967.
7. Gitelson, M.: The emotional position of the analyst in the psycho-analytic situation. *Int. J. Psychoanal.* **33**:1952.
8. Greenson, R.: The non-transference relationship in the psychoanalytic situation. *Int. J. Psychoanal.* **50**:1969.

9. Heimann, P., On countertransference. *Int. J. Psychoanal.* **31**:1950.

10. Kemper, W.: *Problemas de tecnica psicoanalitica,* Siglo XXI, 1972.

11. Klein, V.: *El caracter femenino,* Paidos, B. Aires, 1965.

12. Lampl de Groot, J.: Problems of psycho-analytic training. *Int. J. Psychoanal.* **35**:1954.

13. Lampl de Groot, J.: The role of identification in psycho-analitical procedure. *Int. J. Psychoanal.* **37**:1956.

14. Little, M.: The analyst's total response to his patient's needs. *Int. J. Psychoanal.* **38**:1957.

15. Lopez Ibor, D.: *La agonia del psicoanalisis,* Espasa-Calpe, 1951.

16. Molina-Nuñez, J.: Symposium sobre el problema del tiempo en psicoanalisis. II Forum Int. de Psicoanalisis, Zurich, 1965.

17. Molina-Nuñez, J.: Contribucion a la psicoterapia breve. Congreso Mundial de Psiquiatria, Madrid, 1966.

18. Molina-Nuñez, J.: *About Shortened Psychoanalytic Therapy,* Gottingen, 1968.

19. Nacht, S.: *La presencia del psicoanalista,* Proteo, Buenos Aires, 1966.

20. Prado de Molina, M. and Gallego Meré, A.: Dinamica de la transferencia en los tratamientos en coterapia. III Forum International de Psicoanalisis, Mejico, 1969.

21. Prado de Molina, M.: La mujer y su problematica. *Revista Espanola de Psicoterapia Analitica,* Vol. IV, Num. 3 y 4, 1971.

22. Prado de Molina, M.: Transferencia y contratransferencia e implicacion del sexo en cooterapia. Mesa Redonda de la Academia de Psicoanalisis, V Forum Int. de Psicoanalisis, Zurich, 1974.

23. Rickman, J.: Symposium on the termination of psycho-analytic treatment. *Int. J. Psychoanal.* **31**(3):1950.

24. Searles, H.: Oedipal love in the countertransference. *Int. J. Psychoanal.* **40,** 1959.

25. Sechehaye, M.: *La realizacion simbolica,* Fondo de Cultura Economica, Mejico, 1958.

26. Thompson, C.: *Interpersonal Psychoanalysis,* New York, Basic Books, 1964.

CHAPTER NINE

AFRICA WITH SPECIAL
REFERENCE TO NIGERIA

TOLANI ASUNI, MA, MD, DPM, FRCPsych, FNMCPsych

Africa is a vast continent with peoples of different colors, ranging from near White in the North to Black in the area south of the Sahara. Even though Islam appears to be the dominant religion in many countries of Africa, Christianity of different denominations is also very strong. There are also many traditional and syncretic religious sects. The cultures of the people are different, as is the climate. It is because of these and other differences that it is often oversimplification to generalize about Africa.

Yet there are similarities of importance that allow for some cautious generalization. Most of the countries in Africa have at one time been under colonial domination. This has had very great impact on the psychology of the people. Even with this colonization, there were some differences. The impact of French colonial power is somewhat different from the British; the French attitude was assimilation while the British was not. Perhaps the most common denominator is the poverty and little or no technological development. It is for this reason that Allen German[6] in his review of psychiatry in Africa called the situation "psychiatry of poverty". This description was factual rather than derogatory.

Another common denominator is the relatively young age of the total population and the very low proportion of old people. This factor can also lend support to the description of psychiatry in Africa to be "psychiatry of the young".

A large part of Africa is still traditional or at most transitional in practically all aspects of life. This factor of traditionalism and the extreme dearth of Western trained doctors, especially psychiatrists, have made traditional methods of healing flourish. Perhaps it is because of this that it has been suggested by Prince,[14] Ari Kiev,[9] and others that the traditional psychiatric practice may be better suited to the people than western psychiatry. Torrey[15] even went further to equate the North American psychiatrists with witch doctors.

The problem with both Prince's and Kiev's views is that psychiatry cannot be isolated from the tempest of change going through Africa. While their views sound attractive from the point of view of shortage of trained man power, and the retention of factors that are not only psychotherapeutic but also giving strength to mental state, these factors are being eroded by the rapid social, economic, and cultural changes. Wherever possible, however, some of the factors are being utilized by some psychiatrists in Africa. A good example of this is the Village System in Aro; see Lambo[11] and Asuni.[1, 4]

The problem with Torrey's idea is that he sees psychiatry where the African does not see it, and because in North America, where psychiatry deals with what the African does not see as psychiatric, he equates psychiatrists with those in Africa who deal with the same problem. In other words, what are regarded as social problems in Africa are sometimes regarded as psychiatric problems in North America. This problem is deeper and more fundamental. Where does psychiatry begin and social action end? Because the line of demarcation is so vague, some psychiatrists have advocated more social action within, and in the context of, their profession, especially in technologically developed countries.

ATTITUDE TO PSYCHIATRIC DISORDER

The attitude to psychiatric disorder varies from rejection to veneration, depending on the nature of the disorder and the place. Indeed some people use some of their less-disturbing psychotic symptoms, like delusions and hallucinations, to attain the role of priest-healers who command great respect and fear from the people. On the other hand, the total rejection of the epileptic in Uganda has been well described by Orley.[13]

What are generally regarded as psychiatric disorders are the psychoses, and it is only those that are very disturbing and disruptive of the system that are thus regarded. In other words, the depressed patient may not be regarded as a psychiatric case if the symptoms are tolerable. Neurotic conditions are not usually regarded as psychiatric, and this may well account for the very few neurotic patients seen in modern psychiatric facilities. Psychiatry in Africa may then be justifiably described as "psychiatry of the psychoses" as of now.

This does not mean that the discomfort or dysfunction or impairment caused by the less-disturbing psychotic conditions or neuroses are not recognized. They are, but are not regarded as psychiatric, and some other agencies, especially the syncretic religious organizations, are consulted[3, 6] with these problems. Since the stigma of mental illness is very strong in some areas, it is understandable that psychiatry will not be used as frequently as it could be. It does not appear, however, that it is the stigma that plays the major role in this connection, but rather, the attitude.

There is also the high *level of containment* of dysfunction and impairment caused by mental illness. A depressed farmer, for instance, who does less at his work because of his illness is tolerated. His enervation may be the result of anemia, malnutrition, or other physical illness prevalent in Africa. Paranoid interpretation of phenomena in the person or society is so common and is shared by members of the family that it is sometimes difficult to define when it becomes a delusion.[10] Even the vagrant psychotic is tolerated—perhaps a bit less than the village idiot.[5] Some are seen walking stark naked and no attention is paid to them.

The unfortunate aspect of this high level of containment is the conviction of a mentally ill accused person when the offense is a reaction to his psychotic experience or even a manifestation of his mental disorder. Since his impairment or dysfunction has been well tolerated, the fact that he may be mentally ill and that his offense is related to his illness is very seldom raised in court.

Containment sometimes goes to the other extreme of veneration of the psychotic if his symptoms fit him into the role of healer or religious leader.

It has to be stated, however, that this high level of containment is being eroded. The social and economic changes on the continent are making impairment more difficult to tolerate. The anergia or absenteeism of the self-employed cannot be tolerated in a paid-employment situation. Concern is now being expressed by people about the vagrant psychotics, not because they are disruptive to the system, except by wandering on roads and constituting a danger to motorists, but because they are being regarded as eye sores in the cities. The temptation to build places of confinement for these vagrant psychotics is very strong, and it is hoped that the authorities will appreciate that it will be inhuman to confine them if they cannot be given the privilege of available modern treatment.

In any case, it has been observed[5] that these vagrant psychotics do not regress and disintegrate in their personality while roaming on the streets as much as they might have done if incarcerated in a psychiatric hospital for a long time.

In spite of the alienation often described of the schizophrenics (and most of the vagrant psychotics were schizophrenics), they were found to be in places where a large number of people congregate and move around like market places, lorry stations, and commercial centers, hardly ever in remote isolated areas. Even the mute catatonic schizophrenics were found in similar places. They were not found in residential areas. This observation suggests that while schizophrenics still need contact with other people, they cannot stand the close contact with people to which they will be exposed in residential areas, but they can stand the contact with those who are on the move in such places as markets and lorry stations. It also suggests that they are still trying to communicate with other people, but in their own peculiar way. If they are deprived of this opportunity that they have on the streets and are forced to be in closer contact with others for a long period without adequate treatment, they disintegrate as they do in the old type of psychiatric hospitals.

It was also observed that they responded to treatment in a remarkably short time when taken into a psychiatric hospital with a planned short intensive treatment programme. Most of the patients were discharged within a few months.

In contrast to the schizophrenics, it is the depressed who tend to alienate

and isolate themselves. It is they who have the urge to, or do hear hallucinatory voices telling them to walk away into the bush or forest. They may
not have any conscious intention of suicide, yet their response to the urge or
the hallucinatory voices may be suicidal. In fact a number of depressed
patients have been known to walk away never to be found again. They
might have died of inanition and dehydration, or have been bitten by
snakes. It is this observation that has led to the use of the phrase "suicidal
equivalent" for such a behavior. To be alive is to be with people; to be dead
is to be without people. Walking away from people into the bush, not on
beaten tracks where other people may be encountered, is in itself death. In
addition to this symbolic death there is the veritable danger of getting lost
and not being able to find a way out, even during some degree of remission.

Fortunately for some, they have been able to find their way back to a foot
path or a main road, hungry, dehydrated, bedraggled, beaten, and tired
after days of wandering in the forest without food or water.

FORENSIC PSYCHIATRY

The extreme shortage of psychiatrists in Africa makes the practice of
forensic psychiatry a challenging one. It leads one to look for answers to
problems not from established practices in economically developed countries, but from the circumstances of the poor situation. Usually, there is only
one psychiatrist available, if the area is lucky at all to have one. Even though
he may be called by the prosecution or defense to give expert evidence, his
sole objective is to assist the court, rather than either side of the case. This
situation calls for a very high degree of moral integrity on the part of the psychiatrist. It has the advantage of not putting psychiatry to ridicule as is often
the case in situations where two psychiatrists oppose each other, each giving
an interpretation of a phenomenon to suit his or her side of the case, thus confusing the case rather than assisting the court.

This leads to the problem of interpretation and the problem of diminished
responsibility. It is held by a number of psychiatrists in Africa that it is not
for them to decide on the level of responsibility. The diagnostic label is not
important either. What is important is the relationship between the
symptoms and the offense. Quite often, this relationship can be established.
An accused person who has the paranoid delusion that some people are
plotting to destroy him reacts to this delusion by killing members of the
plot. The relationship between his symptom of delusion and the act of
homicide is quite clear. On the other hand, the relationship may not be so
clear. It is in such a situation that the psychiatrist has a problem. The
answer to the problem has been found not to be in terms of diagnostic label,

but in giving an account of the patients' symptoms and the observation of his behavior, and relating this to the pattern of the particular type of illness as is generally accepted. The criminal behavior may or may not fit into the pattern, and this is for the psychiatrist to say.

This down-to-earth approach may appear simple and unsophisticated. It does not work on assumptions and interpretations. It is not tied to any schools of psychiatric thinking which may conflict. It does not tie down the psychiatrist to the use of legal jargon.

There are no special psychiatric hospitals for offenders in Africa to speak of. The attitude now is to treat a mentally ill offender or prisoner, especially if he is psychotic, in the usual psychiatric hospital. If he constitutes a security risk, rather than convert the hospital into a maximum security institution (which may militate against effective treatment), he is kept and treated in prison. Fortunately in some areas like Nigeria, there are very few of such dangerous prisoners. The prisoners with minor psychiatric problems who are not dangerous are treated as outpatients, attending the outpatient service like any one else. It is argued that the prison is their environment, no matter what we may think of prisons generally; and it is logical to treat them there while they are living in that environment.

This attitude and practice allow the prisoner to distinguish between the custodial and the therapeutic agents. The therapist cannot be fully effective if he is identified with the custodial agents by the inmates.

The treatment of the psychopath who has violated the law is a great problem. Can psychiatry truly claim to be able to do much for them? Even if it can be claimed by some that much can be done for them, in the reality of the situation in Africa with the extreme shortage of psychiatrists, it is not possible to support this claim. Psychiatrists in Africa cannot afford to dabble in areas where they cannot be effective. The trend, therefore, is not to accept criminal psychopaths for treatment in a psychiatric hospital. Even where one tries to do so, the situation often arises that the criminal is sent back to prison from the hospital, as he cannot be safely contained there. This is the trend, at least, in Nigeria.

REHABILITATION

In technologically developed countries where the work ethos is very strong, there is more paid employment; and where emphasis is placed on the individual standing on his own feet rather than affiliation to his group, it is understandable that rehabilitation is seen essentially in terms of occupation. The dignity of a person lies solely in his ability to earn a living. In developing countries of Africa, where paid employment is in much shorter supply, and where group affiliation is of greater importance, we have found that social rehabilitation is far more important than occupational rehabilitation.

With adequate social rehabilitation, that is, resumed social acceptance and affiliation, the gentle social demand and pressure are often enough to get a patient to work. If it is the social expectation that he follows his father or his peers to farm or fish or trade, he goes with them primarily as a fulfilment of his social obligation and in the process of fulfilling this, he resumes work with them. Work is important, but a man's dignity lies not solely in his working, but also in his acceptance by his group. If he is able to work and he is working but not affiliated to his group or accepted by his group, he is isolated and lost.

Fortunately, there are few relatively large psychiatric hospitals where patients are kept for years and years. Even in these few psychiatric hospitals, the patients are made to work on farming and looking after the grounds of the hospital. The point has often been made that they could be trained for employment in factories, so that on discharge they can get paid employment. The problem is that such paid employments are in short supply, and there are large numbers of people who have not had any serious psychiatric illness and are also looking for such jobs.

Occupational rehabilitation has been found to be much easier with traditional rural patients than with educated urban patients. It is easier for the rural patient to be carried along into working in traditional occupations like farming, for he has acquired this skill for traditional occupations, than have to learn a new skill for paid employment that might not be available. What makes the situation even more serious is that the needs of such displaced urbanized patients are greater, while the needs of the rural patients are much simpler.

Emphasis on occupational rehabilitation requires other social services and support to be effective. These social services and support include availability of active labor offices, lodging houses, adequate social service agencies, and personnel. All these are not well-developed in African countries to make occupational rehabilitation a priority. On the other hand, the family is still a strong supportive factor in terms of accommodation, food, and group affiliation. It has to be admitted, however, that this is being eroded especially in the big cities.

Traditional Healers

Not to say a few words about traditional healers while discussing psychiatry in Africa would be disappointing. It has often been recommended that in view of the shortage of psychiatrists in Africa, in view of the long time it will take to train an adequate number of psychiatric personnel, and in view of the effective role of the traditional healers, their acceptability, accessibility, and relatively large number, they should be incorporated into the official health delivery services. Some even quote the example of barefoot doctors in China to support this recommendation.

Asuni[7] in a review of "existing concepts of mental illness in different cultures and traditional forms of treatment" in Africa found wide differences. For instance, he had this to say from Orley's[13] report about Baganda doctors of Uganda: "Some practice only the giving of herbs or blood cupping; a large number are also possessed by the spirit. There is no recognized period of apprenticeship to healing art, since in such case it is the spirit speaking through the doctor who diagnoses and orders the treatment, and so the doctor himself does not need to learn anything. In practice this results in there being no well defined body of Kiganda belief about the origin and treatment of illness."

This is in contrast to Prince's[14] report on indigenous Yoruba psychiatry in which he described the Yoruba concept of illness, training of the healer, and some of their techniques. He summarized the psychotherapeutic techniques as follows: suggestion, sacrifice, manipulation of the environment, ego-strengthening elements, abreaction, and group therapy. He observed that none of these factors involves the patient's insight into his own deeper motives, with resulting expansion of self-awareness and personality maturation. The herbalists use medicines.

Turner[16] describes the practice of the Ndemba doctor in what was then Northern Rhodesia, where the concept of disease is not individual but group based. Therapy is a matter of sealing up the breaches in social relationships simultaneously with ridding the patient of his pathological symptoms. Ndemba do not know of natural causes for diseases. The diagnosticians are diviners and their therapists are in effect masters of ceremonies. Divination is a form of social analysis, in the course of which struggles among individuals and factions are brought to light, so that they may be dealt with by traditional ritual procedures.[7]

On the other hand, according to Whisson,[18] the Luo of Kenya considered organic disorders to have supernatural or mental origins. The Luo sought the motive and social causes of all disorders, rather than organic causes. As a result, their appreciation of social causation and their ability to cope with functional disease were probably well-developed.

Some traditional healing systems recognize physical causes of mental illness; others do not. Some use physical methods of treatment; others do not. Consequently, in some cases, greater emphasis is placed on social order and integration than on the individual. Some help the patient to live with his dysfunction rather than to attempt a cure. Some exorcise the offending spirits; others do not, but make use of the spirit to the benefit of the patient.

Some confine themselves to the psychoneuroses; others treat all psychiatric disorders. In general, it can be repeated that each system is geared to the sociocultural needs of its society, and it cannot be transferred effectively to another society. This is also true to a considerable extent of modern psychiatric schools.

Perhaps the most important question regarding the official recognition and use of traditional healing is relating to the changing sociocultural scenes. To what extent is it possible or even wise to try to retain a practice of traditional healing and integrate it into modern psychiatric practice when the sociocultural basis from which the traditional healing derives is changing? The argument in favor of integration is that even those who seem to have moved away from the traditional way of life often resort to traditional methods of treatment when in serious trouble.[17] This is a strong argument, but then is the situation going to remain the same, with the rapid sociocultural changes taking place?

Lambo[12] who has been frequently quoted as making use of traditional methods of treatment along with modern psychiatry, limits this to traditional procedures like sacrifices, confessions, and other magicoreligious techniques. "These techniques are not different from prayers offered by priests and clergy men for sick people, or thanksgiving services for those who have recovered. They do not interfere with the procedure of modern psychiatric practice. In fact it will be poor psychiatry to interfere with the religious beliefs, tradition and culture of patients."[7]

Supplementing modern with traditional methods does not create much of a problem. It is integrating the two that is fraught with difficulties. The only way to resolve the issue is to study the traditional methods in depth. Unfortunately, this has not been done to a sufficient extent, and most accounts available are impressions and anecdotes. Even with the neuroses, which are expected to respond to traditional methods of treatment, no sufficient empirical study has been done to confirm this expectation. Until thorough and reliable studies of traditional healers are done, it will be a waste of time, and it will be unreasonable to continue to talk about how to incorporate and integrate them into the system.

Modern Psychiatric Practice

Modern psychiatric practice in Africa is generally eclectic. In spite of the subtle criticism of Western-trained psychiatrists in Africa for using Western methods and not exploring traditional systems, it has to be said that just as traditional systems make use of positive factors in the sociocultural setting so does the modern psychiatrist. For instance, he does not see his patients alone, in isolation from the patient's relatives. He involves them as much as possible in his diagnostic exercise and treatment procedure. True enough he does not practice deep insight psychotherapy, but this does not mean that he does not practice psychotherapy. In any case, how relevant is deep insight psychotherapy of the different Western schools to the African scene, where most of the patients seen are psychotic? How economical in time is the practice of deep insight psychotherapy when there are so few psychiatrists?

In any case, it is the medical model of the practice of psychiatry that appears to be relevant and acceptable to Africans, as stated by Kiev[9] who went on to explain that the British, the orientation of whom a large number of psychiatrists in Africa share, do not hypothesize an organic etiology for all psychiatric illness. Rather, they differentiate between personality, the illness, and the environment. Each of these, while they are all interdependent, can thus be examined independently, because the illness is viewed as occurring to an individual, rather than being synonymous with him—that is, a patient has a schizophrenic illness but is not a schizophrenic. He gave the example of the University of London's Institute of Psychiatry of Maudsley Hospital where psychotherapy is not applied across the board, and it is only rarely that one will find someone who feels that schizophrenia can or should be treated with psychotherapy.

What he says of the use of the Medical Model in England applies also to Nigeria and other parts of Africa—that it seems to produce a greater tolerance of psychiatric abnormality in the community as well as an inclination to differentiate between psychiatric disorder and social functioning. Thus a diagnosis of schizophrenia does not automatically confer a poor prognosis on the individual, as indicated in a study of vagrant psychotics who were suffering mostly from schizophrenia.[5]

The psychiatrists in Nigeria and other parts of Africa use physical treatment including electroconvulsive therapy (ECT), the often dramatic result of which convinces the people of the efficacy of modern psychiatry, to the extent that some patients and their relatives ask for it to be given to the patients. The abhorrence of ECT by psychiatrists in technologically developed countries appears to be a culture-bound phenomenon. Superficial psychotherapy is given to every patient, but it is taken for granted, as it is inconceivable that a patient can be treated without some level of psychotherapy. The milieu of at least one hospital—the Neuro-Psychiatric Hospital, Aro, Abeokuta, Nigeria, is considered to be therapeutic.

The patient is not deprived of his clothing; he wears his own clothes and not hospital uniform or pyjamas. There are no stated visiting hours, and relatives are encouraged to visit as often as they can. The time of the patient in hospital is not tightly programmed. He goes to the Occupational Therapy Department in the morning, and he is free to do what he likes for the rest of the day. He participates in informal activities on the wards if he likes. The atypical group psychotherapy that takes place once a week has been described by Asuni.[2]

Family therapy is practiced as a routine, and the depth of this is determined by the individual case. It has not been institutionalized. Where it is obvious that family dynamics are strongly involved in a particular case, the appropriate intervention is made. Unnecessary probing is not done, but, on the other hand, the involvement of relatives in the diagnostic exercise and treatment program often reveals the type of family dynamics that operate in each case, and appropriate steps are taken during the interview between the therapeutic team, the patient, and members of his family.

Some patients are also involved in the treatment of other patients. The therapeutic role is shared by all who have contact with patients, and it is not concentrated in the hands of professional people alone. The level of psychotherapeutic involvement varies according to the function of the personnel, but it is specialized in the psychiatrists and nurses.

A lot goes on in the psychiatric hospital which is of therapeutic value, but the staff have little or no time to sit back and conceptualize what they are doing; or to carry out research into what they are doing spontaneously. From time to time, a penny drops and gives cause for reflection, as in the following case. A highly educated man was admitted into the closed unit of the hospital because he was very disturbed and could not be contained in the open unit. The closed unit is most inferior to the open unit in physical facilities. When his condition improved, it was suggested to him that he would be transferred to the open unit, which he knew to be more comfortable. He refused to be transferred. The psychiatrist immediately thought that the patient might be having a residual personality defect which did not make him want to take advantage of the "attractive" suggestions. To clarify the point, the patient was asked why he did not want the transfer. He explained that while he had been in the closed unit he had made friends with other patients and staff, and he was familiar with the environment. If he was transferred he would have to start all over again to make friends. He preferred to remain in the closed unit until his discharge home.

This incident made us realize that we, the psychiatrists and the nurses, use our own values on our patients—that we tended to value physical comfort more than emotional and personal relationship in our hospitalized patients. This realization has been confirmed several times by patients' requesting to be admitted to the closed unit which we had thought to be very poor physically and about which we had been apologetic. It made us wonder how the closed unit was more comfortable as compared with the natural environment of some of the patients.

This raises the question—to what extent should the hospital environment be different from the environment of the patient, having regard for adequate decency and human concern. It is reasonable to expose the patient to a better environment if he comes from an extremely poor one; this hopefully will stimulate him to improve his own environment. However, the differences in quality should not be so large that the better one cannot be within his reach.

Psychiatric Hospital and the Community

Over the years, the Neuro-Psychiatric Hospital of Aro, Abeokuta, has been regarded as a hospital more and more. The psychiatrist is seen to be first and foremost a doctor and only secondarily as a specialist in his own field. This is in keeping with traditional attitude to healers who are all-purpose therapists. When the mentally ill person comes to the hospital, he expects a medical model approach to his problems, and it will be failing him not to use the approach he understands and appreciates. This is another strong point in favor of the medical model. He is not likely to come to hospital with problems which are essentially social and which will need mainly psychotherapy.

In addition to this, the objective in treatment is directed toward the total personality of the patient. Where he has a physical illness as well as his psychiatric illness, or where some physical pathology is found during his contact with the hospital, this is treated by the psychiatrist. It is only in cases which require more investigation than we are equipped to carry out, or special expertise that we do not possess, that he is referred to the appropriate specialist.

The relatives of patients who live in the village while the mentally sick ones are receiving active and intensive treatment also use the hospital for their physical complaints; so do the villagers and other neighbors near the hospital. Perhaps the most striking scene is on Saturday mornings when the children from neighboring schools usually troop into the outpatient clinic for their physical complaints like fever, ulcers, wounds, and such. This practice of treating physical cases in our psychiatric hospital is deliberately and actively pursued to make the hospital a part of the community. It helps to remove the stigma that may be attached to a psychiatric hospital. It is also believed that it is educational. Those children who have been treated for their physical complaints in the hospital will think nothing of it if they are later in life referred to a psychiatrist.

On the hospital grounds, one finds some women seated under the shade of a tree selling fruits and other wares that may be needed by patients. They are allowed by the hospital administration to continue to do this in the belief that this is what happens in the general community where people congregate, and there is no reason to discourage it. This practice not only serves some needs of the patients and presents to them a familiar scene, but also helps the trading women to accept a psychiatric hospital as part of the community where they can carry on their trade. Of course, the acceptance of psychiatric service is implied.

In the proposal to use a new village to board our patients and their relatives some years ago, the villagers were told that it would be in their interest if the road to the village were made motorable to enable us to get there quickly in case of crisis. They made the road motorable. They were also told that it would not be in the interest of our patients and their relatives to get physical diseases due to lack of public health facilities while staying in the village. They provided the labor and material to sink a well, for the first time, and build salga lavatory pits, again for the first time, and even build a mud incinerator, under the guidance of public health personnel. The response of the villagers was so impressive that it was thought that public health personnel can borrow a leaf from the exercise in promoting public health in villages.[1]

In summary, it will be observed that psychiatry in Africa, especially in Nigeria, is being made acceptable to the people, and it is utilizing sociocultural factors within the community in the management of patients. These factors will change in time, and of course, the practices that have been described will also have to change. In changing the practices, it is hoped that innovation rather than imitation will be the guiding principle— innovation of systems that will be relevant and appropriate to the situation, rather than imitation of systems that are in practice in a different environment.

REFERENCES

1. Asuni, T.: Community development and public health by-product of social psychiatry. *West Afr. Med. J.* **13**(4):151–154, 1964.

2. Asuni, T.: Nigerian Experiment in Group Psychotherapy. *Amer. J. Psychother.* **21**(1):95–104, January 1967.

3. Asuni, T.: Religious conversion and psychoses. *Int. Ment. Health Res. Newslett.* **9**(4):6–8, Winter 1967.

4. Asuni, T.: Aro hospital in perspective. *Amer. J. Psychiat.* **124**: December 1967.

5. Asuni, T.: Vagrant psychotics in Abeckuta. *Amer. J. Med. Assoc.* **63**(3):175–180, May 1971.

6. Asuni, T.: Socio-Medical Problems of Religious Converts. *Psychopathol. Afr.* **9**(2):223–236, 1973.

7. Asuni, T.: *Existing Concepts of Mental Illness in Different Cultures and Traditional Forms of Treatment in Mental Health Services in Developing Countries.* T. A. Baasher, G. H. Castairs, F. Griel, and F. R. Hasoler, (Eds.), W.H.O., Geneva, 1975.

8. German, G. A.: Aspects of clinical psychiatry in sub-saharan Africa. *Br. J. Psychiat.* **121**:1972.

9. Kiev, A.: *Transcultural Psychiatry.* The Free Press, New York, 1972.

10. Lambo, T. A.: The cultural factors in paranoid psychoses among the Yoruba tribe. *J. Ment. Sci.* **101**:239–266, 1955.

11. Lambo, T. A.: A plan for the treatment of the mentally ill in Nigeria: The village system at Aro. In *Frontiers in General Hospital Psychiatry,* L. Linn, (Ed.), Int. V. Pr., New York, 1961.

12. Lambo, T. A.: Innovation not imitation. *World Health,* May 1973.

13. Orley, J. H.: *Culture and Mental Illness.* East African Publishing House, 1970.

14. Prince, R.: Indigenous Yoruba psychiatry. *Magic, Faith and Healing,* A. Kiev, (Ed.), Free Press, New York, 1964.

15. Torrey, L. F.: *The Mind Game: Witchdoctors and Psychiatrists.* Bantam Books, New York, 1973.

16. Turner, F.: A Ndemba doctor in practice. In *Magic, Faith and Healing,* A. Kiev, (Ed.), Free Press, New York, 1964.

17. Tumasi, F. A.: *Medical Systems in Ghana,* Ghan Publishing Corporation, 1975.

18. Whisson, M. D.: Some aspects of functional disorders among the Kenya Luo. In *Magic, Faith and Healing,* A. Kiev, (Ed.), Free Press, New York, 1964.

PART TWO

NEW AND UNUSUAL THERAPIES
AND RELATED ISSUES

CHAPTER TEN

CREATIVITY AND MENTAL HEALTH

E. PAUL TORRANCE

As a person grows psychologically and copes with his everchanging environment and self, his creativity is called into play. Every time he meets a problem for which he has no learned or practiced solution, some degree of creativity occurs. This is a health-engendering process and as long as it continues there is growth and psychological health. If it stops or is distorted, sickness begins to occur. If this process continues and therapeutic forces fail to revive the natural health-engendering processes, breakdown occurs.

As new problems, difficulties, and challenges are met, and creative solutions occur, the solutions must somehow be communicated to keep this health-engendering process going. Since this involves bringing something new into being or awareness, a certain amount of anxiety is aroused. Thus a potentially successful new solution requires a courage that even unsuccessful old solutions do not require.

To explore this conceptualization of the problem of mental health and creativity it is necessary that we examine two key concepts—the role of communication in the creative process and the nature of creative courage. Such an examination is attempted in this chapter.

COMMUNICATION, AN ESSENTIAL PART OF CREATIVITY

I have insisted that communication is an essential part of the creative process.[58, 59] Although I have found instructive a great variety of definitions of creativity, I have found the following process definition most helpful in generating and testing hypotheses, designing learning and therapeutic experiences, constructing tests of creative thinking abilities and achievements, and designing experiments to study creative functioning:

Creativity is a process through which a person becomes sensitive to or aware of and concerned about problems, deficiencies, gaps in information, missing elements, and disharmonies for which he has no learned solutions; brings together available information and asks questions; defines the difficulty or identifies the missing information; searches for alternate solutions; makes guesses or formulates hypotheses about possible solutions; tests and retests these hypotheses; modifies and retests them; and communicates the results.

I prefer this definition because it describes a natural, healthy, human process, and strong motivations are involved at each stage. An examination of these motivations helps explain why communication is of great importance in mental health.

Awareness of problems and concern about their solution may be aroused by an almost infinite number of conditions. Regardless of the source or sources of arousal, sensing of an incompleteness, conflict, or unsolved problem arouses tension. When this happens, we say that the person is "curious," "has a divine discontent," or "recognizes a need." Whatever label we use, the person is aroused and cannot rest. He searches both in his own memory storehouse and in other resources such as books and the experiences of others, trying to understand the nature of the difficulty. From this effort, he may be able to define the problem or identify the gap in information. This done, he cannot rest until he produces possible alternative solutions, trying to avoid the obvious unworkable solutions by investigating, diagnosing, manipulating, rearranging, and making guesses or approximations. Still he is unable to rest until he has tested, modified, and retested his hypotheses or approximations. He is still motivated to attain successively closer approximations until his solution is aesthetically as well as logically satisfying. The tension remains unrelieved, however, until he communicates his results. If the process is a lengthy one and the problem is difficult, few people can withhold communication until there is a logically and aesthetically satisfying solution.

Observations of children and adults during creative activities, the personal accounts of eminent creative people, and experimental studies leave little doubt that the need to communicate in the creative process is a strong force. If we could understand better why this motivation to communicate is so strong and what function it plays in facilitating or inhibiting creative behavior, we might have the key to important problems of maintaining and cultivating mental health.

The misunderstanding of the creative person's need to communicate by the "man on the street" can be observed in such common statements as, "he just wants to show off," "he wants attention," or "he just wants everybody to know how smart he is." Such misunderstandings, moreover, are not limited to the "man on the street." I recall how hurt and angry I became during one of the presentations at the 1966 Utah Creativity Research Conference.[56] The speaker ridiculed all of the previous presentations at the Conference although he had not heard them. Mostly, however, he ridiculed the people who had made the presentations. The essence of his message was that the participants had really not accomplished anything, that all they wanted was to "show off" and be admired for their cleverness. In the discussion, I attempted falteringly to explain something about the role of communication in creativity, saying:

> If we go back into history, even back to primitive man, every year since primitive man existed, when he finds out something, he wants to tell somebody about it (p. 147).[56]

The speaker's immediate retort was:

> Yes, and if there were nobody to tell, many of them wouldn't do it. They
> want to be admired for their ingenuity (p. 147).[56]

Usually in a more charitable vein, scholars of the dynamics of creativity
have included the need for recognition as a motivating influence. For
example, Storr[55] explained that the creative person attributes a place of
greater importance to inner reality than to the external world but that a
part of his satisfaction from his creative achievement may be the feeling
that, at last, a part of his inner life is accepted by others. Such scholars,
however, have seen this need for recognition as only one of the underlying
motivations for communication in the creative process.

Alternative Motivations for Communication

Let us examine some of the possible alternative motives that serve at different times to encourage communication and facilitate the creative
process.

Perhaps one of the most persistent and recurrent of these motivations as
described in creativity literature is simply the discharge of the excitement
that results from creative discovery. The classical example is that of Archi-
medes running through the streets of ancient Syracuse shouting, "Eureka!
Eureka!" when he discovered how to determine the amount of gold the
king's crown contained. Repeatedly the author has observed this
phenomenon in both children and adults when they make their creative
leaps and communicate them. This is perhaps a major reason why most
children and adults enjoy taking creativity tests and participating in
creativity experiments. It may also help explain why they enjoy such
activities more in dyads than when they perform them individually or in
large groups.[65] In discussing their indepth interviews with highly creative
people, Rosner and Abt[48] noted that excitement seems to have been a common force in facilitating and sustaining creativity in their subjects. They
stated that this excitement was usually associated with arriving at new
insights, seeing new principles, and discovering new relationships.

Perhaps one of the most fundamental of all needs of man is to maintain
anchors or contacts with reality. An understanding of this need is especially
crucial in understanding the dynamics of creativity, since the creative
person places great importance on inner realities and since the production
of a truly original idea makes the person who produces it a minority of one,
at least for a time. This problem has been noted by a number of students of
the creative process but rarely if ever emphasized by them. Herbert Read[44]
wrote, "What man always desires is a firmer grasp on reality" (p. 27).

Storr[55] saw this as one of the contributions of creative writers, artists, and musicians. Their productions (communications) give themselves and others a firmer grasp of reality.

Storr[55] has seen the young child's unsuccessful attempts to communicate his discoveries as the source of what he has termed the "divine discontent" that spurs much creativity. He has pointed out that most people can recall their frustration in not being able to make adults understand because they do not have the words to do so. He has maintained that very young children understand the meaning of what is said to them long before they master the use of language and suffer frequent humiliation from being unable to communicate their insights. As a result they need and develop an inner world of fantasy. Storr has maintained that man's prolonged and unsatisfactory infancy is itself adaptive, since it leaves him with a "divine discontent" that spurs him on to creative achievement.

Storr[55] has also maintained that the tensions of the great creators of our society have been universal rather than personal and that this has enabled them to communicate with others when they find new paths to reconciliation. He has contended that the need to link the real and the ideal is a perpetual tension but that it has always been productive of new, attempted solutions.

There is much in the creativity literature concerning the role of pathology of personality in creativity. For example, Storr[55] has pointed out some of the dynamics of both schizoid and depressive tendencies in creativity. He insists that "creativity is a peculiarly apt way for the schizoid personality to express himself . . . since most creative activity is solitary, . . . the schizoid person can avoid the problem of direct relationships with others" (p. 57). If the schizoid person writes, paints, or composes, he communicates of course, but the communication is entirely on his own terms. Storr believes that in artists of all kinds there is an inherent dilemma in the coexistence of two trends—the urgent need to communicate and the still more urgent need not to be found out. He cited Einstein as an example of a person who was able to communicate and express himself without coming into close contact with others. Storr believes that it is highly probable that part of Einstein's intense desire to create originated from his lack of close contacts with other people and the consequent threat of finding the world devoid of meaning.

Other writers have also described the phenomena Storr pointed out in Einstein. Rosner and Abt's[48] subjects described such phenomena in several ways. For example, Bonnie Cashin, the noted fashion designer, described her experience as follows:

> I often have a difficult time communicating my feelings and thoughts in the spoken word. . . . I think this is a hangover from my shyness as a child.

I've outgrown the shyness, but I can communicate best in my work, whether it's design, painting, or writing, to say whatever it is that is to be said (p. 245).

Storr[55] has hypothesized that the depressive temperament may drive a person to create as a means of self-justification and that communication is an essential element in this process. A principal concern of the depressive person is to protect himself from the danger of loss of self-esteem. Since self-esteem depends on receiving love from others, Storr has contended that the recurrent production of creative work, if at all successful, brings recurrent injections of self-esteem. Unfortunately, the self-esteem, reassurance, and elation produced by successful creative achievement is generally short-lived in the depressive person.

Henry Murray's[38] taxonomy of needs suggests a number of alternative needs that may motivate communication in the creative process. The needs that seem most obviously to be linked with communication in creativity include:

1. Dominance: to influence or control others.
2. Autonomy: to resist influence or coercion.
3. Play: to relax, to amuse oneself.
4. Cognizance: to satisfy curiosity.
5. Exhibition: to attract attention, to excite, to amuse, to shock, to thrill others.
6. Infaavoidance: to avoid failure, shame, ridicule.
7. Counteraction: proudly to overcome defeat by restriving and retaliating.
8. Recognition: to excite praise and commendation, to demand respect.
9. Achievement: to overcome obstacles, to exercise power, to strive to do something difficult as well and as quickly as possible.

In summary, to understand the role of communication in creativity requires the examination of multiple motives, as well as recognition that at different times and with different people, quite different motives may be operating. It is certainly doubtful that fixation on any single motive such as "getting attention" or "showing off" will produce genuine understanding of the dynamics of communication in creativity.

Deterrents to Communication in Creativity

The very fact that the production of an original idea makes the producer at least for a time a minority of one is a deterrent to communication in creativity. Being a minority of one is dreadfully uncomfortable. Yet indications are that when communication ceases or becomes distorted (dishonest, inaccurate), creativity ceases, becomes distorted, or diminishes.

Along with the need to communicate is the need to communicate the truth. Yet there are many deterrents to honest communication. In her book, *Killers of the Dream,* Lillian Smith[53] presents a disturbing picture of the influence that the way of life in the southern region of the United States has had on the creative search for truth. She maintained that much of the creative writing and art done in the rural South has been marred by a fear of finding out and telling the truth. She commented that our creative artists and writers have dreamed so many dreams that they feared, if written or put in color or clay, would seem to the people they loved terrifying nightmares, and to those they did not know but with whom they had identified so profoundly would seem an act of treason. Writers and artists created the official version or did not create at all lest they be regarded as disloyal to the South. According to Lillian Smith rarely did a poet put other than his carefully censored thoughts on paper, sifting them through layers of taboos.

Lillian Smith[53] also pointed out the paradox that it was among the dominant free of the rural South that creative talent was so fettered by anxiety that it could not be expressed, while among the segregated Blacks creative talent burst forth and found expression in the artisan trades, music, dance, football, basketball, baseball, track—things that they could do with their bodies. Apparently most of the verbal creativity of Southern Blacks had to "go underground" and is only now being recognized through creativity tests[63] and through studies of Black English.[24] There has been a great deal of inventiveness in the development of the Black vernacular, the purpose of much of which is to keep Whites from understanding what they are communicating.[15] Once Whites learn and communicate to one another the meaning of this Black vernacular it loses its value and new words and expressions must be invented. Susan Houston[24] found that even among poor Black children there is constant language play and verbal contests. She found that they placed high value on creativeness and she rated the stories they told her as highly inventive.

Original ideas in all fields are frequently met with unmerciful criticism. Two important factors must be understood: (1) original ideas, when first communicated, usually do have imperfections, and (2) many critics seem prone to misunderstanding. In his interview with Rosner and Abt,[48] Sidney Hook, the noted philosopher, commented on this matter from his experience. He stated that in looking back over some of his earlier works he was surprised at their liveliness and freshness. He explained that when he was younger he was not so much concerned about "covering his flanks against criticism." He continued, "It took me some time to learn that there was a will to misunderstand in controversial fields. I am not so sure that I am better understood today despite my precise and carefully qualified way of stating what I believe to be true. I feel today more cramped . . ." (p. 299).

Children generally are more vulnerable to criticism and rejection than are established scholars such as Sidney Hook. Toynbee[68] has written that children are even more sensitive to hostile opinion than adults are and are even readier to purchase, at almost any price, the toleration that is society's reward for "poor-spirited conformity." Barkan,[6] a researcher in art education, has observed that children are attentive to the reactions of other people when they communicate their ideas. If their ideas and inventions are viewed with interest, children create more ideas. If their efforts are unnoticed or rejected, children lose confidence in their ability to create and depend on the ideas of others. Pauline Pepinsky[41] came to a similar conclusion as a result of intensive studies of three natural organizations—a college campus, a research organization, and a planned community. She pointed out the need for patrons or sponsors who can protect the creative person whose ideas are ignored or rejected until he can work them out and make them productive.

Communication in Sustaining Creativity and Mental Health

Regardless of the underlying motivations for communication in the creative process, it seems clear that communication is an important force in keeping creative processes "going" and maintaining mental health. Thus to facilitate healthy growth, it is necessary that the environment somehow encourage the communication of creative ideas and discoveries. While a stimulating environment may be important, a responsive environment is equally or more important. This is especially important if inner realities and experiences have an important role in creativity. This why the author has stressed the importance of being respectful of the questions and imaginative ideas of children, showing them that their ideas have value, and the like.[58, 59, 67]

The following are examples of ideas for keeping open the kind of communication that seems essential to creative growth and mental health:

1.   Deliberately provide a time, place, and atmosphere that encourages rather than discourages the communication of creative discoveries and ideas. This might be something like the class meetings described by William Glasser in *Schools Without Failure.*[17]

2.   Provide highly creative children and young people with sponsors, patrons, or mentors. Wherever independence and creativity occur and persist there is almost always some person or agent who plays this role. Such a role is played by someone who possesses prestige and power in the

same social system. He does several things. He encourages and supports the young person in communicating and testing his ideas. He protects the young person from the reactions of peers long enough for him to try out some of his ideas, modify them, and achieve some degree of success. This seems to have occurred in the experiences of many of the eminent creative people described in such investigations as those of Cox,[11] Goertzel and Goertzel,[18] Roe,[46] and Rosner and Abt.[48]

3. Provide opportunities for collaboration in dyads or other small group formations for creative activities. In a number of experiments, I[61, 64, 65] have shown that in dyads children and young people seem more willing to attempt difficult tasks, produce more original ideas, appreciate the quality of their ideas more, and enjoy the experience more than in large groups or alone. Communication seems easier in dyads and other small group formations than under other conditions.

A number of the contemporary creative people interviewed by Rosner and Abt[48] attributed much of their success to dyadic or other small group collaboration. For example, David Krech, the psychologist, commented as follows:

> My research for the past two decades has been done in collaboration with other people. When one of us gets an idea, each one of us plays with it himself, each after his own fashion; but before we *do* anything with it, we discuss it with everybody else. . . . It is in these discussions where a lot of errors are caught (p. 64).

4. Encourage the development of communication skills through authorship. A promising practice in many schools is encouragement of children to become authors. Even kindergarteners and first graders can dictate their stories, poems, songs, and ideas to a recorder (human or electronic). One such experience has been described by Smith and Willardson.[54] This program was guided by the idea that the purpose of language arts instruction is to develop students' abilities to communicate their feelings and ideas to others. Smith and Willardson believed that asking a child to write a story to no one in particular sets up a false situation.

Many creative adults have mentioned the power of writing their ideas as a facilitator of creativity. Wilder Penfield,[48] for example, described his experiences as follows:

> . . . when I write and rewrite, and restate the evidence and the information in trying to prepare it for publication. Then, very often once I get my thoughts truly expressed, I see things I never suspected before. Although each one of them brings a thrill, that's a far more creative thing than stumbling on accidental discoveries (p. 106).

Many creative people have commented that once they drew a picture, photographed an object or event, wrote something, or rewrote something, they have seen solutions that had not occurred to them previously.

Conclusion

In conclusion, the need for communication in the creative process is a powerful one, and communication plays an essential role in the dynamics of creativity. Not one motive but a variety of motives seem to underlie the need to communicate creative ideas and discoveries. Important among these are excitement and need for anchors or contacts with reality. There are, however, many deterrents to honest communication in the home, school, and society in general. Whenever honest communication is not possible or is punished harshly, creativity is bound to suffer.

COURAGE TO COMMUNICATE

From the arguments that have been presented concerning the necessity for communicating one's discoveries and creations and the problems and threats attendant to doing so, it seems obvious that courage is essential to creative functioning and mental health. Rollo May's recent book, *The Courage to Create*,[34] has called attention to this problem. May believes that creativity represents the highest degree of emotional health and as the expression of healthy persons in the act of actualizing themselves. He described the particular kind of courage needed in creativity and mental health as:

1. The capacity to move ahead in spite of despair.
2. The willingness to express one's own original ideas.
3. Commitment with openly admitted doubts and openness to new learning.
4. A centeredness within one's own being.
5. Ability to act without rashness.

Such courage, May maintains, is essential to the creative dramatist, poet, musician, dancer, painter, minister, scientist—everyman.

There are many reasons why the communication of creative ideas or products requires courage. As W. J. J. Gordon[19] has emphasized, the production of creative ideas involves the emotions, the irrational, admitting that once a breakthrough occurs, the ideas must be submitted to the tests of logic. May refers to this process as a "suprarational" one rather than an "irrational" one and this term seems to be more appropriate. The elements of commitment, doubt, intensity, total involvement, heightened consciousness, and subjectivity also emphasize the need for courage. Simply and powerfully stated, however, producing a truly new idea immediately makes the producer a minority of one—at least for a time. And being a minority of one is uncomfortable—it takes courage.

Scholars who have analyzed what is required in outstanding achievement, especially creative achievement, are in general agreement that courage remains one of the most essential requirements. Outstanding creative achievement always involves a step into the unknown. Such achievement involves being different, testing known limits, attempting difficult tasks, making honest mistakes, and responding to challenge. All of these behavior patterns require courage.

Studies of the lives of people who have produced ideas and inventions that have changed the world indicate that one of the truly important characteristics has been the courage to stick to one's original ideas in the face of ridicule and disagreement.

Instead of merely adapting or adjusting to his environment, the creative person deliberately goes about changing that environment. He commits himself to goals that require sustained expenditures of intellectual, emotional, and physical energy, plus continued changes in behavior. This commitment characteristic abounds in studies of eminent people whose work has changed the world.[11, 18, 25, 46, 48]

Peer Pressures

Kurt Lewin[30] through his research revealed some of the reasons why the creative researcher must have courage. To Lewin, research meant taking the next step from what is known. This means that the researcher must have a clear insight into the present state of knowledge surrounding the subject. This helps him maintain contact with the rest of the world. But it also means that he must free himself from the scientific prejudices of the present developmental stage of knowledge in his field. Here lies the difficulty surrounding the creative person's problem.

Lewin explained that scientific taboos, like social taboos, remain intact not so much by rational argument as by common attitude among scientists. He warned that "any member of the scientific guild who does not adhere strictly to the taboos is looked upon as queer; he is suspected of not adhering to the scientific standards of critical thinking" (p. 7).[30] Similar taboos exist in almost every field of human endeavor. Certainly the field of psychiatry is rich in examples of thinkers who have had the courage to pioneer new ideas, Sigmund Freud being a prime example.[25]

Studies of Creative People

Since psychologists have given little attention to the measurement of individual differences that appropriately might be labeled "courage," it becomes necessary to synthesize results concerning the complex variables involved in courage.

D. W. MacKinnon and his associates at the University of California at Berkeley[32] found that the eminent architects whom they studied described themselves as imaginative, active, inventive, independent, individualistic, and progressive. The psychologists who observed them described them as enterprising, independent, assertive, energetic, and individualistic. All of them expressed a desire to be adventurous, and 80% or more of them said that they would like to be courageous, daring, enterprising, and energetic. Their early life histories, compared with those of their lower-achieving peers, were characterized by greater freedom of exploration, more frequent changes, and self-assertive independence. If these behavior patterns did not indicate the possession of courage, they certainly indicated they were getting good experience, or preparation, for courageous behavior.

In a study of D. C. Dauw and the author[66] students identified by tests as highly creative in their thinking were differentiated from similar, unselected individuals by characteristics that appear to be associated with courage. The highly creative young people in this study comprised 115 high school seniors, identified by tests in a population of 712 seniors in a single metropolitan high school. They compared these 115 creatively gifted seniors with a sample of unselected young people with similar background characteristics on a test of attitude patterns. The creative students demonstrated high patterns on the Experimental, Intuitive, and Resistance to Social pressures scales, far more frequently than did the comparison group. They less frequently showed high patterns on Rules and Tradition, Structure and Plans, and Passive Conformity. An examination of the items making up these patterns indicates that there is a strong element of courage in the scales favoring the highly creative students.

Factors Involved in Courage

Although social scientists have not developed very extensive information about what causes individual differences in courage and what conditions facilitate courageous behavior, a number of useful facts seem fairly well established. Several experiments have shown that most people behave more courageously, attempt more difficult tasks, and take more risk in small groups than they do alone or in large groups.

In studies involving survival,[60] I found that group leaders chose solutions that required greater personal risk and courage when sharing with the group, rather than personally shouldering all of the responsibility. When the entire group became involved in problem-solving and decision-making, they considered a larger range of alternatives. Also, there were fewer misunderstandings, all of the members were more willing to accept the decision, and each worked harder to carry it out.

The author also found in working with children 5 and 6 years old playing a target game, that those working in pairs consistently attempted more difficult tasks than those working singly or in large groups.[61] Additionally, the author has found that 5-year-old children and college students alike produce more original ideas working in pairs than when working alone.

Apparently, two important factors are operating. Knowing where others stand clears up misunderstandings and encourages the choice of more demanding, though superior alternatives. Knowing that the group supports him, a leader, teacher, or supervisor takes courage in making the more demanding and risky decision.

A basic requirement for personal courage of almost any kind is self-confidence—especially confidence in ability to think. The underconfident person desperately may want to suggest something, but fears it will be rejected, or that he may be ridiculed. In an unpublished study by the author among 90 junior high school students from disadvantaged backgrounds, it was found that 95% answered "Yes" to the question, "Do you think that many times your suggestions and ideas are not taken seriously by the rest of the class?" These youngsters were actually afraid to think, or they felt that there was no point in their exerting the effort to think.

Honesty also seems inseparable from courage. Adults, perhaps unconsciously, condition children to be dishonest. This conditioning exists in the home, school, church, and community. Certainly, independent judgment, courageous convictions, emotional sensitivity, intuitive questioning, and openness to experience are all important attributes of being oneself. Each of these is impaired seriously by subtle conditioning to dishonesty. The productive, creative thinker must be able to make independent judgments, stick to his conclusions, and work toward their achievement. It is this singleness of purpose that so often makes him a minority of one.

Implications for Educational and Psychotherapeutic Methods

Numerous educators and psychotherapists have called attention to the implications for educational and psychotherapeutic methods of what is known about the roles of communication and courage in creativity and mental health. In 1958, L. S. Kubie[28] in his book, *Neurotic Distortion of the Creative Process,* described this challenge. He argued that the goal of education and psychotherapy should be to free the preconscious processes from the distortions and obstructions imposed by unconscious processes and from the pedestrian limitations of conscious processes. He maintained that the unconscious can spur the process on and that the conscious can criticize, correct, and evaluate it.

The past 15 years have witnessed many promising efforts in both education and psychotherapy to meet this challenge. In education, I and my associates have worked persistently at this task.[59, 62, 63, 67] Other notable contributors to this effort in education include Paul Baker,[5] G. A. Davis,[67] Edward de Bono,[12, 13] Elizabeth Drews,[14] W. J. J. Gordon,[19, 20] J. C. Gowan,[21] S. J. Parnes and his associates,[39, 40] Joseph Renzulli,[45] Calvin W. Taylor,[56, 57] and F. E. Williams.[69] All of these workers have combined in various ways creative expressive and creative problem solving activities with conditions that provide opportunities for communicating creative ideas and other productions and help in finding the courage to do so.

A number of psychotherapeutic methods have long attempted to deal with these problems among those who have to some extent become ill because they their courage to communicate their creative ideas in healthy ways. One good example of these methodologies is Moreno's[37] psychodrama and sociodrama. S. R. Slavson's[51, 52] activity group therapy, Fritz Perls'[42] gestalt therapy, play therapy,[3, 8] and even the methods of Freud,[25] Adler,[1] and Rank[43] to some extent attempted to deal with these problems. Recently, more direct attacks on these problems have been made by Transactional Analysis,[22] the Encounter Movement,[31, 49, 50] Creative Aggressiveness Training,[4] and similar methodologies. Less spectacular but equally promising have been psychotherapeutic methods that have grown out of the arts.

A great deal has been written about poetry therapy, art therapy, music therapy, dance therapy, and the like. In the past, these therapies have been regarded as methods to be used along with more traditional methods. However, a recent trend seems to be to accept them as psychotherapeutic methods in their own right. For example, Molly Harrower[23] has taken the position that poetry *is* therapy. She has pointed out that long before there were therapists there were poets who composed poetry to cope with their inner turmoil. Once expressed in words, "all engulfing feelings become manageable" (p. 3). Through the use of her own poetry she has illustrated how poetry has served for her both developmental and therapeutic purposes. Specifically, she showed how each of Erikson's developmental stages was "worked through" in poetic efforts at the time each stage emerged. Among the therapeutic functions of poetry she identified the following:

1.   To solve a conflict.
2.   To clarify thoughts and feelings.
3.   To create order from inner chaos.

4. To make feelings manageable when flooded or overwhelmed by feelings.

5. To wring something positive, at least temporarily, from defeating experiences.

6. To set thoughts and feelings in order to emerge triumphant from difficulties.

7. To ward off paralyzing depression when there are negative pressures, despair, and anguish.

8. To communicate, to share, not in an exhibitionistic way, but as an integral part of experience.

9. To utilize or convert emotional shock from its negative content to something positive and constructive.

10. To restore an inner balance that has temporarily been lost.

11. To achieve or maintain personal integrity.

Reflected in this listing of therapeutic and growth functions is the need to communicate, even if only to oneself. Persons who are already sick need the help of a therapist and/or group to find the courage to communicate. Some of the methods therapists and teachers use to accomplish this goal are illustrated in the works of Frank and Theresa Caplan,[8] Dan Cheifetz,[9] Natalie Cole,[10] Richard Gardner,[16] Edith Kramer,[27] Kenneth Koch,[26] Helene Lefco,[29] and many others.

REFERENCES

1. Adler, A.: *New Leading Principles for the Practice of Individual Psychology*, Littlefield, Adams & Co., Patterson, N. J., 1959.

2. Arieti, S.: Creativity and its cultivation: Relationship to psychopathology and mental health. *Amer. Handb. Psychiat.* 3:722–741, 1966.

3. Axline, V. M.: *Play Therapy*, Houghton Mifflin, New York, 1947.

4. Bach, G. R., and Goldberg, H.: *Creative Aggression: The Art of Assertive Living*, Doubleday, New York, 1974.

5. Baker, P.: *Integration of Abilities: Exercises for Creative Growth*, Temple University Press, San Antonio, Texas, 1972.

6. Barkan, M.: *Through Arts to Creativity*, Allyn & Bacon, Boston, 1960.

7. Blatner, H. A.: *Acting-In: Practical Applications of Psychodramatic Methods*, Springer Publishing Co., New York, 1973.

8. Caplan, F. and Caplan, T.: *The Power of Play*, Doubleday, New York, 1973.

9. Cheifetz, D.: *Theater in My Head*, Little, Brown, Boston, 1971.

10. Cole, N. R.: *Children's Arts from Deep Down Inside*, John Day, New York, 1966.

11. Cox, C. C.: *The Early Mental Traits of 300 Geniuses*, Stanford University Press, Stanford, Calif., 1926.

12. De Bono, E.: *Lateral Thinking*, Harper & Row, New York, 1970.

13. De Bono, E.: *Thinking Course for Juniors* (*Ages 5-12*), Blandford Forum, Dorset, UK, Direct Education Services, 1974.

14. Drews, E. M.: *Learning Together,* Prentice-Hall, Englewood Cliffs, N.J., 1972.

15. Folb, E.: Rappin' in the Black vernacular. *Hum. Behav.* **2**(8):16-20, 1973.

16. Gardner, R. A.: *Therapeutic Communication with Children: The Mutual Storytelling Technique,* Science House, New York, 1971.

17. Glasser, W.: *Schools Without Failure,* Harper & Row, New York, 1969.

18. Goertzel, V., and Goertzel, M. G.: *Cradles of Eminence,* Little, Brown & Co., Boston, 1962.

19. Gordon, W. J. J.: *Synectics,* Harper & Row, New York, 1961.

20. Gordon, W. J. J.: *Making It Strange,* Harper & Row, New York, 1968.

21. Gowan, J. C.: *The Development of the Creative Individual,* Robert R. Knapp, San Diego, Calif., 1972.

22. Harris, T. A.: *I'm OK—You're OK,* Harper & Row, New York, 1969.

23. Harrower, M.: *The Therapy of Poetry,* Charles C Thomas, Springfield, Ill., 1972.

24. Houston, S.: Black English. *Psychol. Today,* **6**(10):45-48, 1973.

25. Jones, E.: *The Life and Works of Sigmund Freud,* Basic Books, New York, 1953.

26. Koch, K.: *Wishes, Lies, and Dreams,* Vintage Books, New York, 1970.

27. Kramer, E.: *Art as Therapy with Children,* Schocken Books, New York, 1971.

28. Kubie, L. S.: *Neurotic Distortion of the Creative Process,* University of Kansas Press, Lawrence, Ks., 1958.

29. Lefco, H.: *Dance Therapy,* Nelson-Hall, Chicago, 1974.

30. Lewin, K.: Frontiers in group dynamics. *Human Relat.* **1**:5-41, 1947.

31. Lieberman, M. A., Yalom, I. D., and Miles, M. B.: *Encounter Groups: First Facts,* Basic Books, New York, 1973.

32. Mackinnon, D. W.: *The Creative Person,* University of California General Extension, Berkeley, Calif., 1961.

33. Maslow, A. H.: *Toward a Psychology of Being,* Princeton, N.J., 1962.

34. May, R.: *The Courage to Create,* W. W. Norton, New York, 1975.

35. Mead, M.: Where education fits in. *Think,* **28**:16-22, 1962.

36. Mearns, H.: *Creative Power,* Dover Publications, New York, 1958.

37. Moreno, J. L.: *Psychodrama,* Vol. I, Beacon House, Beacon, N.Y., 1946.

38. Murray, H. A.: *Explorations in Personality,* Oxford University Press, New York, 1938.

39. Parnes, S. J.: *Aha!: Insights into Creative Behavior,* D. O. K. Publishing Co., Buffalo, N.Y., 1975.

40. Parnes, S. J. and Noller, R. B.: *Toward Supersanity: Channeled Freedom,* D. O. K. Publishers, Buffalo, N.Y., 1974.

41. Pepinsky, P. N.: *Originality in Group Productivity. I: Productive Independence in Three Natural Situations,* Research Foundation, Ohio State University, Columbus, Ohio, 1959.

42. Perls, F.: *Gestalt Therapy Verbatim,* Real People Press, Moab, Utah, 1969.

43. Rank, O.: *Will Therapy and Truth and Reality,* Alfred A. Knopf, New York, 1945.

44. Read, H.: *Icon and Idea,* Faber and Faber, London, 1955.

45. Renzulli, J. S.: *New Directions in Creativity. Mark 1,* Harper & Row, New York, 1973.

46. Roe, A.: *The Making of a Scientist,* Dodd, Mead & Co., New York, 1962.

47. Rogers, C. R.: Toward a theory of creativity. In *Creativity and Its Cultivation,* H. H. Anderson, (Ed.), Harper & Row, New York, 1959.

48. Rosner, S. and Abt, L. E., (Eds.): *The Creative Experience,* Dell, New York, 1970.

49. Schutz, W. C.: *Joy: Expanding Human Awareness,* Grove Press, New York, 1967.

50. Schutz, W. C.: *Here Comes Everybody,* Harper & Row, New York, 1971.

51. Slavson, S. R.: *Creative Group Education,* Association Press, New York, 1937.

52. Slavson, S. R. and Schiffer, M.: *Group Psychotherapies for Children,* International Universities Press, New York, 1975.

53. Smith, L.: *Killers of the Dream,* W. W. Norton, New York, 1949.

54. Smith, L. and Willardson, M.: Communication skills through authorship. *Elem. Engl.* **48:**190–192, 1971.

55. Storr, A.: *The Dynamics of Creativity,* Atheneum, New York, 1972.

56. Taylor, C. W., (Ed.): *Climate for Creativity,* Pergamon Press, New York, 1972.

57. Taylor, C. W.: Developing effectively functioning people—The accountable goal of multiple talent teaching. *Education,* **94:**99–111, 1973.

58. Torrance, E. P.: *Guiding Creative Talent,* Prentice-Hall, Englewood Cliffs, N.J., 1962.

59. Torrance, E. P.: *Rewarding Creative Behavior,* Prentice-Hall, Englewood Cliffs, N.J., 1965.

60. Torrance, E. P.: *Mental Health and Constructive Behavior,* Wadsworth Publishing Co., Belmont, Calif., 1965.

61. Torrance, E. P.: Peer influence on preschool children's willingness to try difficult tasks. *J. Psychol.* **72:**189–194, 1969.

62. Torrance, E. P.: *Dimensions of Early Learning: Creativity,* Adapt Press, Sioux Falls, S.D., 1969.

63. Torrance, E. P.: *Encouraging Creativity in the Classroom,* William C. Brown, Dubuque, Iowa, 1970.

64. Torrance, E. P.: Influence of dyadic interaction on creative functioning. *Psychol. Rep.* **26:**391–394, 1970.

65. Torrance, E. P.: "Stimulation, Enjoyment, and Originality in Dyadic Creativity." *J. Educ. Psychol.,* **62:**45–49, 1971.

66. Torrance, E. P. and Dauw, D. C.: Attitude patterns of creatively gifted high school seniors. *Gifted Child Quart.* **10:**53–57, 1966.

67. Torrance, E. P. and Myers, R. E.: *Creative Learning and Teaching,* Dodd, Mead, New York, 1970.

68. Toynbee, A.: Is America neglecting her creative minority? In *Widening Horizons in Creativity,* C. W. Taylor, (Ed.), John Wiley, New York, 1964.

69. Williams, F. E.: *A Total Creativity Program for Individualizing and Humanizing the Learning Process,* Educational Technology Publications, Englewood Cliffs, N.J., 1972.

CHAPTER ELEVEN

POETRY THERAPY

ANTHONY PIETROPINTO, M.D.

We do not know for sure what therapy the first designated healer on earth used, but we can take our clue from the medicine men and shamans of the earth's most primitive tribes today.[41] Whether we seek out Mexican or American Indians, Africans, Polynesians, or Eskimoes,[4] we find the use of incantations or rhythmic invocations used to treat illness, particularly emotional disorders.[7] Shamans and witch doctors in many tribes believe that there is a psychic phase to every disease and seek to remove this causative agent from the patient's mind. Words are powerful medicine, and in some Arctic tribes, the shaman has a poetic vocabulary that encompasses three times as many words as are known by the rest of his community.[7, 23]

From the inherent rhythms in man's vital organs, such as the hormonal variations of the menstrual cycle, the respiratory rate, and the iambic heartbeat, to the psychic pleasure and comfort adults and children obtain from rhythmic activities such as copulation, masturbation, rocking, and dancing, there is a universal language in rhythm[27, 28] that undoubtedly led earliest man into an appreciation, if not an understanding, of its power.

Plato advocated the use of religious rites accompanied by rhythmic music and drums for relief of emotional distress, and Aristotle not only acclaimed the traditional incubation rites, but went on to advocate poetic drama as an effective means of emotional catharsis.[5] Soranus, a Roman physician of the First Century A.D., encouraged mentally disturbed patients, during their lucid intervals to read and to participate in dramatic performances, employing tragedy to counteract mania and comedy to counteract depression.[30]

"I don't know why it has taken the healing professions so long to discover the connection between poetry and the cure of souls," S. I. Hayakawa lamented in a postscript[13] to Jack J. Leedy's pioneering volume, *Poetry Therapy*. It hasn't really taken long; we've known it all along. The Greeks must have known it before Hippocrates, when the same god, Apollo, was given domain over both poetry and medicine. Perhaps poetry therapy for emotional illness was medicine's first effective treatment.

Poetry therapy is, nevertheless, new in the sense of being a formalized ancillary therapy, in comparison with occupational, recreational, and art therapies. Only in the last decade have poetry therapy groups been springing up in abundance at psychiatric hospitals, clinics, universities, and artists' workshops in this country and abroad; yet, previously, every psychotherapist who was ever presented with a poem by a patient became involved in poetry therapy, willingly or not. We have known for ages that people in distress found solace in poetry; it is only recently that we have begun to understand the mechanisms by which poetry helps and how the therapist can most effectively use it as a therapeutic tool.

One of the prime problems that has confronted psychotherapists, regardless of their therapeutic orientation, has been the limitations of verbal communication in conveying emotional feeling and unconscious material. Our ordinary spoken language is reasonably adequate for conveying factual information, asking questions, and making corrections in the listener's misperceptions of what we have already tried to convey. In such communication, we are using words as signs. A sign tends to establish a one-to-one relationship between the word and some object, action, or attribute in the real world. As Jung notes, a sign is always less than the concept it represents.[15] Signs are used in secondary-process communication, where the highly personalized, rich associations of primary-process concepts are modified to conform with the rules of adult logic to make communication as unambiguous as possible.

Yet all thought starts as primary process, and this involves symbols. A symbol always involves more than the concept it represents. It encompasses all of those associations with the concept based on our past experiences, observations, and fantasies. For example, as a sign, the word father denotes simply one's male parent. As a symbol, it is a highly charged indicator that comprises all the positive and negative experiences, feelings and fantasies associated with one's own male parent and others bearing that designation or those characteristics. We experience emotion on this primary-process level. The child first thinks on this level, and it takes him many years to learn to modify his thoughts so that his highly subjective world and those of others may find some common boundary where thoughts can be exchanged with the greatest degree of mutual understanding.

It is the aim of the psychotherapist to establish contact with the primary-process material, often hopelessly adulterated by the time it emerges from the patient, for language as thought is quite different from language as spoken communication.[40]

Rollo May notes that we usually learn more about psychology, in terms of man and his experience, from literature than from the science of psychology, because literature cannot avoid "dealing with symbols and myths as the quintessential forms of man's expression and interpretation of himself and his experience."[26] Theodor Reik similarly observes that "the metaphors of the poet are often more meaningful than technical scientific language with all its precision and clarity."[36] Precision and clarity, to the extent they are attainable, are qualities of secondary process, not primary-process thought.

Psychoanalytic theory gave the therapist two potential tools for exploring the unconscious, the realm of primary process. One was free association; the other was dream interpretation. Even here, the drawbacks were formidable. Some patients are too guarded to acquire the knack of free association, and some are rarely able to recall and recount dreams. The skill of the therapist is vital. Without his ability to interpret capably, the patient will gain virtually nothing from his own efforts. Moreover, the primary-process communication is unilateral; even though the therapist may use his own unconscious in understanding the patient, his responses to the patient are in the form of secondary-process communication. In group therapy, free association and dream interpretation are rarely used, since the group members cannot be expected to participate with the therapist in skillfully analyzing one another's productions.

Poetry thus emerges as the most effective way to express emotional experience as communication. It is defined as writing that formulates a concentrated imaginative awareness of experience in language chosen and arranged to create a specific emotional response through its meaning, sound, and rhythm. The eliciting of an emotional response is the *sine qua non* of poetry; if it is present, we can dispense with rhyme, meter, and form, as many good poems have done.

Poetry is essentially primary-process communication, for in its use of the metaphor and simile, it follows the Von Domarus principle of establishing identity between subjects by virtue of a single shared attribute.[42] In the line, "The road was a ribbon of moonlight . . . ," the poet is noting that roads and ribbons are flat and much longer than they are broad; this is enough to justify saying the road *was* a ribbon, something we would not be permitted to do in secondary-process communication. Similarly, the relative brightness of the road compared to its surroundings and the brightness of the moon establishes an identity between these dissimilar objects, making the road a ribbon of moonlight.

Curiously, more than half a century before Freud advocated the use of free association in psychotherapy, at least two authors had encouraged using the process as a means of facilitating the writing of original, creative poetry.[29]

Because poetry is free from many of the restrictions imposed by conscious thought, it shares many attributes of the dream, the royal road to the understanding of the unconscious mind, where primary process rules the realm. Dreams abound in symbols, analogous to the poetic metaphor, and in free association between concepts, giving dreams their rapidly shifting, illogical quality.

In dreams, distortion occurs in the interest of evoking strong emotional feelings, the "censor" using the dream work to disguise conflict-laden material and permit it to emerge in a more tolerable form. Poetry likewise offers the patient the opportunity to express contradictory emotions in a complex, secret language, where direct expression of such feelings and thoughts might not be dared.[10] Poems, like dreams, have their latent as well as manifest content, and poets in therapy often find deeper levels of meaning in their works, not consciously recognized at the time the poems were written. Condensation, displacement, synthesis, and symbolization are all part of the poetic process, just as they are elements of the dream work. If dreams have inherent therapeutic qualities, it would not be surprising to find these same qualities in poetry.

The poet usually writes for the same reasons that the dreamer dreams: to resolve an emotional conflict, to provide vicarious wish fulfillment, and to supply emotional catharsis. Robert Frost says that a poem "begins in delight . . . and ends in a clarification of life—not necessarily a great clarification, such as sects and cults are founded on, but in a momentary stay against confusion."[12]

The poem, like a symptom, often embodies both a conflict and the defense against that conflict, these elements existing in a disguised form.[38] In his work, the poet not only finds relief from anxiety, but also is often able to progress toward a resolution, rejection, or acceptance of his conflict. Thus the poem bears kinship to the psychotherapeutic process, as well as to the dream and to the symptom itself.

In his paper "The Relationship of the Poet and Daydreaming,"[11] Freud stated that adult fantasies are wish fulfillments that are usually concealed by the daydreamer because of their childish and regressive nature. The poet is able to give these adult fantasies a pleasurable form, overcoming the repulsion or guilt feelings we usually associate with them. The poet too is motivated by an intense desire originating in the present, the memory of an earlier experience in which this wish was fulfilled, and anticipation of a future situation representing the wish fulfillment. He has sufficient sensitivity of awareness of his own and others' impulses, dreams and fantasies to be able and daring enough to express them verbally. A truly creative artist must have a strong instinctual drive, an extraordinary capacity for sublimation, a laxity of repression, and an ability to verbalize. The origins of art, Freud maintained, lie in neurosis, even though creativity and poetry are similar to neurosis but not in themselves neurotic.

Carl Jung, in a lecture entitled "On the Relation of Analytic Psychology to Poetry,"[16] said that "in order to do justice to a work of art, analytical psychology must rid itself entirely of medical prejudice; for a work of art is not a disease, and consequently requires a different approach from the medical one. Since art derives from psychic motives, it is a proper subject for psychology, but by its very nature art is not science and science by its very nature is not art." Although, Jung conceded, it is an undeniable fact that a work of art arises from much the same psychological conditions as neurosis, he will not put a work of art on the same level as a neurosis: "If a work of art is explained in the same way as a neurosis, then either the work of art is a neurosis or the neurosis is a work of art." In treating a work of art in a scientific manner, we reveal personal threads that the artist has, intentionally or unintentionally, woven into his work; but this kind of analysis does not truly concern itself with the work of art itself, for the work escapes from the limitations of the strictly personal and soars beyond the personal concerns of its creator.

Jung distinguishes two types of artistic products, one "introverted," wherein the artist has a definite aim, makes a conscious effort to create, and chooses his words with complete freedom, and the other "extraverted," wherein the work of art arises spontaneously from the poet's subconscious and resists any conscious alterations. Jung considered the extraverted type of creation an autonomous complex: "a psychic formation that remains subliminal until its energy-charge is sufficient to carry it over the threshold into consciousness. Its association with consciousness does not mean that it is assimilated, only that it is perceived; but it is not subject to conscious control."[16]

Jung's observations have special relevance to poetry therapy, for the poems produced by most patients are of the extraverted type, written with little conscious planning and subjected to little correction and polishing. They tend to be products of powerful conflicts and emotions, taking their form on a subconscious level and erupting into consciousness when the pressure for their release reaches a critical threshold. The therapist cannot regard these poems strictly as expressions of pathology, or hope to reduce them to simple expressions of common psychodynamic conflicts. Whereas there are some analogies between symptoms and poetic inspirations, and the poet does reach some resolution of his inspiration in the completed poem, poetry is often a means of self-exploration and development rather than an expression of pathology, just as psychotherapy is often more a vehicle for personal growth than cure of symptoms. Jung viewed therapy as an approach to living one's life in a creative and evergrowing way, integrating the conscious and unconscious so as to develop a unique personal identity in a never-completed process which he called "individuation."

In a sense, Jung was founder of the art therapies, since he encouraged his patients to use their creative talents and to find and establish the special meanings of their work. "Whether or not something is a symbol," he wrote, "depends primarily on the attitude of the consciousness that contemplates it."[14] The poet is responsible for stating the meaning of his poem, since the symbols have reference to him in a personal way. The interpretation of poems, therefore, gives the patient a more active and healthy role than does interpretation of dreams or symptoms by the therapist.

This does not imply that the meaning of a poem is always entirely clear to a poet. As Kris stated, poetry may tolerate or require ambiguity, and multiple meanings do exist in the unconscious of both artist and audience.[18] The poet, in contrast to the scientist, may explore the full range of responses to language, including imagery. Communication with others lies not so much in the artist's prior intent as in the consequent recreation by his audience. Yet much of the poetry produced by patients in therapy is not written for an audience and, unlike the creations of the professional writer, their poems are highly personal, with interpretations to be left solely to their creators.

Frederic Perls, the leader of the gestalt therapy school, sees poetry as the antithesis to the neurotic verbalizing in which patients often engage.[33] "The speaking activity of the poet is," he maintains, "an end in itself; that is, just by the behavior of overt speech, just by handling the medium, he solves his problem. . . . His content is not a present truth of experience to be conveyed, but he finds in experience of memory or fancy a symbol that in fact excites him without his (or our) needing to know its latent content." In having a beginning, middle, and end, the poem avoids the morass of neurotic repetitions and interminable obsessions; it finishes the situation.

It is not necessary for the poet to know the latent content of his poem, Perls states. The act of writing is, in a sense, a solution to his problem. The poet finishes it with a feeling of his having, for the moment, come to a resting place, a solution. Further poems may follow, but their content is bound to differ, and this makes them unlike the neurotic obsession that shows little progress or change in its repetition. (Robert Frost once answered the question, "Why do you write poems?" with the reply, "To see if I can make them all different."[39])

The goal of therapy, Perls reminds us, is not for the therapist to become aware of something about the patient, but for the patient to become aware of himself. In traditional Freudian psychoanalysis, the therapist focuses on his unaware patient who is in the process of free association, so that the therapist can learn about the patient. In poetry therapy, the therapist encourages the patient to explore for himself, to listen to his own words and learn from them. For the poet embroiled in his own conflicts, the vocabulary will be idiosyncratic and initially incomprehensible, but not chaotic. For the poet dealing with problems he can recognize in others, the words will be less obscure. In either case, poetic language is unique and expressive of true feelings.

The past decade has seen a vast expansion in the number of schools and therapists expounding humanistic or existential modes of treatment, in contrast to the traditional Freudian approach. Whether we speak of Rogerian, gestalt, transactional analysis, rational emotive therapy, psychodrama, or any of the art therapies, we are dealing with a philosophy whereby the patient is seen less as someone with an illness to be cured and more as a peer with a therapist who will facilitate his emotional development along a lifelong continuum.

Rollo May points out the folly of seeking final solutions through creative writing: "'The need to express one's self in writing,' Andre Maurois tells us, 'springs from a maladjustment to life, or from an inner conflict, which man cannot resolve in action.' No writer writes out of his having found the answer to the problem; he writes rather out of his having the problem and *wanting* a solution. The solution consists not of a resolution. It consists of the *deeper and wider* dimension of consciousness to which the writer is carried by virtue of his wrestling with the problem."[25]

There were, of course, psychiatrists who gravitated instinctively to poetry therapy long before it had burgeoned into its full-bloomed multibranched status among the art therapies. Dr. Smiley Blanton, cofounder of the American Foundation of Religion and Psychiatry, stated in his book, *The Healing Power of Poetry,* "I write from long experience in using poetry as a specific means of therapy."[3] Similarly, Dr. Milton M. Berger, past president of the American Group Psychotherapy Association, claimed in 1968 that he had used poetry therapy in individual sessions for nearly 20 years.[2]

The major contribution to the development of poetry therapy as an organized, effective group therapy for the emotionally disturbed came from an alliance between Eli Greifer and Dr. Jack J. Leedy.[21] Eli Greifer was a lawyer by education, a pharmacist by profession, and a poetry therapist by avocation. Plagued by a variety of psychophysiologic ills, he found relief in poetry, and published volumes of "therapeutic poetry," including *Poems for What Ails You* and *Psychic Ills and Poemtherapy,* in an attempt to help others find similar solace. In the 1930s, Greifer opened the Remedy Rhyme Gallery in New York's Greenwich Village, where poems were kept on file, catalogued to befit specific complaints, and ready to be dispensed as one might prescribe medication. From this naive beginnning, Greifer brought his remedial rhymes to psychiatric patients as a volunteer group therapy leader at Creedmoor State Hospital. It was then Dr. Leedy encountered him and invited him in 1959 to start a group at Cumberland Hospital in Brooklyn.

Dr. Leedy was able to bring the needed psychiatric insight and therapeutic skills to Greifer's enthusiastic but simplistic, somewhat didactic approach. "Poemtherapy" became "poetry therapy." While Greifer went on to form groups at Willoughby Settlement House in Brooklyn and the Staten Island School for Retarded Children, Dr. Leedy was founding the Association for Poetry Therapy to provide communication among the nation's poetry therapists. Leedy and Greifer collaborated on a series of publications, emanating from the Poetry Therapy Center in the East Village section of Manhattan, in which principles of poetry therapy were laid down to guide new practitioners. Greifer died in 1966, 3 years before the publication of Leedy's *Poetry Therapy,* a volume that concluded with a memorial tribute to the visionary pharmacist.

By 1971, poetry therapists from as far away as California, South America, and England, in a group comprising psychiatrists, psychologists, social workers, teachers, librarians, and poets, were assembling annually in New York to present papers and exchange views. Now there are so many poetry therapy groups at mental hospitals, clinics, private therapy centers, and training institutes that one tends to forget the apathy which Greifer and Leedy initially had to overcome. Yet the lineage of an untold number of today's poetry therapy groups undoubtedly stemmed from the unpretentious and droll Remedy Rhyme Gallery.

POETRY IN INDIVIDUAL THERAPY

Poetry is a remarkable tool, but it takes technique as well as tools to achieve optimal results. There are almost as many techniques as there are therapists, and each therapeutic craftsman will impart his own individual stamp to the process, but we can begin by dividing poetry therapy into individual and group therapies, and poems into those by poets other than the patient and those written by the patient himself.

Where poetry is used in individual therapy, the initiative usually arises with the patient. It is not uncommon for people to write poetry in times of stress, and once a therapist is presented with a poem, he is thrust into the field of poetry therapy, whether he wishes it or not. A dream brought into session might be passed over, although not easily; a poem is virtually impossible to ignore. Patients bring their poems to a therapist or a group for a variety of reasons, sometimes as a gift, reflecting an increased trust and decreased fear of criticism, sometimes as a desire to bring out a previously forbidden feeling, or even as their only means of breaking through a state of self-isolation.[1] Under duress, some people express themselves more easily in writing than in speaking, not only in poems, but also in letters and even suicide notes,[43] which may, in delineating the conflict, provide enough catharsis and insight to abort the suicide attempt. Writing may make the patient slow down and organize his thoughts (although some poems may represent a more spontaneous, unstructured expression), and often gives him the opportunity to evaluate details and attain self-understanding.

Not only will patients frequently write poems to or about their therapists as a means of dealing with transference feelings, but some therapists have even written poems to and about patients to service their own countertransference needs.[6]

Not everyone writes poetry; however, a surprising number of people, particularly those who have experienced deep emotional conflicts, have written poetry at some point in their lives. Adolescence tends to be the most productive period, primarily because of the stresses of this tumultuous period, with its growing awareness of adult sexuality and the conflicts between expressing independence and regressing into the fading security of childhood dependency. As intrapsychic conflicts are resolved, as the adolescent enters into mature sexual relationships and formulates his life goals and philosophies, many a teen-aged poet puts aside his pen forever.

I would encourage every therapist early in his encounters with a patient to ask directly whether that person writes or ever has written poetry. The poetry may have been written as a compulsory school assignment, as a way of gaining prestige and reward through publication, as a means of communicating love or other emotions to someone, or even as a seductive attempt to win another's favors. Even poems written under these conditions will reveal much about the writer's psyche. But, in most cases, a patient will tell you he simply felt like writing the poem—that it flowed under an emotional pressure that was relieved in the act of writing. Poetry has the remarkable capacity of capturing and preserving emotional feelings, as a block of amber can preserve a leaf throughout the years unchanged and resistant to the ravages of time. A patient may be able to tell you that he had a "nervous breakdown" many years ago, but might not remember what he was experiencing at that time. If he had turned to writing poetry at that critical time, however, his poems will be able to convey forcefully the agonies, struggles, and hopes of that period with all of the original intensity. Patients who have written poetry throughout their lives can present the therapist with an emotional chronology, their works recreating the emotional highs and lows, the crises, and the spiritual growth or deterioration that occurred over the years.

One of my patients, Cathy, had a history of schizoaffective depressions since her midteens. She presented me, early in my course of therapy, with a number of poems written in her adolescent years. One poem particularly conveyed the horror that accompanied her faltering attempts to maintain her psychic equilibrium:

> In a room I walk between
>   the ceiling and floor,
>   but never touch either.
> Warm rug—cold ceiling,
>   which is the best place
>   of refuge?
> If possible lip service
>   can be paid to both,
>   being lonely in one,
>   free in the other,
>   but never really
>   anything in either.

In flight I knocked
over a lamp—a
frightening scream!
Then the ceiling collided
with the floor.

After 3 years of individual therapy, including group poetry therapy, Cathy's poems were lighthearted and joyous, reflecting her new confidence in herself:

Of spring time ground
invites running feet
and pounding hearts.
Outside scents
and slices of soft warm air
seep through cracks
and taste of adventure . . .
Succumbing to a serene smile
of a yellow balloon
floating in the free breezes
mingling with glee
of a dog jogging with his master
streaks of pink and blue kites
of the children . . .
And popcorn and glacier cold vanilla ice cream cones
that drip softly
onto hands
with the bases loaded . . .
And I think I hear someone laughing.

Memory is a notorious falsifier, especially with regard to emotionally charged material, but the poems will survive unchanged. Nor should we think of poetry's preservative powers in terms of the remote past. A patient with a Friday office appointment may experience an intense emotional upheaval on a Tuesday night. If he turns to writing poetry at this crucial moment, he can present his therapist with the essence of that moment in its original, not reconstructed, form. Some patients intuitively "write out their feelings" at times of crisis and do not consider it poetry. While their finished products may lack the polishing, the elaboration of symbolic transformation, and the conciseness of a conventional poem, their ability to convey and elicit an emotional response through words that erupt unbridled by the restrictions of syntax, grammar, and logic qualifies these writings to be therapeutic poetry, with all the inherent advantages to the therapist and the patient.

Jo-Ann, a 36-year-old nun who had recently left the convent on a trial basis, joined our poetry therapy group at my invitation, even though she made it clear that she had never written poetry before. She brought several original poems to the group, but they dealt with general, rather than personal topics, and those of a personal nature were about pleasant experiences only. Then while visiting her parents during the Christmas holidays, in a distant city, she was overcome with depression. On her return, she showed me what she had written in the depths of her despair:

> I want to die . . . die . . . die
>   echoes sad feelings
>   at a joyful holiday time.
> These the tones
>   that tend to steal o'er me
>   as I slip deeper and deeper
> Into my own chamber of depression and self-inflicted pain.
> Death, o death. . . . for you I wish
> To die and thus
>   to end *this* life
>   of mere appearance
> For, if depth perceived,
>   disclosure'd be. . . . long time life deceased
>   For freedom *to be*
>   *to err*
>   *to just plain let down one's hair*
> Had ne'er been allowed to enter in and share
>   the "real" reality to life and living.
> And now—too late—me thinks
>   to turn the wheel of fate
>   so as to redirect a course
>   that life might take
> "Pessimism," hope holds no sway,
> And so a plea, "death do not delay."

Jo-Ann was able to discuss her depression with her father the following day, and left her hometown with the feeling that the chronic alienation from her parents that she had always experienced was not as severe as she had recently believed. When I told her of my surprise that someone who had only written poetry during the last few months would turn to it in a time of great stress, Jo-Ann answered simply that she had no other alternative; there was no one she could have turned to at that hour, so she put her emotions on paper. There had been earlier periods in her life when solutions did not come as easily, when depressions were deeper and lasted for many weeks. Here her poem was not only the means of giving vent to her frustration, but it helped her open channels of communication to father and therapist. Jo-Ann would have had great difficulty conveying the feelings she had experienced to me 2 weeks afterward, but the poem made it possible to recapture the crisis and proceed to deal with the issues that precipitated it.

Even patients who have written poetry in the past may need a direct invitation to share it. A poem is such a highly personal thing that the writer may feel too painfully vulnerable to risk its presentation in therapy without encouragement and reassurance. Just as therapists must often initiate discreet but direct inquiries about sexual behavior, suicidal ideation, aggressive feelings, and fantasies, so must they often be the ones to broach the subject of poetry if they do not wish to risk leaving a potential treasure trove unearthed. I do not ask patients to write poetry, even if they have done so in the past. Poetry should flow spontaneously, and any specific request, even in the form of a strong suggestion, may take on the aspect of a classroom assignment. Poetry produced under such conditions is apt to be stilted, guarded, excessively concerned with style and format, and impoverished in relevant content, as the patient attempts to please the therapist. However, a casual inquiry often provides the impetus for a patient to begin to write poetry or return to it after a long absence.

The therapist should be aware of the potential value of a poetic creation and accept a proferred poem with the appreciation it deserves. He should recognize the difficulty many patients will experience in sharing their work, and refrain from discussing such issues as why the patient is presenting the poem or at what point in the session the poem should be read. I recommend dealing with it immediately, by inviting the patient to read it aloud himself, since his intonations often clarify the meaning and mood of the poem; however, if the patient shows the slightest reluctance to read it himself, I do not press the matter, for many find this experience too stressful, being unable to verbalize directly what they have had the courage to commit to paper. The next step is to ask if the therapist may read it aloud, again respecting the patient's wish to read it silently if he prefers. The therapist may then handle the poem just as he would a dream, usually opening with general questions about the patient's feelings or circumstances at the time he wrote the poem. Just as individual components of a dream are analyzed, individual phrases or lines may be explored.

The therapist will often find the poem arousing feelings within himself and may elect to convey these to the patient. If the therapist opens such statements with phrases such as "This line suggests to me . . ." or "This image might represent . . . ," the patient is encouraged to offer his own associations in return, for the ambiguity of the poetry allows interpretations on many levels. In other therapy situations where the therapist offers interpretations, even in such terms as "Perhaps you feel . . . ," the patient will tend to ignore the "perhaps" and hear the pronouncement as indisputable truth from the mouth of the oracle. Dream interpretation offers no exception, for the dream seems more of a mystery to the dreamer than to the analyst, and interpretation often tends to be a one-sided affair. But since the patient is the conscious creator of the poem, he may feel well justified in sharing in the interpretative process and may engage, with the assistance of the therapist, in stripping the disguises from the conflicts that prompted the poem.

One occasionally encounters a situation in which a poem written by a patient plays a major, if not indispensable, part in providing the therapist with the understanding he needs to formulate an effective treatment plan. One particularly dramatic case occurred when a 17-year-old high school girl was referred to our mental health clinic by her internist. For 2 months, the patient had been vomiting on an almost daily basis, and had lost 20 pounds. She weighed only 80 pounds when she came to us. She was unable to retain even water in her stomach on many days, and had insomnia, nightmares, and menstrual irregularity. Depressive moods predominated, with outbursts of inappropriate excitation and laughter. She was the middle child of the family, having an older sister, 22, and a younger brother, 12. She had been dating a boy her age for several months, but was very concerned about his use of heroin.

Anorexia nervosa occurs in several types of patients, both psychotic and nonpsychotic. When the condition occurs in adolescent girls, it often represents an unconscious attempt to arrest physical growth with the attendant sexual development and new responsibilities adulthood imposes. This patient, fortunately, wrote poetry, and several of her poems dealt with the theme of a helpless child in a young woman's body. One poem read:

I remember "little worlds" where I used to play;
I knew much more back then, than I know today.

I knew, of course, trees made the wind, their branches
    holding up the sky,
And always I would cry so hard when one of them would die.

I knew where all the fairy rings were, and the people of the sea. . . .
Now I cannot go to them and they don't call to me.

Oh, what could I give to be back then?
So very, very small—
How I wish I were not now so very, very tall.

The things I say seem silly now, but once they were so true.
Oh, God! Upon my death-bed, let my cry go up to you!

Now this life is over, let me begin again.
To watch the raindrops dancing, and again the morning sun.

Oh, to be a child, running free and wild—
Fate, be reconciled—let me be born again.

The patient's therapist, whom I supervised, showed me her poems. We agreed that therapy should focus on and support the patient's dependency needs, such as her need for parental attention and her avoidance of plans for marriage. The patient, having shared her poems, was able to discuss openly her needs, her guilt feelings, her ambivalence about sex, and her tendency to cast herself in mothering roles. The vomiting stopped within a month. Her weight reached a low of 73 pounds, but she regained 11 pounds in 2 weeks, and in less than 2 months, she weighed 105 pounds.

There are cases where poetry seems to be the only way patients are able to communicate with us and let us understand the nature of their conflicts and the way in which they perceive themselves. Evie came to us at age 19 with a history of long periods of absence from school associated with anxiety and numerous suicide attempts. Her parents were separated and her mother worked at night, during which hours the patient would have relations with a series of men who were usually married and considerably older than she. Her relationship with her mother was marked by frequent quarrels, after which the patient felt extreme guilt and often attempted suicide.

Evie presented as an obese, listless young woman who dressed in faded work clothes. It was difficult to communicate with her. She said as little as possible, sat apathetically, and only her keeping of appointments indicated she had any hope of benefiting from therapy. Then she confided that she liked to write poetry, and brought in some of the poems she had written. And in those poems were the conflicts, the love, the anger, and the hurts she could not bring herself to talk about. One dealt with her reticence to reveal herself:

"Glass Princess"

I am the glass princess.
You'll not see me cry.
I will walk on the outskirts of your tremor,
Head held high . . .
I will display no emotion . . .
No one will ever know where it's at with me.
My ice gray eyes stare out at the vacant silence.
I am in pursuit of an invisible dream . . .
I am following a rainbow only I can see.
I will fear the daylight . . .
For the sun reveals too much,
And in the velvet night,
I will be me.

In her fantasies, Evie was a princess. She surrounded several of her poems with graceful drawings of handsome young men embracing a long-haired willowy girl clad in diaphenous gowns, the physical antithesis of the plump, ungainly girl who wrote the poems. Her creations explored her ambivalent feelings for her lovers and the turbulent relationship with her mother, always at the center of the vortex.

Evie is still in therapy at our clinic, after more than 3 years. She is thinner, attends college, tends to become involved in healthier relationships with men who are single and close to her own age, and no longer makes suicidal gestures. She still has periods of depression and underachievement, and still lives with her mother in a sometimes tense relationship. There is still work to be done, but the glass princess who displayed no emotion has been shattered, revealing the warm and sensitive girl trapped inside.

I have presented these case illustrations to indicate how the patient's poetry may be involved in the process of individual psychotherapy. When doing poetry therapy in groups, the therapist has a certain degree of control with regard to how he structures the group and he may even elect to choose all the poetry used. In individual therapy, there are no clear-cut techniques, short of those the therapist uses routinely in his treatment approach. Group poetry therapy is an ancillary one, where most patients will be seen concurrently in individual therapy; we may speak of "individual" poetry therapy, but we are not referring to a distinct entity, merely the incorporation of poetry into individual psychotherapy. The poems presented above provided an effective means for the patients to communicate what they were feeling to the therapist, who could further utilize the poems as a springboard for a wider exploration of conflicts, as a guideline for therapeutic strategy or as a means of reintroducing issues dealt with by the poems at later sessions, as reference points.

Patients will sometimes present the therapist with a poem written by a published author, rather than one of their own. Such poems are not less therapeutic, for the patient is acknowledging that the poet has expressed the same thing he is feeling, or, at least, has evoked a sympathetic response. One patient, divorced and having problems with his current loved one, sent her, after a quarrel, a copy of Noel Coward's "I Am Not Good at Loving," and used the poem in therapy as an impetus to a discussion of his painful feelings of inadequacy.

Some psychiatrists, such as Drs. Milton Berger and Smiley Blanton, have made it a practice to introduce poems into sessions, selecting works that relate to a particular patient's feelings and difficulties. This obviously involves some sort of direct intervention on the part of the therapist, yet allows the patient more freedom in dealing with the introduced material than he would have in the case of a comment or interpretation presented in the therapist's own words. The therapist, by enlisting an outside poet, is bringing a third party into the therapeutic relationship; this may strengthen the influence of the therapist, but it also gives the patient the opportunity to explore what the poet is saying and relate to it in terms of his own feelings, or even contradict it, since it does not involve a direct repudiation of the therapist. If the therapist is seeking to reassure the patient, he can resort to the words of an impersonal writer, one who has addressed himself to the world and not to one particular situation; the patient can readily appreciate that the therapist's sentiments are not hollow words spoken to placate him, but have been voiced also by esteemed authors and preserved through the years as universal truths.

Eli Greifer felt that a poem's didactic message has a specific healing power in itself, and many poetry therapists, especially those working with severely disturbed or uneducated patients, have stressed the importance of choosing poetry that has a clear, unambiguous meaning. Other writers have scoffed at such an attitude, and maintain that the value of a good poem lies in its presenting the reader with words that allow a high degree of subjective interpretation and personal involvement, since reality does not actually present us with the series of clear-cut entities that our prose speech tends to imply.[20] Both viewpoints have validity. Direct suggestion or exhortation has always had a place in psychotherapy, even though it is rarely held in highest esteem; the benevolent reforms of William Tukes, the moral therapy of DuBois, the psychoreligion of Mary Baker Eddy, and even the techniques of the modern hypnotherapist attest to the benefit some patients obtain from sympathetic, didactic direction. Yet no matter how simple and direct a poem may seem to be, the patient is bound to bring part of himself into its interpretation. One college professor made a study of the ability of honors students to interpret poetry and reported that "the most disturbing and impressive fact brought out" is that a large proportion failed to understand even the poems' prose sense, their "plain, overt meaning, as a set of ordinary, intelligible English sentences, taken quite apart from any further poetic significance." He estimated that over 70% of university students would misinterpret poetry.[37] What disturbed the professor should be welcome to the poetry therapist. Even "simple" poetry catalyzes highly subjective responses in the reader, and what may be abhorrent to the teacher is a boon to the therapist.

If the therapist presents the patient with a copy of a poem, or if the key lines or sentiment can be easily recollected (such as Henley's "I am the master of my fate,/I am the captain of my soul."), the patient receives something to sustain him between sessions, something to which he can resort when crises arise. For the obsessive or schizophrenic, the poem can supply a bit of useful ritual that has structure and appropriateness, while conveying a suitable affectual tone to the conflicts. For the passive-dependent patient, the poem can be a voice of authority. For the depressed and insecure patient, memorization becomes a form of mastery, increasing self-confidence.

The therapist who plans to introduce specific poems into sessions should select material that genuinely appeals to him. If a poem seems appropriate to the situation at hand, but does not evoke an emotional response in the therapist, it may well also fail to appeal to the patient. Some "great" poems, because of archaic language or complex structure, have not stood the test of time in being able to speak directly to our unconscious. Modern poetry draws on any image, no matter how mundane, repugnant, or bizarre, as long as it can move the reader,[8] and is sometimes more useful in poetry therapy than more venerable acclaimed works. Some of the modern poets and even songwriters have great appeal for the young, but cannot reach those older people who have not updated their vocabularies and opened their minds to, though not necessarily espoused, new styles of living and thinking.

Some great poetry is truly timeless. Cassius' lines in Shakespeare's "Julius Caesar" still have the power to make us confront the possibility of taking a risk involving a substantial change in our life when endless obsessing may carry us beyond the critical point to lose that option forever:

> There is a tide in the affairs of men
> Which, taken at the flood, leads on to fortune;
> Omitted, all the voyage of their life
> Is bound in shallows and in miseries.

Robert Frost's "The Road Not Taken" also has been used to get patients to explore the dilemmas of making a choice. One patient pointed out to me that the less-traveled road is said by the poet to be actually worn really about the same as the other, a line frequently overlooked in interpreting the poem.

Kahlil Gibran's *The Prophet* contains a wonderful section on "Children," in which he admonishes parents that children do not belong to them and must have their own thoughts, "for their souls dwell in the house of tomorrow. . . . You may strive to be like them, but seek not to make them like you." Presenting a meddlesome mother with such a passage opens her mind to a new approach to her parental role, without putting the therapist in the position of condemning her, scolding her, or forcing her to defend herself. For the overly possessive spouse, Gibran's section "On Marriage," with its exhortation to "let there be spaces in your togetherness," extols the importance of individuality within a love relationship.

Professor Morris Morrison, who has provided home instruction to emotionally disturbed schoolchildren, was able to break through the self-isola-

tion of a depressed adolescent girl suffering from a disfiguring skin condition by introducing her to Emily Dickinson's "I'm Nobody."[31] He was also
successful in curbing a preadolescent schoolboy's aggressive behavior by
focusing the child's diffuse hostility via the nursery rhyme "I Do Not Like
Thee, Doctor Fell." Nonsense poetry is often helpful, especially in dealing
with youngsters, because wit is a highly effective way of disguising
aggression; the nonsense language allows the widest possible leeway in sym-
bolizing repressed conflicts while maintaining the security of highly covert
expression.[34]

Occasionally, the therapist may even share his own writing with the
patient. Dr. Berger describes how he motivated a depressed 72-year-old man
with feelings of low self-esteem to write an anniversary poem to his wife by
simultaneously writing a poem himself to his own wife.[2] To persuade the
patient to take the risk of exposing his sentiments, the therapist had to take
the same risk. Therapeutic situations do not often present opportunities that
warrant such a degree of intimacy, but when they occur, the rewards for the
therapist who will dare, and for his patient, can be great indeed.

POETRY THERAPY AS GROUP THERAPY

As a form of group therapy, poetry therapy offers the greatest advantages.
While poetry in individual therapy may provide emotional catharsis, a
means of facilitating communication with the therapist, or comfort through
identification with a poet, a group offers the opportunity for the patient to
share and respond to deep emotional material with others while preserving
as much of his anonymity and privacy as he requires at the time. He soon
realizes, of course, how much he has in common with his fellowmen, and
that he is not alone in his loneliness, his fears, and his dreams. This
encourages him ultimately to share more of his personal life story, as he
would in more conventional types of group therapy.

The uniqueness of poetry therapy lies in its ability to be person-centered,
not pathology-centered. In other groups, patients present symptoms and
problems; here they offer poetry. Patients who resist joining other groups
because they are afraid to talk about their problems with "disturbed"
people may be willing to share their poems with others who share an
interest in poetry. The poems do offer a source of refuge if the patient
should find it too threatening to talk about himself directly, but the
knowledge that this avenue of retreat exists often gives the patient the
courage to express things he would not otherwise dare.

Poetry therapy groups often progress more quickly than other groups. By
introducing a poem, the group is plunged immediately into involvement,

without long periods of awkward warm-ups and false starts that characterize other types of group sessions. There is less tendency for patients to vie for the therapist's attention or to dominate the group, for the poem is heard by all and responded to by all. By stressing the common feelings elicited by a poem, rather than focusing on someone's "problem," a sense of group identity is more quickly fostered. The rapid establishment of interaction, the avoidance of involved analysis of individual case histories, and the inherent flexibility make poetry therapy ideal for open-ended groups, especially where frequent loss of members and addition of new ones are inevitable, as in psychiatric hospitals.

The method of conducting a poetry therapy group varies over a broad range, usually depending on the therapist's level of training, his therapeutic orientation, and the types of patient available to him. A state hospital librarian may gather regularly with a group of severely disturbed patients referred by clinical staff to read them selected poetry in an effort to curb withdrawal tendencies and convey a feeling of concern; any comments by patients in such a group will be apt to relate strictly to the poem read, and the leader will not attempt to analyze personal problems. At the other extreme, an analytically oriented psychiatrist may conduct his group in a manner no different from other forms of group therapy, wherein patients are encouraged to share all personal details of their conflicts, to relate to poetry in terms of distinct past life experiences, and to explore transference phenomena that arise within the group. Even though most poetry therapy groups serve as ancillary therapy, in that the patients are simultaneously involved in individual psychotherapy or some other method of treatment, the therapist should bear in mind that the same phenomena that occur in other types of group therapy will appear here, as well: attempts to relate to the therapist rather than other group members, transference formation with other group members based on past relationships with siblings or parents, formation of cliques or subgroups, various forms of resistance, and attempts to dominate or withdraw from the group. Whether the therapist chooses to analyze these phenomena within the group, he must remain aware of their existence and deal with them when they threaten to disrupt the group or impede its effectiveness.

Almost any type of patient may be accepted into a poetry therapy group. I try to avoid patients who have been referred by other therapists who believe the patient would profit from a group experience even though the patient is not motivated; a procession of members who drop out after one or two sessions can be demoralizing to an already established group, which has the usual difficulties coping with the arrival of any new member. An initial screening interview is helpful in eliminating coerced patients and in allaying the anxieties of prospective members by introducing them to the concept of a therapy that is not pathology-centered. Patients who are currently writing poetry or who have written it in the past are excellent candidates, but many who have never written or even liked poetry have become enthusiastic writers and group participants.

Patients who are grossly inappropriate in their behavior can be disruptive, particularly if they try to dominate the group and interrupt other members; however, a diagnosis of schizophrenia or a past history of severe pathology should not automatically discourage the therapist from accepting patients. The poems written by ambulatory schizophrenics in my group do not differ significantly from those written by "less disturbed" patients, and the poetry therapy group seems to accentuate similarities in feelings and thoughts rather than differences in mental status.

Women seem to predominate as readers and writers of poetry. Our culture often stereotypes activities and attitudes as belonging to one sex or the other, and the poet has been envisioned as an asthenic, effeminate figure. The emergence of rock music bandleaders and folk singers who write their own lyrics, such as Bob Dylan and John Lennon, has begun finally to counter poetry's past unmasculine image.

I prefer to keep the age of the group members within a 20-year range. Younger patients relate well to modern song lyricist-performers, such as Dory Previn, Judy Collins, and Justin Hayward, and they occasionally cassette tape recorders to sessions to share songs with the group. Older patients prefer more conventional poets and may not consider the street language of the folk-lyricist as true poetry. While poetry therapy, especially in a large group, may be effective in narrowing the generation gap and exploring youth-parent conflicts, the therapist must, in striving for such results, insure an age balance so that the older patient does not become isolated or the target of focalized parent-directed negative transference.

Even though some therapists routinely work with groups as large as 20, I feel maximum benefit can be obtained with smaller groups, preferably 6 to 8. A very large group—and some as large as 55 have been cited—will be dominated by the therapist, who usually selects all the poetry, reads it, and then invites discussion. This does not allow all members to participate meaningfully and is hardly a true group therapy; a small subgroup of more aggressive members may take over the group, reducing the rest to spectators. Six members plus the therapist and possibly a cotherapist will constitute an efficient group, small enough to give all a chance to speak or read their works in a limited time period and large enough to allow subgroup formation and group interaction. Since regular attendance may pose a problem with some members, especially if the poetry therapy group is held to be secondary to their individual psychotherapy, a total of eight patients will insure a reasonably adequate turnout, although I have read poetry with as few as two members present and shared a pleasant and profitable hour. It may no longer be group therapy at that point, but it is still poetry therapy.

Since poetry therapy sessions can usually circumvent long warm-ups, an hour is adequate for a group. Many therapists prefer to allot 90 minutes or 2 hours, especially when the patients are encouraged to spend time in the group actually writing poetry.

How the group is actually conducted will depend on several variables, but essentially the therapist should decide the relative emphasis he wishes to place on writing poetry versus reading poetry written by established authors, and how he himself wishes to relate to the group. Poetry therapists today include not only psychiatrists and psychologists, but social workers, teachers, librarians, theatrical performers, and writers. Some of these, obviously, have had a minimum of training in psychotherapy, and their groups tend to consist of people without severe psychiatric problems, such as schoolchildren, senior citizens, college students majoring in education and behavioral science curricula, or drama students. A few "non-professionals" are employed or serve as volunteers in psychiatric hospitals, where they reach out to otherwise neglected chronic patients or help fill the long daily hours of more acute patients with constructive and enjoyable activity. While hospitalized patients may have severe pathology, the poetry therapist has the security of support and guidance from the psychiatrists and nurses who assume ultimate responsibility for the patients' therapy.[19]

The influx of paramedical and paraprofessional therapists into the field of poetry therapy has resulted in the majority of therapists' assuming a less detached role than that of the classical analytic therapist, who would be benignly nondirective in an effort to encourage the development of transference and to stimulate the patients into initiating interaction. Even among psychiatrists and psychologists, those most attracted to poetry therapy are usually from the "humanistic" schools and tend to be more directive or, at least, less remote. Thus there is a tendency among therapists to promote an atmosphere of egalitarianism and occasionally abdicate their roles as group leaders as they get caught up in the heady atmosphere of the poetic process. I do not mean to discourage therapists from getting caught up in the spirit of the poetry; in fact, they must be susceptible to its magic if they wish the patients to engage themselves with any enthusiasm. Yet they must not lose sight of the extreme vulnerability felt by a patient who has shared one of his own creations, and the leader must sometimes intervene when another patient responds to the poem in a critical manner by redirecting the critic's response toward personal experience, not the poem itself. Similarly, "dissection" of a poem or line-by-line analysis, quite permissible in a classroom, can ruin the therapeutic value of a poem and can be traumatic to the poet. Poems should be launching points for discussion of feelings and experiences, and should not be rephrased and clarified in prose language, for this reduces the rich symbolic communication to mere sign exchange[32] and defeats the whole purpose of poetry. Too often, the therapist feels obligated to focus his attention on the patient who has just read a poem, exploring feelings in an intense one-to-one interchange, while the rest of the group becomes reduced to spectators. Actually, since the poet has already formulated his creation, the response initiated in others is often more valuable to pursue.

And so, the poetry therapist is perpetually faced with the dilemma of how much direction and leadership he should exert in order to encourage spontaneity and creativity without letting the group drift aimlessly. Even in state hospitals, therapists have been able to conduct free-flowing groups by employing minimal direction while encouraging maximum participation of the patients.[9] Yet in early sessions or in an inpatient setting, the therapist may be in a position of having to select all the poems to be read by the group. He should choose poems that come to grips with basic problems, such as depression, loneliness, fear, alienation, and need for love, but which contain a note of optimism or, at least, the will to carry on the struggle. Some therapists, including Dr. Leedy, advocate the "isoprinciple,"[22] using poems most akin in feeling tone to the mood of the patients. This is, paradoxically, the reverse of the method employed by the ancient physician, Soranus, who used comedy for treating depressions and tragedy for mania. However, since the melancholy poems recommended, such as Cowper's "Light Shining Out of Darkness" or Henley's "Invictus," end on notes of hope and encouragement, perhaps they are more analogous to comedy than tragedy in the classic sense.

Whenever possible, I prefer to use poetry written or selected by the patients in the group. The clinic's duplicating machine has been an invaluable aid for quickly making copies of poems brought in by the patients. Each patient receives a copy, which enables him to follow and refer back to the poem being read. Most group members, like myself, save copies of all poems read in the group and bring many back to subsequent sessions, so that we will occasionally return to a previously discussed poem if it seems relevant to a current discussion. Patients often write poems that they are reluctant to share, but carry them to the session and may become motivated to volunteer them after the progress of the session gives them sufficient courage.

Having collected and duplicated all poems offered by the members at the start of a session, I usually select as an opener a poem by a patient who has been in recent crisis, although I try to avoid letting any members dominate the group week after week. Patients are generally willing to read their own

creations, although I will defer to their wishes that I read their poem
instead. The ensuing discussion may be led by the poet or by one of the
other members who wishes to respond to it. Having read the poem itself, the
poet usually finds it relatively easy to discuss the circumstances that
prompted his writing it. Sometimes we have spent the whole hour on one
poem; other sessions have consisted of a rapid-fire succession of poems with
little discussion, the members becoming inundated by an invigorating flood
of poetry.

The therapist should be prepared for those inevitable days when no one
comes bearing poems. My selections at such trying times have varied from
Byron's "Don Juan and Haidee," which deals with issues dear to the hearts
of women's liberationists, to Dory Previn's song lyric, "listen," which says
most movingly that we all contain the heroic and absurd elements of
humanity within us and must ultimately find the answer to life's meaning
within ourselves.[35] I once turned to Ogden Nash's whimsical "Song to be
Sung by the Father of Infant Female Children" and triggered a bold discussion of incestuous feelings between parents and children. If Robert
Frost's poems are "all different," so are poetry therapy sessions.

A cotherapist, particularly a paraprofessional, can be very effective in
breaking down therapist-patient barriers by providing the patients with a
less authoritarian, more peer-like figure. The mental health assistant who
conducts seesions with me has helped draw out patients by introducing
poems, asking questions and offering comments in an egalitarian interaction with patients and me. The presence of a cotherapist, especially one of
the opposite sex, offers great opportunities for therapist-patient
transference, while avoiding too much transference to one leader, especially
during the early phases of a group when transference bonds between
members are not easily formed.

Finally, there are poetry therapists who put emphasis on actually writing
poetry in sessions.[24] They may ask patients to free associate to common
stimuli, such as a piece of fur or a small aquarium or a key-ring, building
poems from whatever words or phrases occur to them. Some therapists use
specific exercises, asking patients to complete certain phrases, such as "I
feel strange when . . . but I feel at home when. . . ."[17] Others try to facilitate
interaction among members by having group members write poems about
one another or asking them to compare other members to animals, colors,
literary characters, or inanimate objects. Round-robin techniques may be
used, whereby each patient adds a line to a poem in turn, making the completed work a true group achievement. Therapists may open a session with a
poem, a recorded song, or a short film, and then ask the patients to respond
in writing.

Writing during sessions has advantages and disadvantages. It is time-consuming, tends to isolate patients from one another during the actual writing process, promotes free association to external rather than internal stimuli, and produces a more superficial type of poetry. On the other hand, it encourages poetry writing in patients who are not already doing it, promotes group feeling, sharpens sensitivity to the environment, and overcomes inertia and resistance in a group that is not progressing.

Poetry therapy has found its way into prisons, nursing homes, elementary school classrooms, drug rehabilitation centers, and schools for the handicapped. It is the sort of therapy from which one does not need an illness to benefit. Like the rays of Apollo's sun, poetry brings light and warmth—or, more aptly, elicits light and warmth from us, so that we become more aware of what we are and what we feel.

Why do patients write poetry? Why does anyone? One of the best answers I have ever received came from Evie, the "Glass Princess":

To All Those Who Have Touched My Life

Do not feel flattered
or be angered
if your name appears somewhere among my many words.
I write poems of myself
to remind myself that
I am alive.
So it is with all of you.

REFERENCES

1. Berger, M. M.: Nonverbal communication in group psychotherapy. *J. Group Psychother.* **8**:161–178, 1958.

2. Berger, M. M.: Poetry as therapy—and therapy as poetry. In *Poetry Therapy*, J. J. Leedy, (Ed.), Lippincott, Philadelphia, 1969, p. 77.

3. Blanton, S.: *The Healing Power of Poetry*, Cromwell, New York, 1960, p. 11.

4. Bowra, C.: *Primitive Song*, World Publications, Cleveland, 1962.

5. Butcher, S. H.: *Aristotle's Theory of Poetry and Fine Art*, Dover, New York, 1951, p. 255.

6. Cahn, M. M.: Poetic dimensions of encounter. In *Encounter: The Theory and Practice of Encounter Groups*, A. Burson (Ed.), Jossey-Bass, San Francisco, 1969.

7. Eliade, M.: *From Primitive to Zen*, Harper, New York, 1967, pp. 24–25, 30.

8. Engle and Carrier: *Reading Modern Poetry*, Scott, Foresman & Co., Glenville, Ill., 1955.

9. Erickson, C. and Lejeune, R.: Poetry as a subtle therapy. *Hosp. Community Psychiat.* **23**:56–57, February 1972.

10. Ferreira, A. J.: The semantics and contexts of the schizophrenic's language. *Arch. Gen. Psychiat.* **3**:128–138, 1960.

11. Freud, S.: The relationship of the poet and day-dreaming. In *Collected Papers*, Vol. IV, Hogarth Press, London, 1953, pp. 173–183.

12. Frost, R.: The figure a poem makes. In *Complete Poems of Robert Frost*, Holt, New York, 1939.

13. Hayakawa, S. I.: Postscript: metamessages and self-discovery. In *Poetry Therapy*, J. J. Leedy, (Ed.), Lippincott, Philadelphia, 1969, p. 269.

14. Jacobi, J.: *The Psychology of C. G. Jung*, Yale University Press, New Haven, 1951, p. 97.

15. Jung, C. G.: Approaching the unconscious. In *Man and His Symbols*, C. G. Jung (Ed.), Doubleday, Garden City, N.Y., 1964, p. 55.

16. Jung, C. G.: On the relation of analytic psychology to poetry. In *The Portable Jung*, J. Campbell (Ed.), Viking Press, New York, 1971, pp. 301–322.

17. Koch, K.: *Wishes, Lies and Dreams: Teaching Children to Write Poetry*, Chelsea House, New York, 1970.

18. Kris, E.: *Psychoanalytic Explorations in Art*, International Universities Press, New York, 1952, pp. 39–47.

19. Lauer, R.: Creative writing as a therapeutic tool. *Hosp. Community Psychiat.* 23:55, February 1972.

20. Lawler, J. G.: Poetry therapy? *Psychiatry*, 35:227–237, 1972.

21. Leedy, J. J.: In memoriam: Eli Greifer 1902–1966. In *Poetry Therapy*, J. J. Leedy (Ed.), Lippincott, Philadelphia, 1969, pp. 273–274.

22. Leedy, J. J.: Principles of poetry therapy. In *Poetry Therapy*, J. J. Leedy (Ed.), Lippincott, Philadelphia, 1969, pp. 67–68.

23. Lippert, J.: *The Evolution of Culture*, Macmillan, New York, 1931, p. 601.

24. Luber, R. F.: Poetry therapy helps patients express feelings. *Hosp. Community Psychiat.* 24:387, June 1973.

25. May, R.: *Love and Will*, Dell, New York, 1974, p. 169.

26. May, R.: The significance of symbols. In *Symbolism in Religion and Literature*, R. May (Ed.), Braziller, New York, 1960, p. 13.

27. Meerloo, J. A. M.: Archaic behavior and the communicative act. *Psychiat. Quart.* 29:60, 1955.

28. Meerloo, J. A. M.: Mental contagion. *Amer. J. Psychother.* 13:66, 1959.

29. Menninger, K.: *Theory of Psychoanalytic Technique*, Harper, New York, 1964, p. 45.

30. Mora, G.: History of psychiatry. In *Comprehensive Textbook of Psychiatry*, A. M. Freedman and H. I. Kaplan, (Ed.), Williams & Wilkins, Baltimore, 1967, p. 11.

31. Morrison, M. R.: Poetry therapy with disturbed adolescents. In *Poetry Therapy*, J. J. Leedy (Ed.), Lippincott, Philadelphia, 1969, pp. 90–91.

32. Pattison, E. M.: The psychodynamics of poetry by patients. In *Poetry the Healer*, J. J. Leedy (Ed.), Lippincott, Philadelphia, 1973, p. 213.

33. Perls, F. S.: Verbalizing and poetry. In *Gestalt Therapy: Excitement and Growth in the Human Personality*, F. S. Perls, R. F. Hefferline, and P. Goodman, (Eds.), Julian Press, New York, 1951, p. 321.

34. Pietropinto, A.: Exploring the unconscious through nonsense poetry. In *Poetry the Healer*, J. J. Leedy (Ed.), Lippincott, Philadelphia, 1973, p. 52.

35. Previn, D.: *On My Way to Where*, Bantam, New York, 1971, pp. 115–117.

36. Reik, T.: *Fragments of a Great Confession,* Farrar, Strauss & Co., New York, 1949, p. 211.

37. Richards, I. A.: *Practical Criticism: A Study in Literary Judgment,* Harcourt, New York, 1929, p. 292.

38. Rothenberg, A.: Poetic process and psychotherapy. *Psychiatry,* **35:**238–254, 1972.

39. Rothenberg, A.: Poetry and psychotherapy: kinships and contrasts. In *Poetry the Healer,* J. J. Leedy (Ed.), Lippincott, Philadelphia, 1973, pp. 106–107.

40. Sullivan, H. S.: The language of schizophrenia. In *Language and Thought in Schizophrenia,* J. S. Kasanin, (Ed.), W. W. Norton & Co., New York, 1964, p. 9.

41. Trask, W.: *The Unwritten Song,* Macmillan, New York, 1966, pp. x–xiii.

42. Von Domarus, E.: The specific laws of logic in schizophrenia. In *Language and Thought in Schizophrenia,* J. S. Kasanin, (Ed.), W. W. Norton & Co., New York, 1964, p. 111.

43. Widroe, H. and Davidson, J.: The use of directed writing in psychotherapy. *Bull. Menninger Clin.,* **25:**110–119, 1961.

CHAPTER TWELVE

FOLKLORE PSYCHOTHERAPY
IN JAPAN*

AKIHISA KONDO, M.D.

INDIGENOUS JAPANESE UNDERSTANDING
OF THE CAUSE OF DISEASE

Japanese Attitude Toward Nature

In *Japan—A Short Cultural History,* Sansom[7] writes, "In its earliest forms the religion which, much later, came to be known as Shinto, the Way of the Gods, seems to have been a polytheism of a crude and exuberant type. The chronicles tell us of evil deities who swarmed and buzzed like flies, and of trees and herbs and rocks and streams that could all speak. To say that the primitive Japanese conceived of all natural objects as harboring spirits, or that their religion was an animistic nature worship is to apply exact terms to things which are too vague and various for simple definition. But certainly they felt that all perceptible objects were in some way living."

The Spirit of God—"Kami-no-ke"

Though the Japanese, in prehistoric times, did not have a clearly defined notion of "spirit," it was from their basic attitude toward nature that the notion of spirit later evolved. It did so in spite of pressure from and influence by Chinese and Buddhistic thinking. In one of the oldest chronicles, the *Kojiki*[3]—*Record of Ancient Things*—compiled around 712 A.D., rampant epidemics were reported in the reign of Emperor Sujin. He dreamed of a deity (Oh-Mono-Nushi-No-Oh-Kami) who told the emperor that if he arranged to have a man named Oh-Ta-Neko worship him, the evil pestilence (Kami-no-ke) would never arise. Directly translated Kami-no-ke means "spirit of god," for "Kami" is the equivalent of "god," "no" of "of," and "ke" of "spirit." This means that epidemics or diseases were understood to result from provocation of the spirits of gods.

The Evil Spirit—"Mono-no-ke"

Later, rather than Kami-no-ke, the god's spirit, the word Mono-no-ke gradually came to be used more frequently to denote evil spirits that cause disease and suffering. Mono signifies things or perceptible objects on the one hand, and the mysterious or the miraculous on the other. In the latter instance, Mono was used as a sort of abstract noun to hint at something mysterious or a miraculous being. It is interesting to note that Mono has two different meanings. For the ancient Japanese it might indicate that all

---

* Acknowledgments are expressed to Harold Kelman, M.D., for the idea, organization, and editing of this chapter.

perceptible objects or things had the miraculous or the mysterious within them. Ke means a spirit or spirits. Therefore Mono-no-ke, in its direct translation, is the spirit of the mysterious or the miraculous including not only the god's spirit, but also the spirit of every sentient and insentient being, and in its literary sense it did not mean necessarily either a good spirit or a bad spirit. But in its common usage it came to signify the evil spirit, perhaps because of people's fear of its mysterious power to cause diseases and mishaps.

Mental Disorder—"Mono-kurui"

Mental illness was no exception to the common belief of the ancient Japanese that diseases are caused by the evil spirit—"Mono-no-ke." This attitude is etymologically reflected in the ancient word for mental illness or a mentally disordered person, "Mono-kurui." Mono is supposed to be an abbreviation of "Mono-no-ke" and kurui means being out of order or disordered; hence "Mono-kurui" signifies a mental state or a person of such a mental state that became disordered (kurui) by being affected or possessed by the evil spirit (Mono-no-ke). By the end of the tenth century, some diseases seemed to have been differentiated from those which were considered to have been caused by the evil spirit. However, mental disturbances were seen as caused by Mono-no-ke.

Even the modern colloquial Japanese term for an insane person, "Ki-chigai," bears a trace of the characteristic meaning of its predecessor, "Mono-kurui," for Ki, a derivative of Ke, means spirit or spirits, and chigai means different, consequently signifying a person whose ordinary spirit is displaced by a kind of spirit, though people nowadays prefer to interpret it more scientifically as a state of mind that is different from normalcy.

The Living Spirit—"Iki-Ryo"

By the end of the tenth century or at least in the early eleventh century, it seems that a differentiation of the notion of "Mono-no-ke" into two kinds of spirits developed. One of them is the living spirit, the spirit of a person who is alive, which was called "Iki-ryo" or "Ikisu-dama." Iki and Ikisu denote living or live, and Dama means spirit or spirits. People in those days seriously believed that the hostile, angry spiteful spirit of a living person caused trouble, derangement, and sickness to the person toward whom its animosity, anger, or spite was directed even if he was not aware of it. It is suggested by some scholars that the notion of Iki-ryo or Ikisu-dame had been conceived and developed by the ancient Japanese based on their experience of dreams in which they found themselves visiting people in a place distant and different from their own.

The Spirit of the Dead—"Shi-ryo"

Once the notion of a living spirit that could exist apart from the person himself was believed, it is understandable that people would easily develop the notion that when a person dies, his spirit leaves his body. This spirit was called "Shi-ryo," the spirit of the dead. Shi means death or dead, and ryo stands for a spirit or spirits. It will actively cause derangement, sickness, or other mishaps to the person against whom the deceased had a grudge while he was alive. There are quite a number of descriptions, stories, and legendary tales regarding these spirits, including *The Tale of Genji*,[9] a novel written by a court lady, Murasaki, around the early eleventh century. They tell us how strongly these notions were embedded in people's mind at that time. It explains why these notions survive even now in the depths of the modern Japanese unconscious.

The case of Sugawara Michizane will exemplify the spirit of the dead, Shi-ryo. He was a brilliant scholar and an able statesman. In 899 A.D. he was promoted to a top-ranking ministerial position next to Fujiwara Tokihira, the leader of the Fujiwara family, the most powerful clan of that period. But in 901 A.D., he was deprived of his honorable position through Fujiwara's intrigue and exiled to a remote place in the southern district of Japan where he died of grief in 903 A.D. Soon after, Tokihira died at the age of 39, followed by the crown prince at the age of 21, and then the son of the crown prince at the age of 5. Terror-stricken the emperor restored the late Michizane to his former rank but he himself died at the age of 46.

The premature demise, successively, after Michizane's death of those who were connected with his exile, was believed by the people at that time to have been caused by the Shi-ryo of Michizane. In order to soothe the anger of his spirit, a shrine was built in Kyoto. It is easy to see that those people who died a premature death, with the exception of the son of the crown prince who died at the age of 5, had apparently been suffering from guilt-ridden anxiety because of their petty intrigues against Michizane. It is also evident that people's sympathy for Michizane and antipathy against clan members after his death must have aggravated their agony and precipitated their physical death not to speak of the autosuggestive effect of their own belief in the spirit of the dead.

Koto-dama—The Spirit of Words

The ancient Japanese also believed in the existence of miraculous spirits in words, which they called "Koto-dama." Koto stands for words, and dama for spirits. In an anthology of verses titled *Man-yo-shu* (*A Collection of Myriad Leaves*),[5] compiled around the middle of the eighth century, is a poem that praises the land of Yamato (Japan) as the land where spirits of words flourish. People believed that Koto-dama have the power to bestow happiness on the person to whom the happy words were expressed; hence liturgy had an effect. At the same time they were afraid of the power of evil words. They believed they could cause disaster or misfortune to whomever the words were addressed; hence cursing was believed to carry malevolent power.

The Fox Spirit

Once the notion of spirits was established through the belief in Kami-no-ke, Mono-no-ke, Iki-ryo, Shi-ryo, and Koto-dama, there naturally followed from the Japanese attitude toward nature the belief in the existence of spirits in every sentient and insentient being. Particular attention must be paid to the belief in the spirits of foxes and snakes in view of their influence in later days. Foxes were considered by the ancient Japanese as messengers of Inari, the rice god, and as conveying his spirit, on which a fulsome rice crop depended. Since the size of the rice harvest was a matter of great concern to people in an agricultural society like Japan, Inari worship became quite popular. Gradually the worship of Inari extended to his messenger foxes who came to be regarded as having a power of their own to influence human life for better or for worse. It was especially believed that the evil fox spirits were the causes for mental disturbances, and the insane person was often called "Kitsune-tsuki," one who was possessed by the fox spirit. The belief in the fox spirit has been popular in almost every district in Japan, and there are quite a number of books that give information about this belief.

The Snake Spirit

Because of humidity and high temperatures, snakes were found almost everywhere in Japan. Many places still bear the name originally related to the presence of snakes. Their presence was more beneficial than harmful to the ancient Japanese whose livelihood depended chiefly on agriculture. Snakes were fond of rats which caused tremendous damage to grain as crops and in storage. Even in the recent prewar era, when agriculture was still one of the main industries in Japan, farmers hoped that snakes would inhabit their storerooms as protection against damage by rats. Because they are amphibians, they were also believed to have the power to control rain. Since water is vitally important for rice raising, snakes were respected in connection with it. All these factors contributed to snake worship. There is a description in *Nihongi,*[1] *Chronicles of Japan,* from the earliest times

to 697 A.D., an official history compiled in 720 A.D., about snake worship.
It is related to Oh-mono-nushi no Oh-kami, a god whose name appeared
before in connection with Kami-no-ke, the spirit of god.

It tells that Oh-mono-nushi no Kami was a snake god who lived in Mount
Mimoro and whose spirit took a human form to marry a girl. It also
informs us regarding the ancient Japanese belief that an angry snake spirit
could cause mishaps. Later, though not so popular as the case of the fox
spirit, there developed a belief that the snake spirit causes mental derangement.

A HISTORICAL REVIEW OF
JAPANESE FOLKLORE PSYCHOTHERAPY

The Method of Exorcism in Ancient Times

In ancient Japan when people believed that all evils were caused by evil
gods, they had to depend on persons who were believed to possess special
miraculous powers to expose gods who caused evils, to communicate with
and to pacify or subdue them, so that they would be purged of these evils.
To acquire this power a person, called a Shaman, would go into a trance
state during which he would be possessed by powerful gods. The trance was
induced in a special setting using the necessary tools.

It might sound absurd to say that a Shaman's function in ancient society
was analogous to that of a modern psychotherapist. The latter is expected
to be able to determine the causes of his patient's symptoms and to understand and analyze them. The therapist's task is to help the patient develop
or strengthen his ego or his healthy self so that his neurotic tendencies will
be weakened or kept under control. He is expected to put himself in a state
of free floating attention in a setting in which he faces his patient or has him
on the couch. A Shaman believes he acquires his power through being
possessed by gods, while a psychotherapist believes his ability comes from
therapeutic experience, theoretical knowledge, and self-understanding during personal analysis. However strange it may sound, it is on the basis of
their similarities that the term psychotherapy is used in the study of the
Japanese Shamanistic approach used in dealing with mental disorders. It is
actually a form of exorcism.

In *Kojiki—Record of Ancient Things*—there is a chapter on how the Sun
Goddess, Ama-Terasu-Oh-Mi-Kami, concealed herself within the heavenly
cave, how the 800 myriad deities were alarmed because total darkness
covered the world and various evils arose, and how a Shaman goddess
managed to induce the Sun Goddess to come out of the cave. In this

chapter the prototype of the Shintoistic method of exorcism is described. The following quote is from Philippi's[6] modern translation:

> They (the eight-hundred myriad deities) summoned Ame-no-ko-yane-no-mikoto and Puto-tama-no-mikoto to remove the whole shoulder-bone of a male deer of the mountain Ame-no-Kagu-yama, and take heavenly papaka wood from the mountain Ame-no-Kagu-yama, and [with these] perform a divination. They uprooted by the very roots the flourishing ma-sakaki trees of the mountain Ame-no-Kagu-yama; to the upper branches they affixed long strings of myriad magatama beads; in the middle branches they hung a large-dimensioned mirror; in the lower branches they suspended white nitite cloth and blue nitite cloth. These various objects were held in his hands by Puto-tama-no-mikoto as solemn offerings, and Ame-no-ko-yane-no-mikoto intoned a solemn liturgy. Ame-no-ta-dikara-wo-no-kami stood concealed behind the door, while Ame-no-uzume-no-mikoto bound up her sleeves with a cord of heavenly pi-kage vine, tied around her head a head band of the heavenly ma-saki vine, bound together bundles of sasa leaves to hold in her hand, and overturning a bucket before the heavenly rock-cave door, stamped resoundingly upon it. Then she became divinely possessed, exposed her breasts, and pushed her skirt band down to her genitals. Then Takama-no-para shook as the eight-hundred myriad deities laughed at once.

It is evident that Ame-no-uzume-no-mikoto, in her possessed state, as a Shaman, played a central role of inducing the Sun Goddess to come out of the cave. However, various preparatory measures used to bring about a possessed state in Ame-no-uzume-no-mikoto should not be overlooked as they became a sort of prototype for exorcists in later days. The meanings of these preparatory measures are as follows.

Performance of Divination.   Divination was performed by two gods through the burning of the whole shoulder bone of a male deer of the mountain Ama-no-kagu-yama in a fire of heavenly papaka wood from the same mountain. This was done in order to determine the correct method of exorcism. The method of divination was later changed influenced by Chinese thought. However, divination continued to be performed as one of the essential methods of exorcism up to the present.

The Ma-sakaki Tree of the Mountain Ame-no-kagu-yama.   The ancient Japanese believed that the spirit of god descends and abides in a tree, often being old or of majestic appearance. "Ma-sakaki"-ma is a prefix to denote admiration. It is a general term for the evergreen trees around a sanctified area. The ancients believed that mountains were the dwelling place of gods' spirit. Ame-no-kagu-yama was supposed to be one of those sacred mountains. The Kojiki tells that the upper, the middle, and the lower branches of the tree were decorated with jewels, a mirror, and white and blue clothes, respectively, and that these various objects were held in his hands by Puto-ta-ma-no-mikoto as solemn offerings. All this leads to the conclusion that the tree was used to invite the god spirit to descend and abide in it. In connection with the offerings, Sansom[8] writes:

> The offerings were primarily food and drink. Later, cloth was added, and eventually a symbolic offering came into use, by which strips of paper, representing strips of cloth, were attached to a wand and placed on the altar. Then, by a curious development, these symbolic offerings (known as gohei) themselves came to be regarded as sanctified, and even as representing the deity, who was sometimes mystically supposed to descend into them. Thus, in course of time, the gohei themselves became objects of worship and were presented by priests to the devout, who set them up on their domestic altar; while strips of paper, cut in a prescribed way, and attached to a straw rope, to this day confer a special sanctity on places where they are suspended.

I wish to add that gohei are important instruments used by exorcists or Shinto priests for inducing the god spirit to descend into it.

Intonation of a Solemn Liturgy.   The ancient Japanese firmly believed in the power of the spirit of words, Koto-dama. When a liturgy or statement is made in honor of a deity, it is made with the firm belief that they can communicate with and be answered by the deity. The solemn liturgy intoned by Ame-no-ko-yane-no-mikoto sets an example to be followed by exorcists in later days.

The Goddess's Wearing of Sacred Things.   The goddess Ame-no-uzume-no-mikoto bound up her sleeves with a cord of heavenly pi-kage vine, tied around her head a band of heavenly ma-saki vine, and bound together bundles of sasa leaves to hold in her hands. The meaning is that she is sanctified by those sacred items and is prepared for the coming stage of possession. Preparatory purification through contact with sacred things or cleansing body with water continues to the present in the practice of exorcism.

Stamping on an Overturned Bucket Resoundingly.   Stamping on an overturned bucket produces the sound effect of beating on a drum. Such a sound is quite effective for inducing a state of trance if it is skillfully done. In some cases, instead of a bucket, a kind of lute—koto—or a bow string was used for the same effect. The exorcist in later days used one of these instruments or similar ones.

The State of Being Divinely Possessed—"Kami-Gakari" (God-Possession).   The goddess became divinely possessed, exposed her breasts, and exhibited her genitals. She was in a trance or a state of ecstasy. In this state one was supposed to have been possessed by the spirit of god. In this state the spirit of the possessed was believed to be afloat or in abeyance and the spirit of the god, descending into the possessed, expressed himself through the possessed. This seemingly deranged behavior of the possessed must be taken as god's self-expression. In this sense the goddess's exposure of her genitals and breasts has the effect of driving the evil spirits away by virtue of the spirit of god residing within her.

According to my view, the process of possession can be considered as a process of identification of the possessed with the spirit of god. When the person who is supposed to be possessed is a woman, it is perhaps much easier for her to get into the state of identification with the deity than a man, for she can more or less unconsciously experience the process as symbolical sexual intercourse with a god. From this point of view, we can understand more clearly the psychological meaning of breast and genital exposure and the state of ecstasy or trance and of other derangements of the possessed as quite similar to that of sexual orgasm. It is written that in ancient Japan there were quite a number of goddesses, princesses, and empresses who had the experience of being possessed and revealed miraculous powers in one way or another. It also is a fact that most of the exorcists in local communities and founders of so-called new religions in later days were women.

Buddhism and Exorcism

Around 552 A.D. Buddhism was introduced from China through Korea. The introduction of Buddhism caused a severe clash between the progressive and conservative groups. The former favored not only Buddhism but also advanced Chinese culture while the more conservative group preferred to remain with their indigenous beliefs. The final victory went to the progressive group. Concerning Confucianism, supposedly introduced earlier, there was no conflict, perhaps because its teachings had more to do with political and ethical matters than with religious beliefs. The Confucian emphasis on filial piety fostered the idea of ancestor worship among the Japanese. This in turn made one of the most important functions of Buddhism in Japanese social life in this period consoling the spirits of family ancestors, a notion typically Japanese.

Buddhism was propagated and protected by the government under the aegis of the emperors. It became a national religion in the Nara period. In this period two aspects of exorcism are to be considered. One is the status of indigenous Shintoistic exorcists, and the other is the rise of Buddhistic exorcists. Even after the introduction of Buddhism there were empresses who carried out the traditional function of exorcism. For example, when there had been a long drought during the reign of Empress Ko-kyoku, and when all efforts made by the local exorcists had failed, she went to the head-waters of a certain river and prayed to god. The result was a continuous rainfall for 5 days. However, after a scandalous incident involving Empress Sho-toku and a high ranking Buddhist priest named Do-kyo around the middle of the eighth century, the tradition of the ruling empress functioning as an indigenous exorcist ceased to exist. With it went at least officially, a decline in the status of the Shintoistic exorcists. However, they did not lose the faith of the common people.

Buddhism, in those days, was regarded except for a few intellectuals, as a more effective and powerful exorcising method than the indigenous variety. The schools of Buddhism established in this period, such as Sanron, Jojitsu, Hosso, Gusha, Kegon, and Ritsu, were too philosophical and scholastic to be comprehended by the Japanese whose mind was naive but practical. Rather, with their background in the native belief in the spirit of words, Koto-dama, they felt as more mysterious and miraculous the power of the solemn intonation or recitation of the sutras by the Buddhistic priests attired in impressive robes accompanied by the sounds of musical instruments. They took it almost as a sort of incantation. Because of their understanding of Buddhism the common people requested that Buddhist priests recite the sacred sutras to exorcise the evil spirits whenever they became sick or were troubled.

In the *Nihon-Ryoi-Ki* (*Records of Miraculous Stories of Japan*)[2] there were many stories about the miraculous power exerted through the recitation of the sutras. They inform us of their way of understanding Buddhism. Buddhist priests functioned mainly to exorcise evil spirits, to console the spirits of ancestors, to perform rituals, and to carry on scholastic activities in the temple. In this way, despite its alien origin, Buddhism infiltrated the Japanese mind.

Taoism and Exorcism

While Buddhism was accepted because of the traditional Japanese belief in the spirit of words, Koto-dama, hence liturgy, Taoism, supposedly introduced from China in the early seventh century, was accepted also on the basis of the belief in divination. By comparison Taoistic methods of divination were much more advanced, logical, profound, and mysterious than are native ones. Taoistic divination gained such a strong foothold among the general public that there was established, around the middle of the seventh century, an official department in charge of astrology and the teaching of Taoistic methods of incantation and exorcism. Taoistic exorcism was called "On-Yo-Do"—the way of Yin and Yan—and Taoistic exorcists were called "On-Yo-Ji"—the practitioner of the way of Yin and Yan.

Taoistic exorcism lasted a very long time. Its peak was the Heian period. Being anxious to westernize Japan the Meiji government banned them as superstitions. But even today their strong influence can be seen, for example, calendar descriptions which mention fortunes for each day of the year.

Enriched by Buddhism and Taoism, Japanese exorcism continued to maintain its essential characteristics and permeated into the daily life of the common people. In the lapse of time of more than 1000 years until the Second World War, despite periodical suppression by the governments, it was one of the requisites of Japanese social life with some modifications and varieties depending on age and situation.

Exorcism Since the War: 1941–1975 A.D.

During the war the word "Kami-kaze" (god's wind) became world famous. Originally it referred to the typhoon that destroyed the Mongolian's warships which attempted to conquer Japan in 1281 A.D. The populace believed that the typhoon was caused by the spirit of the gods to whom they had offered prayers. Even in a twentieth century war decided by the effectiveness of highly scientific weaponry, the Japanese believed, however unconsciously, that the spirits of the gods had ordained their victories; hence the name kami-kaze was given to a corps of fliers who were ordered to attack the American fleet. Also during the war, Shinto priests performed religious services for the young men who were conscripted. They waved gohei before they departed to ensure that the spirit of god would descend upon them, protect them from danger, and give them power. They were also given amulets, in which the god's spirit was believed to reside. These examples illustrate how the traditional belief in the spirit of god came to the fore on such a critical occasion as a war.

When the War was over, Japan was defeated, the deification of the Emperor denied, the privileged peace of Shintoism as the national religion abrogated, and sheer existence was barely possible in the ruins and debris of postwar destruction, the Japanese felt despondent and dubious regarding the power of the spirits of their native gods. Into this psychological vacuum there burgeoned new religions. Two sects, namely the Sōka Gakkai and the Rissho Kōseikai, gained ascendancy over all others. Both of them are descendants of the Nichiren sect which has a strong inclination toward esoteric exorcism.

Sōka Gakkai

Sōka Gakkai was originally founded by Tsunesaburo Makiguchi in prewar days, but was actually developed by Jōsei Toda after the war. It is an organization consisting of believers of the Nichiren Shōshu (the orthodox Nichiren sect). It claims that the Nichiren Shōshu is the only authentic religion and that others are false and evil. Only those who believe in the mystical inscription of the title of the Lotus Sutra on a piece of wood believed to have been made by Nichiren himself are guaranteed happiness and prosperity in this world. It asserts that since the calling out of the name of the Lotus Sutra itself had the power to dispel all evils or mishaps, the believers should convert people and make them believe it as soon as possible by any means for the sake of the latter's happiness. By so doing the prosperity and happiness in this world of the believers themselves would be promoted. In this manner, in which one can see the traditional belief in the spirit of words (Koto-dama), its membership rapidly increased.

In order to strengthen the faith of the believers, it resorted to mass ecstasy by gathering them in a big hall and having them repeatedly utter the title of the Lotus Sutra, Namu-myo-ho-ren-ge-kyo, in a big chorus, accelerating the tempo of utterance more and more until they come into a state of emotional upheaval and of ecstasy. Sōka Gakkai also encourages believers to pay a visit and do homage to the sacred inscription so that they could have the mystical experience of being vitalized by the miraculous power of the inscription.

The members of Sōka Gakkai are divided into many groups. Each unit of each group is supposed to have a meeting at least once a month at one of the group members' home in rotation. At the meetings, members are expected to participate in discussions regarding problems presented by members. They are usually discussed and clarified according to the teachings of Nichiren. Each small unit of a group is quite active, and sometimes quite aggressive in its activities to gain new members. Actually it is the spearhead of Sōka Gakkai. The president of this organization often gives an interview to the believers. This is considered to be a special honor for the latter. In such interviews he gives advice regarding the latter's problems. In these ways Sōka Gakkai gives its members a definite feeling of belonging and security that they do not find in their daily life. This psychotherapeutic effect is one of the main reasons why it has gained so many followers in such a short time and become a politically powerful organization.

Rissho Koseikai

Rissho Koseikai was founded by a woman, Myōko Naganuma, and her partner, Nikkyo Niwano. Both came from lower-class families. Myōko often seemed to have experienced states of possession, revelation, telepathy, or other occult experiences. She gave advice in the form of oracles to people who came to her for solutions to their problems. She also seemed to have gained people's faith by healing, while Nikkyo gained their trust by divination, especially by onomancy. Their teachings consisted in advising their followers to put great faith in the power of the Lotus Sutra like other Nichiren sects.

What characterizes them is their stress on the importance of ancestor-worship and humility. According to their view, ancestors' spirits exist, and one can communicate with them by invocations reciting the Lotus Sutra, and by calling to mind the names of one's ancestors with the single-minded intention of propitiating them. They assert that when their descendants do not pay respectful attention or extend sincere gratefulness to them, the spirits of ancestors give warning to their offspring by bringing about disease and mishap to indicate their dissatisfaction or anger. Myōko and Nikkyo taught their followers that humility is the basic attitude to be taken by their followers in any human relationship so that they could learn many things and make their relation with others smoother, and as result have a happy life in this world.

The group method they used is more or less similar to that of Sōka Gakkai. In their case, they instructed their followers to gather in their large temple hall every morning. The followers are divided into many groups for meetings. Each member of the group is encouraged to ventilate his problems to his heart's content, while the others listen with a humble and supportive attitude. In contrast to the aggressive and fanatic atmosphere of Sōka Gakkai, there prevails, at least overtly, an atmosphere of gentleness and permissiveness. Therapeutically speaking, the group setting provides the member with an opportunity for psychological catharsis in a permissive atmosphere that is by itself therapeutic, and in addition to the feeling of belonging, he acquires a kind of peace of mind without being too self-assertive.

It should be noted, however, that even though the feelings of belonging and peace of mind the member experiences are due to the effect of the supportive atmosphere and group setting, they are no less related to the feeling that he is closely connected to the generations of his forefathers to which he belongs and that he is safe from evil, since he is protected by the spirits of his ancestors through the reestablishment of his intimate relationship with them. Here we can see the traditional belief in spirits, particularly ancestors' spirits, which survives in the unconscious of the Japanese mind, and has a bearing on the psychotherapeutic effects above. In this connection, exorcism, in the case of Rissho Kōseikai, means to propitiate the angry or dissatisfied spirits of ancestors by invocation, by calling out their names and by reciting sutra. These, in essence, are no different than the traditional method of exorcism we have observed before.

There are many other sects of new religions, which are not as big as Sōka Gakkai or Rissho Kōseikai but, nonetheless, command the faith of the common people, side-by-side with Tenrikyo, Konkokyo, and other sects that had been established around the Meiji era, not to mention the traditional exorcists still active and scattered throughout Japan. Their influence is not negligible.

SUMMARY AND DISCUSSION

The ancient Japanese believed that all perceptible objects were in some way living. On the basis of this belief, their notion of spirits evolved. Those objects that were believed to have miraculous power were called Kami and their spirits were named Kami-no-ke (God's Spirit). They were so awe-struck by the miraculous, mysterious power of these gods' spirit, that they arrived at the belief that when these spirits were offended they caused evils such as disease and mishaps. In such events god spirits became evil spirits which were later called Mono-no-ke. The notion of Mono-no-ke was enlarged to denote evil spirits in general, in which the living spirit, the spirit of the dead, and the living, the fox's and the snake's spirits, were included. The causes of disease, including mental sickness are, according to indigenous Japanese understanding, evil spirits. Therefore therapeutic measures must be taken to drive away evil spirits, namely exorcism.

Japanese exorcism consists of divination, liturgy (invocation, recitation of sutra, or incantation), use of gohei or a sacred tree or a stone as an object into which god's spirit descends and attaches itself, sound effects (by a bucket, drum, lute, or a bowstring), and the state of being possessed (experienced by the exorcist himself, by a medium, or by the sick person himself). Since exorcism makes use of mental or spiritual processes to bring about a healthier state of mind and body, it is to be taken as a kind of psychotherapy. Comparison was made between the exorcist and the psychotherapist. Even teachings of alien origin, Buddhism and Taoism,

were accepted by the common people as the more advanced forms of exorcism and amalgamated with the Shintoistic exorcism. Japanese exorcism,
her folklore psychotherapy, thus formed, preserved its characteristics
through the ages until now, with some modifications according to the situation.

In my view, Japanese exorcism could never have survived through the
ages, particularly after the introduction of Western medicine including psychiatry, if there had been no need or demand for it by the massess through
the ages. In modern Japan where industrialization is reaching its peak and
science and technology are flourishing, we can see a solemn ceremony being
performed to appease the spirit of the land god by a Shinto priest intoning a
liturgy, dressed in a white robe, with gohei in hand, before the foundation of
a huge office building of one of the biggest steel companies in the world, in
the center of the city of Tokyo, with the pious attendance of the president
and his staff. Perhaps their reason would say "no" if asked whether they
believe in such a spirit, but emotionally they are no different from a
farmer's widow, on a desolate mountain plateau called Osorezan in the
northern part of Japan, who listens with tears in her eyes to the mumbling
words of an old woman exorcist who is in a trance and into whom her dead
husband's spirit descended. In short, there is an emotional need for exorcism among the common Japanese people regardless whether they are conscious of it.

The basic reason for this need, I believe, is closely connected with the
Japanese people's agricultural life. Following an agrarian life, people are
close to nature. They see plants grow from seeds, bloom, and bear fruit in
the field and on the mountain. What they see is alive and has the miraculous
power of growth. It is easy to understand how come they arrive at the
notion of spirit as an entity that works to bring about the phenomenon of
growth in plants. This notion is projected and transferred to every perceptible object, so that these objects are no more just objects but have become
spiritual beings with which they can communicate as a sort of fellow being.

In an agricultural economy one's livelihood depends on the harvest, and
that depends on the weather. Therefore, weather is the Japanese people's
chief concern. It is most important for them to know ahead of time what
sort of weather they might have. Hence divination has been fostered.
Furthermore, when they have bad weather, they want to induce good
weather for better crops. For that purpose with their strong belief in spirits,
they pray to the spirit of weather, or the weather god, to give them good
weather. They do so through intoning solemn liturgies and preparing offerings before a divine tree or a sacred stone or gohei to induce the descent of
god's spirit. Trance or ecstasy, a possessed state, which may be considered
to be psychopathological by modern psychiatrists, is an evident indication

for them of the divinity's presence in the exorcist or the medium as well as of the superhuman power of the exorcist. For more than 2000 years at least, the Japanese had no other way of controlling weather on which their life depended than that of exorcism. Exorcism thus has been an integral part of Japanese life and permeated not only into their way of thinking but also into the deepest layers of their emotions. If psychotherapy is a therapeutic measure for helping patients achieve emotional stability, Japanese exorcism has apparently helped the Japanese who were anxiety-ridden to regain their feeling of security. Therefore it can be considered as a form of psychotherapy which has been efficacious at least for the common people, especially in the rural districts. When Western psychotherapy is used for patients in rural areas, due consideration should be given to this cultural aspect. No psychotherapeutic approach can be effective without understanding the uniqueness of each patient's personality in the matrix of his culture.

Recently Kuba[4] reported on his experience with patients who had a possession syndrome. He stated that in the early phase of his treatment of a female patient who had been possessed by a fox spirit, he used a Western psychiatric approach. The patient's condition worsened so he changed his method and acted as an exorcist, and put himself in the same cultural context as his patient. He told her that he would give her an injection that would definitely exorcise and kill the fox spirit 10 days after the injection. After he injected a placebo, he found that she was entirely relieved of her symptoms on the very day he had promised. His experience seems to support my view.

It is my contention that the basic attitude of Japanese exorcism toward the mentally abnormal is worthy of our attention. It assumes that such a person's mind is more or less temporarily attached to or replaced by some spirit and is not fundamentally sick or different from others. It depends on the kinds of the spirit attached to him whether he becomes a sick person or a person who becomes gifted with such miraculous powers as that of prophesy, divination, healing, telepathy, or clairvoyance, which so often are so useful and beneficial to his fellowman. Therefore, this attitude permits the Japanese to be rather understanding and sympathetic toward madness, at least among the common people. Actually literary works were made of mentally disturbed heroes or heroines, with sympathy and aesthetic appreciation. The serious and devotional attitude of exorcists who appeared often in the form of founders of the so-called new religions gained the people's trust and their ardent following even recently.

However, industrialization and Westernization of Japan are being promoted more and more, and the agricultural countryside that used to be the cradle of Japanese exorcism is rapidly dwindling. The Japanese mind probably has to experience more conflicts and crises before it establishes its identity by integrating the differences between its ancient traditional culture and the culture of the West. Last but not least, it must be added that Japanese culture, as indicated in the description above of Japanese exorcism, has the advantage of having been in close contact with nature, communing with and relating to it so that it helped the Japanese be sensitive, aesthetic, alive, and human, though often naive and emotional. Industrialization and too much Westernization, I fear, may deprive the Japanese of these qualities and create the dangers of alienation from nature and of dehumanization and devitalization.

REFERENCES

1. Aston, W. G.: *Nihongi, Chronicles of Japan from the earliest times to A.D. 697,* 2nd ed., Charles E. Tuttle Co., Vermont, 1973, pp. 158–159.

2. Keikai: *Nihon Ryoi-ki* (*Records of Miraculous Stories of Japan*), 15th ed., Kadokawa Shoten, Tokyo, 1973.

3. *Kojiki,* 10th ed., Kadokawa Shoten, Tokyo, 1974, p. 92.

4. Kuba, M.: Hyoe Shokogun no Seishin-byori gakuteki narabini Shakaibunka Seishin-igaku-teki Kenkyu (A psychopathological and sociocultural psychiatric study of the possession syndrome). *Psychiat. Neurol. Jap.* **75**(3):183, 1973.

5. *Man-yo-shu,* 36th ed., Kadokawa Shoten, Tokyo, 1974, p. 186.

6. Philippi, D. L.: *Kojiki,* University of Tokyo Press, Tokyo, 1968, pp. 82–84.

7. Sansom, G. B.: *Japan, A Short Cultural History,* rev. ed., Charles E. Tuttle Co., Vermont, 1973, p. 25.

8. Ref. 7, p. 57.

9. Waley, A.: *The Tale of Genji,* Vol. 1, 5th ed., Charles E. Tuttle Co., Vermont, 1974, pp. 161–162.

CHAPTER THIRTEEN

PSI [PHENOMENA] IN PSYCHIATRY AND PSYCHOTHERAPY

JAN EHRENWALD, M.D.

Parapsychology is the modern experimental approach to telepathy, clairvoyance, psychokinesis, and related "psychic" or psi phenomena. Until a few years ago, they had been relegated to the lunatic fringe of our culture, but three recent developments have brought about a dramatic change in the status of parapsychology among the behavioral sciences. One is the accumulation in scores of university centers and research laboratories of a wealth of experimental findings which can no longer be explained away as artifacts, statistical errors, or the results of a bizarre international conspiracy of fraud and collusion. The second is the changing attitude of modern theoretical physics and quantum theory toward the classical concepts of time, space, and causality, with an attending greater readiness to accept the spatiotemporal and causal anomalies implied by the occurrence of psi incidents. The third factor is the growing number of observations of apparent telepathic incidents in the psychotherapeutic situation.

As a result, parapsychology has in 1969 been admitted to the American Association for the Advancement of Science, and such prestigious technical journals as *Nature, The New Scientist,* or the *Journal of Nervous and Mental Disease* in this country have opened their columns to publish pertinent clinical and experimental contributions along these lines.

The story of experimental research in telepathy, clairvoyance, psychokinesis, and apparent precognition has often been told and need not be repeated here.[2, 18, 19] More important in the present context is that laboratory tests of the card-calling or dice-throwing type are concerned with an altogether different "psychic" reality than so-called spontaneous incidents seen in everyday life, in crisis situations, in clinic, or in consulting room. Laboratory tests have the advantage of being amenable to quantifiable statistical treatment. But they tell us little about the interpersonal configurations or the psychodynamics involved in a given incident. By contrast, spontaneous occurrences of telepathy in the doctor-patient relationship—and its original prototype in mother-child symbiosis—are eminently suitable for the study of their underlying psychodynamics. I pointed out elsewhere[4] that the mother-child symbiosis can in effect be described as the "cradle of ESP," while the doctor-patient relationship tends to reenact the early relationship between parent and child and can serve as a model of its interpersonal dynamics. That observations of this order are not amenable to mathematical treatment is another matter.

There is a wealth of reports of telepathy in the psychoanalytic situation since Freud's early contributions to the field.[5, 10, 12, 22] Most of them are focusing on telepathy in dreams, although some include various other productions by the patient in the treatment situation. Recent experiments with dream telepathy by Ullman, Krippner, and their associates[24] at the Maimonides Dream Laboratory in Brooklyn have provided valuable confirmatory evidence of earlier clinical findings. They are based on monitoring a subject's eye movements and EEG during the REM state of sleep, while an agent, situated in another room, tries to transmit the impression of a pictorial target he is looking at during the subject's dream phase. The subject is awakened after each dream and asked to record his dream on tape. Two or more independent judges are then called upon to match the dream protocols with a supposedly corresponding number of pictorial targets which were exposed during the experimental nights. The results of the Ullman-Krippner series were highly significant. They have the advantage of combining the quantitative approach with psychodynamic inquiry, and in so doing bridge the gap between so-called forced choice and freely chosen, spontaneous—or semi-spontaneous—psi incidents during analysis.

TELEPATHY IN THE PSYCHOANALYTIC SITUATION

A typical example of telepathy in the psychoanalytic situation is as follows:

Mrs. D., age 30, is a professional woman with an obsessive-compulsive trend and a marked ambivalent attachment to her domineering father. In her third year of analysis she had made considerable progress and was ready for termination. On September 24, 1972, she reported the following dream: "I was back at school and had to recite a poem. But I had lost the page—or I could not remember it. Also, the poem was not finished; I tried to figure out the last verse." Preceding this dream fragment, she saw herself on a vacation trip with her boss who had, in the past, been the object of her guilt-laden Oedipal fantasies but with whom she had since developed a more realistic working relationship.

There was nothing in her associations to account for the second fragment. She felt it was quite uncongenial to her, since she never had a knack for poetry. Where, then, did the reading of poetry in the dream come from?

As it happened, it had originated from me. On September 28, 1972, that is, on the night her dream occurred, I attended the Annual Dinner Meeting of the Schilder Society in New York. The members were invited to report some highlights of their travel experiences during the summer. Instead of doing so I decided to treat my colleagues to my translation of a humorous poem by the German poet Christian Morgenstern. I had translated its first two verses a few years back, had lost the draft, and tried hard to reconstruct it from memory. Worse still, the lost verse had never come off to my satisfaction and I spent half the night preceding the banquet to finish the poem.

On Thursday night it was ready for my recital and it was well received by my colleagues, for its brevity, if not for other reasons. Comparing Mrs. D.'s dream with what happened on my side of the picture, the correspondence of five features in reality and dream is unmistakable:

1.   The dreamer is reciting a poem—as I did.
2.   She is at a loss to find the text—as I was.
3.   The last part or verse of the poem is somehow missing—as was the case with my own script.
4.   She manages to produce the missing lines—and so did I.
5.   The temporal coincidence between dream and real event is likewise unmistakable.

There are thus five distinctive features supporting the telepathic interpretation of the dream. The "mandatory" recital of the dream constitutes what I described as a specific telepathic tracer effect.[5] It comes close to the criterion of *uniqueness* that can be found in the manifest content of a few "striking" dreams reported in the psychoanalytic literature. The multiplicity of distinctive features common to both dream and reality can be described as the second criterion. The third criterion on which the telepathic reading of such observations can be based is less apparent. It can be described as the criterion of psychological, as opposed to statistical, significance, used in the natural sciences and experimental parapsychology. By contrast, psychological significance is based on the meaningful nature of the telepathic reading of the dream fragment under review.

Clearly, the telepathic interpretation indicates that in this case the dreamer tries to take the analyst's place or to reach for the missing part of the poem, and her ultimate success in retrieving it dramatizes her identification with her therapist as the once hated—and secretly beloved—father figure. At the same time, it lifts her positive transference on her therapist— her identification with him—to the level of aritistic sublimation, stripped of the more sensuous aspects of her earlier neurotic fantasies. Another fringe benefit of the telepathic interpretation derives from the fact that it is wholly consistent with the thinly veiled Oedipal significance of the first dream fragment in which she allows herself to go on a trip with another father surrogate. It is through introducing the telepathic interpretation that we can fill a gap in the dynamic understanding of the dream. Like the missing piece of a jigsaw puzzle, it suddenly falls into place: it is "psychologically significant." To this we may add the gain in our clinical understanding of the progress made by the dreamer in the course of the preceding years of analytic treatment. It shows her readiness to be on her own, while at the same time emulating some of her therapist's personal interests, values, and preoccupations.

I submit that in the end, it is the criterion of psychological significance which tips the scale in favor of a telepathic reading in cases of this order. It should be noted, however, that as a general rule, one criterion alone does not suffice to carry conviction. This is true even for mass experiments of the ESP type. Despite their attending criterion of statistical significance—or what amounts to clear-cut tracer effects—they do not seem to "make sense." They are not, in themselves, psychologically significant. On the other hand, the criterion of psychological significance alone may likewise be misleading. In the extreme case, its "meaningful" nature may turn out to be a rationalization of ideas of reference or a delusion in disguise.

TYPES OF INCIDENTS

Using these guiding principles, four types of psi incidents can be encountered in the therapeutic situation—and in psychiatric practice at large. The first are incidents characterized by tracer effects, that is, specific and well-defined bits of information found in the manifest dream content or other productions of the patient. If so, they are often artifacts due to the therapist's preoccupation with matters unrelated to his main therapeutic objectives. In effect, they are telltale signs of countertransference. A second manifestation of psi in psychotherapy is less readily apparent but has nonetheless major significance to both theory and practice.

The basic observations have long been familiar to students of the history of psychotherapy. We know that virtually every school finds a wealth of confirmatory evidence to bear out its thesis. Freudian patients are said to be in the habit of dreaming "Freudian" dreams, Adlerian patients, "Adlerian" dreams, Jungian patients, "Jungian" dreams—at least as far as the manifest content is concerned. More generally speaking, we find that the patients' productions tend to meet the therapist's wishes and expectations concerning the validity of his doctrine or of the school of thought to which he owes his allegiance. This is what I have described as doctrinal compliance by the patient with the therapist's emotionally charged theories.

Yet doctrinal compliance should not be confused with suggestion. Freud noted long ago that the pure gold of psychoanalysis is often alloyed with the copper of suggestion originating from the analyst. Doctrinal compliance, as it is conceived here, is another matter; it is unintended suggestion emanating from the therapist who is unaware of its operation. Yet I submit that for this very reason, it is particularly apt to serve as a vehicle for telepathy between doctor and patient.

A third face of psi in psychotherapy is of an altogether different order, though it has close dynamic affinity to doctrinal compliance. If doctrinal compliance is derived from the therapist's emotionally charged wishes to have his pet scientific hypotheses confirmed by his patients, it is only fair to expect that his own therapeutic motivations, conscious and unconscious, including faith in his much maligned omnipotence or personal myth, may likewise have a direct telepathic impact on the patient. This is all the more likely to occur when they are meeting halfway, as it were, the patient's corresponding hopes and expectations to be cured.

There is far-reaching consensus among therapists of diverse schools of thought that it is precisely patterns of circular feedback involving therapist and patient, reinforced by the culture or subculture in which they are immersed, that are responsible for cures affected by charismatic personalities or faith healers of all denominations.[10]

It should, however, be noted at this point that the question whether a genuine psi element is involved in such situations is difficult to decide. The doctor's therapeutic motivations and the patient's corresponding hopes to be cured are lacking the specific tracer elements on which such a claim would have to be based. The part played by telepathy in the faith healer's— and indeed any therapist's—ministrations is certainly suggestive. But in the absence of clearcut tracer effects, the verdict has to be: "unproven."

This condensed survey of the salient features of psi incidents in the laboratory and in the psychotherapeutic situation, coupled with a wealth of older observations of telepathy in crises or related emotionally charged conditions, should suffice in the present context. It provides us with two contrasting models of psi phenomena in general. One is the model of trivial, emotionally indifferent and biologically irrelevant events of the card-calling or dice-throwing micropsychological type; the other is the paradigm of emotionally charged biologically relevant occurrences involving interpersonal configurations and symbolically meaningful relationships.

I have pointed out elsewhere[6] that the first class of such incidents is largely due to temporary flaws in the screening functions of the ego, of Freud's *Reizschutz*; or to minor snags in the individual's perceptual defenses. Neurologically speaking, they are under the control of the reticular formation in the brain stem which helps to regulate arousal and the access of external stimuli to thalamic and cortical centers. The capricious and dynamically unaccountable incidents of this type can be described as *flaw*-determined.

The second major class of psi phenomena is essentially *need*-determined. It is due to the individual's reaching out for symbiotic closeness and intimacy with his fellowmen, with parental or sibling figures, and, in the last analysis, for mystical union with the universe at large. These need-determined psi incidents are far from erratic. They are subject to the familiar laws of psychodynamics, such as repression, reaction formation, symbolic representation, and the like, and are part of a teleological series. They have to be contrasted with the flaw-determined incidents which do not seem to serve any apparent purpose and are due to structural or organic inadequacies in the individual's defensive posture vis-a-vis stimuli impinging from his social and physical environment.

Viewed in isolation, our distinction between the two classes seems to be of little heuristic value. But the proposed dualistic concept of psi functions helps to understand a paradoxical feature of the syndrome. It gives a reasonable account of our tendency to ward off the intrusion of ESP into consciousness. By the same token, it explains why we put a brake on the potential release of biologically just as undesirable PK impulses: PK must be prevented from getting out of hand and exploding in a paroxysm of unbridled psychokinetic acting out, spending itself like a Roman candle.

These inhibitory mechanisms are in striking contrast to the fact that many individuals—both patients and nonpatients—are anxious to break out of the confines of the "splendid isolation" of personal existence. They seem bent on relinquishing the grip of their "uptight" egos in search of ecstasy, nirvana, or peak experiences, or in mind-bending exercises of the contemporary drug culture. They tend to do so even at the price of the loss of self, of surrender to the lure of Plato's Divine Madness—of mental disease. Yet it is needless to say that complete insulation from psi, or else total Dyonisian surrender to it, are hypothetical cases. In everyday life we are more likely to encounter a blend of both existential positions, with the prevalence of either flaw- or need-determined psi elements in a given case.

CLINICAL VIGNETTES

What then is the relevance of these observations to the theory and practice of modern clinical psychiatry? A few clinical vignettes should illustrate the point.

The first on the list are the implications of the telepathy hypothesis on the clinical picture of schizophrenia. The delusions of our paranoid patients show an embarrassing similarity with some of the basic propositions of parapsychologists. Both take for granted the possibility of thought and action at a distance, both subscribe to certain prelogical or paleological patterns of thinking, and both tend to elicit in their fellowmen much the same tendency to denial, resistance, and what can be described as cultural repression. Yet there is a growing number of observations that indicate that there may be a grain of truth in the patients' delusional claims.[1, 7-9, 15, 21] The patients are indeed able to ferret out repressed hostility in their social environment. Some of their delusional ideas can readily be recognized as pathological distortions of purported persecution by introjected parental figures or "introjects."

It is interesting to note, however, that in experimental ESP tests of the card-calling type they do not score better than nonschizophrenics. This apparent inconsistency can, however, readily be accounted for when we realize that it is precisely the heightened sensitiveness of the paranoid which is also conducive to his frantic attempts to ward off the influx of psi stimuli into his consciousness: he mobilizes a variety of perceptual or ego defenses, including Freud's *Reizschutz* or screening function of the ego, to preserve his mental balance. I noted elsewhere[6, 7, 8] that this tendency may in effect be responsible for the familiar withdrawn shut-in personality of the paranoid patient. Indeed, his dual reaction to psi may amount to a paradoxical blend of the Princess on the Pea and of the Indian yogi resting serenely on his bed of nails.

Similar considerations apply to the possession syndrome.[25] Possession is the product of mental dissociation, coupled with the emergence of one or more highly organized secondary personalities, dramatized, staged, and interpreted in paranormal terms. Its cast of characters is usually recruited from an array of benign or malignant deities, worshipped or feared by the subject and his tribe, by his culture or subculture. In the Christian middle ages, it was the devil or his minions who were usurping or invading the bodies of their victims, transforming them into evil demons, witches, or werewolves.[7]

In modern times, the picture of hysterical dissociation has assumed a new coloring. Cases of demoniacal possession have undergone a striking transformation into mediumistic trance, losing their malignant, demonic qualities. The tendency to paranoid projection has given way to hysterical dissociation, with the emergence of secondary personalities, so-called spirit controls, direct voice communicators, or what not. A classical example is the case of a young lady studied by C. G. Jung[13] who produced the personality of the medieval knight, Friedrich von Grebenstein, in the mediumistic trance. Jung interpreted his appearance in terms of the subject's repressed unconscious complexes or instinctual drives.

Yet by contrast to the familiar clinical picture of paranoid delusions or the possession syndrome, there are a vast number of clinical and experimental observations indicating that the mediumistic trance may at time serve as a veritable breeding ground for the origin of genuine psi phenomena. If this is true, the altered states of consciousness in the mediumistic trance may well serve as collateral evidence of potential psi involvement in the frankly pathological, psychiatric versions of altered states of consciousness as well.

There is a fourth picture familiar to cultural anthropologists and students of diverse esoteric cults that has recently attracted the attention of parapsychologists, although it has as yet remained outside the scope of clinical psychiatry. They are so-called out-of-the-body (OOB) experiences. A typical example is that of a Siberian shaman, claiming that his soul can leave his body and visit far-away places in search of immortality or of remedies for an ailing tribesman. Modern accounts of so-called astral projection or traveling clairvoyance are variations on the same theme, shorn of its indigenous cultural trappings.

OOB experiences may occur in the waking state presenting the familiar picture of depersonalization and derealization. They are more frequent in sleep, dreams, hypnosis, and trance conditions. Some are associated with organic brain damage or are induced by psychotropic drugs. Sufi or Kundalini mystics may bring them about through prolonged fasting, self-flagellation, and other severe physical or spiritual disciplines. They often impress the observer as attempts made by the subject to deny, to challenge, or to experiment with death itself. The fact is that OOB experiences often occur in the wake of severe stress, in illness, or in crisis situations.[8]

However, these clinical-psychiatric observations do not tell the whole story of OOB experiences. There are a growing number of reports about apparent telepathic or clairvoyant concomitants of purported OOB travel—hence the rather prejudicial term "traveling clairvoyance." Experimental observations, including EEG studies, by Tart,[23] Palmer,[17] Osis,[16] and others, stress that the OOB subject is occasionally capable of catching a glimpse of scenes or objects located at places he was supposed to visit or of specific experimental targets he is instructed to "view."

The controversy of such alleged "direct viewing," versus telepathy or clairvoyance "pure and simple," is still undecided. But there is a far-reaching consensus among parapsychologists that the OOB syndrome goes far beyond the clinical picture of mere delusional reactions, distortions of the body image, or other forms of psychopathology.

The list of psi phenomena making their appearance in the lunatic fringe of our specialty would be incomplete without at least a passing reference to what is described as purported poltergeist disturbances. They consist of mysterious rapping noises, erratic movements, or breakages of objects in seeming defiance of the laws of gravitation. They are attributed to psychokinesis (PK) occurring in the presence of, or emanating from, disturbed children or adolescents.

Psychological studies usually reveal a marked tendency to the aggressive acting out of repressed hostile-destructive impulses in such youngsters.[3, 14, 20] My own limited case material indicates that they are expressions of rebellion against overly authoritarian, controlling parent figures who seek to prolong their symbiotic grip on their offspring. (By the same token, it could be argued that the much quoted case of Jung's poltergeist in Freud's bookcase was subject to the same psychodynamic principles).[13]

Observations of this order, if confirmed, would represent a psychomotor counterpart to—or rather reaction formation against—the part played by psi phenomena in the early parent-child relationship that was described as the "cradle of ESP." It should be noted that similar considerations apply to observations of this order regardless of whether genuine PK or ESP is involved in the clinical picture. Above all, they prepare the ground for a dynamically oriented approach in the small but apparently growing number of cases that have come to the psychiatrist's notice.

The same applies to OOB experiences, to the possession syndrome, and even to the potential telepathic factor involved in schizophrenic reactions. It is true that the patient—or his family—usually could not care less what diagnostic label is being attached to his affliction. But he expects the therapist to understand and to speak his language, and to give what to the patient appears as a reasonable account of his harrowing experiences. Failing this, he may turn to an exorcist, a witch doctor, or a charlatan.

The therapist, on the other hand, should be aware of the hidden restitutive potential that is inherent even in some of the more bizarre delusional claims of such patients. More often than not, the patient's insistence on an esoteric—and in effect parapsychological—explanation of his plight is indicative of his groping attempts to counteract his threatening mental disorganization, to "make sense" of his experiences, and to prove his sanity: they are defenses in the Freudian sense. Yet if and when evidence suggestive of a genuine psi element being included in the clinical picture comes to his notice, the therapist is duty bound to approach it in the spirit of the same sober reality testing that he is wont to promote in his patient. Needless to say that such a contingency is in turn bound to have a profound influence on the therapeutic management of his case.

THERAPEUTIC IMPLICATIONS

What, then, are the therapeutic implications of these observations?

The first implication involves therapeutic technique. Once the therapist is satisfied that a genuine psi incident has made its appearance in the treatment situation, he will have to probe into his own countertransference as its potential source. He will have to decide whether to apprise the patient of its occurrence, and to evaluate its diagnostic and prognostic relevance to the total clinical situation. Ibsen once stated that writing means to sit in judgment over oneself. The same is true for the therapist's activity sitting in the glasshouse of an analytic situation made transparent in the light of the telepathy hypothesis. If he finds his own attitudes to be wanting, he may or may not share this with his patient. Either way, his new insight may amount to a salutory educational experience. He may avoid confirming the suspicions of a paranoid schizophrenic by revealing "self-incriminatory" information to him. Alternatively, he may find him receptive to interpretations that are apt to restore his sense of sanity, while proceeding in carefully measured steps toward more inclusive reality testing. He may concede the "reality" of a patient's apparent telepathic experience, but he may pare it down to the response of an unduly sensitive monitoring instrument—the patient's excessive awareness of "freefloating" hostility—in society at large.

An intriguing problem is the prognostic significance of the emergence of psi phenomena in the course of psychotherapy. More often than not they are indicative of a wholesome, positive transference configuration. Jule Eisenbud[9] and Montague Ullman and colleagues[24] have noted that in the schizophrenic they may signify an apparent need to establish—or reestablish—better communication with the therapist or with the patient's fellowmen. This may in turn open the door for a new psychodynamic evaluation, interpretation, and working-through of his underlying conflicts and transference distortions.

More important than problems of technique are the broader existential aspects of the new findings. First and foremost, they cannot but have a profound impact on the existential position of the therapist himself. They are apt to alert him to the reality of human experiences that have in the past been beyond the pale of the psychiatrist's purview, or have at best been pressed into the Procrustean bed of traditional psychiatric nosology. Yet we have seen that schizophrenic or other psychotic reactions, drug-related or otherwise, in addition to being maladaptive, may nevertheless be valid in their own right, even though they are not amenable to consensual validation in terms of the *koinos kosmos* of the existentialists. Such a conclusion does not necessarily call for melodramatic gestures of vindicating or endorsing a paranoid patient's ideas of grandeur or persecution. But they should enable the therapist to approach him in the spirit of respect and understanding, hitherto lacking among his peers. He will perhaps come to realize that the patient's paranoid delusions, though patently maladaptive, need not necessarily be "false beliefs" in terms of the traditional textbook definition. He may be ready to grant that a parental introject may be more real than meets the psychiatrist's eye, and that out-of-the-body experiences, or even the bizarre manifestations attributed to disturbed poltergeist children may contain a grain of truth.

A few more fringe benefits may accrue from such an expanded clinical frame of reference. The therapist will be able to relate to the patient as one "expert" to another—not as a specialist ignorant of the latter's deepest concerns and preoccupations. If so, he will arrive at a better understanding of what on an earlier page was described as the potential restitutive value of a delusional patient's own "paranormal" interpretation of his experience. The therapist will recognize it as the patient's desperate attempts to fit it in with his overall outlook on the world, and should be able to help him to arrive at a new, properly balanced position of reality testing. He should be led to recognize a delusional experience for what it is: an experience containing a kernel of truth that has nevertheless to be dislodged and removed like a noxious foreign body. Yet it is readily understood that the therapist can do this only if and when he has himself attained a properly balanced picture of the newly expanded psychic or psychiatric "multiverse."

In my own experience, such an open-minded attitude prepares the ground for a more authentic therapeutic alliance between analyst and patient. The patient no longer feels that he is "nothing else but mad." Concurrently, he will be more amenable to interpretations that help to put whatever paranormal incidents he has experienced in the proper perspective. Such a perspective is apt to show them up for what they usually are: "noise" in his channels of communication, or else a breakthrough of signals uncalled for in the ordinary business of living. Aided by the therapist, the patient may then be in a better position to dissociate himself from the delusional elements in his experience—or else to integrate them with a more broadly defined multidimensional psychic reality.

REFERENCES

1. Arieti, S.: *Interpretation of Schizophrenia*, R. Brunner, New York, 1955.

2. Beloff, J.: *New Directions in Parapsychology*, Elek Science, London, 1974.

3. Bender, H.: Modern poltergeist research—A plea for an unprejudiced approach. In *New Directions in Parapsychology*, J. Beloff (Ed.), Elek Science, London, 1974.

4. Ehrenwald, J.: Mother-child symbiosis, cradle of ESP. Psychoanal. Rev. **58**.3:455–471, 1971.

5. Ehrenwald, J.: *New Dimensions of Deep Analysis*, Grune & Stratton, New York, 1954.

6. Ehrenwald, J.: The telepathy hypothesis and schizophrenia. *J. Amer. Acad. Psychoanal.* **2**(2):1959–169, 1974.

7. Ehrenwald, J.: Possession and exorcism: Delusion shared and compounded. *J. Amer. Acad. Psychoanal.* **3**(1):105–119, 1974.

8. Ehrenwald, J.: Out-of-the-body experiences and the denial of death. *J. Nerv. Ment. Dis.* **159**(4):227–233, 1974.

9. Eisenbud, J.: *Psi and Psychoanalysis*, Grune and Stratton, New York, 1970.

10. Frank, J. D.: *Persuasion and Healing*, John Hopkins Press, Baltimore, 1973.

11. Freud, S.: *Dreams and Occultism*. In *New Introductory Lectures on Psycho-Analysis*, Hogarth Press, London, 1964.

12. Hollós, I.: A summary of Istvan Hollos theories by George Devereux. In *Psychoanalysis and the Occult*, G. Devereux (Ed.), International Universities Press, New York, 1953.

13. Jung, C. G.: *Memories, Dreams, Reflections,* A. Jaffé (Ed.), Pantheon Books, Random House, New York, 1963.

14. Mischo, J.: Personality structure of psychokinetic mediums. *Proc. Parapsychol. Assoc.* **5**:35–37, 1958.

15. Niederland, W.: Schreber: Father and son. *Psychoanal. Quart.* **28**:151, 1959.

16. Osis, K.: Perspectives for out-of-body research. In *Research in Parapsychology,* Scarecrow Press, Metuchen, N.J., 1974.

17. Palmer, J.: Some new directions for research. In *Research in Parapsychology* W. G. Roll and R. L. Morris, (Eds.), Scarecrow Press, Metuchen, N.J., 1973.

18. Pratt, J. G., Rhine, J. B., et al.: *Extra-Sensory Perception after Sixty Years,* Holt, New York, 1940.

19. Rhine, J. B.: *Hidden Channels of the Mind,* William Sloan, New York, 1961.

20. Roll, W. G.: A new look at the survival problem. In *New Directions in Parapsychology* J. Beloff, (Ed.), Elek Science, London, 1974.

21. Schatzman, M.: *Soul Murder in the Family,* Randon House, New York, 1973.

22. Servadio, E.: Psychoanalysis and telepathy. In *Psychoanalysis and the Occult* G. Devereux, (Ed.), International Universities Press, New York, 1953.

23. Tart, Ch., (Ed.): *Altered States of Consciousness,* Wiley, New York, 1969.

24. Ullman, M., Krippner, S., and Vaughan, A.: *Dream Telepathy,* Macmillan, New York, 1973.

25. Yap, P. M.: Mental disease peculiar to certain cultures: A survey of comparative psychiatry, *J. Ment. Sci.* **97**:313, 1951.

CHAPTER FOURTEEN

PSYCHODRAMA IN A HOSPITAL SETTING

FERRUCCIO DI CORI, M.D.

P sychodrama is stagecraft that, in its full psychological depth, is applied to everyday living. The web of events, feelings, and memories in which a person is enmeshed in his life are visualized, objectified, and projected in a mirrorlike fashion on the environment. Hence the individual can emerge from a psychodramatic course of therapy with a heightened perception of what his own behavior is, was, and could be. If in the reenactment of events appropriate modifications are introduced, it is then within the realm of possibility that the psychodramatic experience will open a new avenue of approach, and will contribute to a better understanding of the personality when other means have failed.

THE CONCEPT OF PSYCHODRAMA

The emoting individual is an undepletable source of stimulation and contribution to his own amelioration or defeat. Under the stimulus of psychodrama he reveals, reports, and reappraises through a process of creating. Ultimately, he relearns simply by reenacting.

Psychodrama is conducted according to techniques that have the clinical ability to modify the course of a disturbance and accelerate its resolution. It is a therapeutic method of choice in cases where a partial or total modification of behavior is desired in the patient, and where the elements of time and action could be a positive coadjutant in the resolution of a repressed or active conflict that keeps the patient from performing successfully in his life course.

But occurring as it does in a milieu of a multifaceted society, psychodrama is subject to polyvalent assessment at different levels and open to different interpretations. And if psychodrama, as stated, is stagecraft applied to everyday living, the stage can as easily be a sidewalk or a bedroom as a hospital ward. In short, the psychodramatic encounter may occur spontaneously anywhere. Brief psychodramatic exchanges in the one-to-one dialogue between psychiatrist and patient are common occurrences with which we are all familiar. And at times psychodramatic episodes of a bizarre nature are played out in society at large.

In a southern town in Italy, for instance, every year on the feast day of the village's patron saint, the children are dressed as angels and sent flying in the air, tied to laundry ropes strung from window to window on either side of the local streets. Their annual angel flight—a source of great pleasure for the children and deep pride for their elders, who feel themselves in communion with God through the intercession of their offspring—was forbidden a few years ago by the local bishop who, suddenly recognizing the potential danger to life and limb of the unusual practice, put a stop to any further flying by means of an ecclesiastical edict. When the day of the angel flight arrived, the church doors were flung open and, before the astonished eyes of the anxious priest, the population thronged through the street, refusing to enter the church or carry the consecrated effigy in procession. As an expression of further and total rejection, a new edition of the saint had been carved to carry on the street instead of the holy patron. The wrath of the bishop culminated in a mass excommunication of the town which spontaneously exiled itself *in toto* to a neighboring village to pray and resume their Catholic obligations. After long and laborious intercession, the village was finally "pardoned," and the children flew again in a psychodramatic heaven made of laundry ropes. Thus the stage of life sets up a series of circumstances that favor the proclivities of the individual for acting out his own motivations and his own repressed impulses regardless of the reality or fantasies involved.

I have myself witnessed in another Italian hamlet the case of a man who leaves for his job as a clerk each morning playing the part of a train. This would perhaps be not so remarkable were it not for the fact that he has the complicity of the entire neighborhood acting out on his behalf. Outside his home at 8:30 each morning he whistles and puffs, and the neighbors gather around to wave goodbye to him. On his return home in the evening, shuffling and chugging, his neighbors are there once more to welcome him back. The man, a conscientious worker and upstanding father of three, escapes reality twice a day by identifying himself with a toy memory of his childhood, while still retaining, within "acceptable" boundaries, the responsibility of his social commitments.

Accordingly, the stage is set in life for spontaneous psychodrama wherever it springs up, sustained and tolerated by a benevolent environment. In a psychotherapeutic setting, psychodrama has more definite boundaries. Fundamental elements of time, space, reality, and fantasy merge or approximate in a mode of action whose goal is the improvement of the patient within a milieu that must operate for his benefit. A favorable setting for therapeutic psychodrama is the psychiatric ward of a hospital, where interaction can be utilized as a form of therapy, making possible the penetration of defenses and, through enactment, the modification of behavior with a view toward partial or even total resolution of conflicts.

A NEW APPROACH TO PSYCHODRAMA

The psychodrama with which this chapter deals differs in a number of respects from the "classic" psychodrama of D. J. Moreno, which is practiced in various centers, primarily in this country. Some of the differences, imposed by the demands of circumstance, were unavoidable. For example:

1. Moreno worked primarily with neurotics. The population with which I work is 95% psychotic—the inpatients of a psychiatric ward at Kings County Hospital in Brooklyn.

2. The Moreno approach requires an elaborate physical setting, an actual theater with a multilevel stage construction. The psychodrama I direct takes place in a large room of the hospital, architecturally unaltered for the performance of psychodrama.

3. The director of Moreno psychodrama works with a number of professional auxiliary personnel, trained to play the roles of the so-called important others (spouse, parent, employer) in the patient's life. I work with a fluctuating staff of students and other hospital personnel, none of whom has any professional training in psychodrama, but who are nonetheless able to play the different roles assigned to them.

The differences so far itemized are obviously quite fundamental, and were I to attempt in every other respect to reproduce classic psychodrama, these differences alone could be expected to lead to a qualitatively different result. In fact, I have made no such attempt. Following are further departures from the Moreno approach, applied to psychodrama at Kings County.

4. The stage of Moreno's psychodrama theater is surrounded by an audience of nonparticipating observers. In the psychodrama room at Kings County, everyone—staff, patients, some 25 to 30 individuals—is a participant.

5. More often than not, Moreno psychodramas are preplanned. Their oft-mentioned spontaneity is, for the most part, spontaneity of action within the framework of a restrictive plot. By contrast, psychodrama at Kings County is as freeform and unstructured as possible.

6. A Moreno psychodrama generally focuses on a single patient or a single family. Psychodrama at Kings County can focus on one, two, or several patients, and occasionally on the entire community.

7. Classic psychodrama rarely ventures very far from a reality situation. The psychodrama I direct ventures into reality and away from it as well, into fantasy, poetry, abstraction.

8. A highly significant technological innovation, unavailable to Moreno when he was developing psychodrama, is the videotape machine, which provides exposure for performing patients to the inescapable objectivity of instant replay.

These innovations and their effect on the patient population under study are the subject of this chapter.

PSYCHODRAMA IN A HOSPITAL SETTING

Kings County Hospital is part of the Teaching Center of the Downstate Medical School, State University of New York in Brooklyn. The patient population living in the ward is exposed to various therapeutic approaches—drug therapy, sports activity, outings, and individual psychotherapy. Psychodrama is one form of approach. It is held early in the morning, twice a week, for a period of 45 minutes. The age of the population ranges from 18 to 60. Most of the community comes from a relatively low socioeconomic stratum, since Kings County is a city hospital.

The Physical Setting

Psychodrama at Kings County Hospital takes place in a large, well-lit room (Figure 1) that is at other times used by the patients as a recreation or group therapy milieu. For the psychodrama session, chairs and sofas are pushed back against the four walls, leaving the center of the room empty except for a pair of overhead microphones. At one end of the room a technician mans a video camera, recording the proceedings.

The Moderator

Psychodrama is a delicate therapeutic vehicle. It requires a skilled moderator/therapist who can direct and control with sensitivity, flexibility, and responsiveness to the mood and messages of the patients, observers as well as players. The moderator is the promoter and catalyst who must "reani-

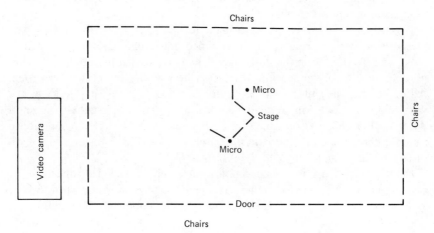

Figure 1.   Setting of psychodrama in hospital.

mate the unconscious" and bring it, through a process of creativity, to the surface. (Arieti) Any anxiety he may experience during the course of the session must be rigorously concealed. In a room full of anxiety the therapist cannot afford his own.

The following illustrates the swiftness, adaptability, and resourcefulness a moderator of psychodrama is called upon to display.

Breaking the silence that typically initiates a session, the moderator says, "Well?"

One of the patients replies, "Wishing well." The moderator ignores it, and the patient says again, "Wishing well." At this point the stimulus is accepted.

"All right," the moderator says, "there, in the middle of the room, there is a wishing well." Four patients are chosen. They move their chairs into the center of the room, engaged by the notion of an invisible wishing well and caught by their own production stimulus. "What do you wish for, Charles?" the moderator asks one of them.

"Money," Charles answers promptly.

"Good," says the moderator, "you have just found $1000 on the street." At once Charles begins to behave in a grandiose manner: he has become a man of wealth and power. "Now, what are you going to do with it?" the moderator asks.

The other performers appeal to Charles for loans and gifts of money; and with the distribution of wealth, richer material begins to emerge. The behavior of the patients becomes sibling-like, with Charles the favored child, the powerful, enviable one. When the situation is sufficiently saturated, the moderator increases the tempo with a further development. He is a poor cashier, he announces, and on his way to the bank he lost $1000. "Did anyone find my $1000?"

Now Charles is forced into the realistic role of the decision-maker. The pleasure principle is reluctantly abandoned and replaced by a reality principle, and Charles is on the defensive. When he calls on his siblings for support, there is a reorganization of relationships within the performer group. Allied at last, they turn upon the authority figure. "How do we know it's your money?" one of them challenges. "Let's call a cop," suggests another. After further convolutions, the plot finally settles on the collective desire to retain a percentage of the found money as a reward for honesty while restituting the larger portion to its rightful owner.

In this way a productive psychodrama emerged and developed simply because the moderator, by chance, opened the session with the word "well", and then instantly exploited the material that spontaneously emerged.

The Population

An average of 25 to 30 persons participate jointly in a session. Eight to ten of them are staff members: resident physicians, psychologists, nurses, medical students, aides. No one but the moderator is trained in the theory or methodology of psychodrama. For this reason, the moderator is compelled to exercise extreme care in avoiding material that the staff may not be able to handle. Nevertheless, the results are surprisingly positive. Untrained, the staff is thoroughly spontaneous in its responses and receptive to the unpredictability of the outcome.

The performer patient is permitted to freely choose his own fellow performers from among the patients and staff members attending the session. He is as likely to choose staff members as patients. Only his own therapist is barred from the psychodrama in which he himself figures.

Patients find the moderator a natural choice to play parental roles. The quality of authority attaches itself so tenaciously to him that even the dictates of gender are sometimes suspended, so that a patient may select a male moderator to play his threatening mother and proceed to interact with the masculine mother smoothly and satisfactorily.

Most of the patients are of schizophrenic type, but affective disorders, organic psychoses, drug addiction, and alcoholism are represented. Ninety-five percent of the group is diagnosed as psychotic.

There is no physical separation between patients and staff. Chairs are lined up against the walls, every seat is taken, and patients and staff are randomly interspersed with no uniforms or other identifying insignia to distinguish one from the other.

Participation in psychodrama is universal. The formal separation between the players in the center of the room and the audience along the walls is deliberately minimized. Comments and suggestions from the onlookers are permitted, at times solicited. Occasional derisive or abrasive remarks are tolerated. From time to time, empathetic outbursts of sorrow or rage occur as well.

Obviously it would be possible to preclude interruptions of this kind. But inasmuch as individuals must interact not only with individuals but with a sometimes judgmental society too, the intervention of the audience—unless it is totally disruptive—is seen as sociologically valid and therapeutically sound. In response to a derogatory remark from a nonparticipating patient, the performer will perhaps modify his behavior in the psychodrama, or ignore the comment, or occasionally cut short his performance. Regardless of his reaction, however, he realizes that his performing does not isolate him from the community. On the contrary, there is continual interaction between the performing patient and the onlookers.

Patients who are exhibitionistic or those with marked narcissistic trends are more willing to participate actively. Those who are resistant and negativistic usually are led in during the middle of a session when the atmosphere is more positively oriented.

THE STRUCTURE OF THE PSYCHODRAMA SESSION

The session starts, quite often, in deep silence. If the moderator permits it, the stillness will continue unbroken for upwards of 5 minutes. It is not a silence pregnant with resistance, and the patients foster it in an almost playful fashion. It is in some respects very much like the anticipatory silence of an audience in a theater whose houselights have just been dimmed. A community ready for psychodrama represents a society in miniature. The behavior of the patients during these initial moments forms a foundation for the structure of the session, and it is incumbent upon the moderator to assess the dominant mood of the community, the quality of its silence, delicate details of indifference or interference. At the opening, he may ask for volunteer players or select from the group himself. Patients who display exhibitionistic trends with dramatic leanings are able to attract and magnetize to the center of the room those who tend to hide at the periphery (see Figure 2).

Improvising a Psychodrama

The session lasts 45 minutes, and may include two, three, or more separate skits. The plot of the psychodrama to be performed is not necessarily confined to significant events in a patient's life. It may be based on an incident just occurred in the ward, or it may be pure fiction of the most melodramatic sort. The subject can be abstract rather than concrete. It may take the form of a monologue, a dialogue with a friend or a staff member of

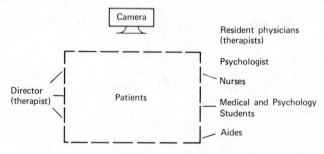

Figure 2. Types of population attending a psychodrama session.

the patient's choice, even a plot that involves the entire community, such as a subway scene or a city in the grip of panic over some threatening disaster.

Most Frequently Selected Topics

1. Memory or event leading to hospitalization.
2. Structured plot by moderator.
3. Structured plot by a patient.
4. Spontaneous plot.
5. Poetry.
6. Proverbs.

Techniques of Staging Plots

1. The patient alone (monologue leading to various involvements).
2. Patient with one opponent playing assigned events which may or may not lead to others.
3. Patient with several members of the community.
4. Patient alone against the community.
5. Patient together with and within the community.

The success or failure of the session turns on a number of factors in addition to the close assessment of the milieu during the crucial early moments. Cultural and social levels of the community prevail in dictating a choice of actual life situations (parental rejection, object loss, aggression, isolation, etc.) when the levels are low; whereas the presence of a dominant group of a higher education level permits performances that deal with such abstract subjects as:

1. The sky and the earth (the former turbulent, controlling, overpowering, rewarding; the latter productive, violent, realistic, frustrating).
2. Cosmic elements—fire, water, earth, air—into which the patient population assigned such embracing symbols projects its own personality molds and inherent conflicts.
3. Shades of affect: rage, tenderness, euphoria, sadness, to be expressed in terms of body language (miming).

ILLUSTRATIVE MATERIAL DEPICTING
VARIOUS CATEGORIES OF PSYCHODRAMA

"When in Rome"

A middle-aged male patient, diagnosed as schizophrenic, paranoid type, with a background of professional activity as a writer and stage director, volunteers to direct and produce rather than perform in a skit of his own devising.

A few days before the psychodramatic event, the patient has asked the moderator for the equivalent in Italian of the English vulgarism "ass." The skit he produces he calls "When in Rome." He outlines a plot wherein several couples are strolling in the streets of Rome. One of the husbands begins to harangue a loiterer for failing to pinch the buttocks of his wife. The patient even supplies dialogue: "What's the matter? Isn't my wife pretty enough for you to pinch?" He indicates that the enraged husband should then set upon the loiterer, throw him to the ground, poke him in the eye with an umbrella—in short, beat him mercilessly. One of the residents in the audience ventures to question the appropriateness of the punishment. Surely an offense as minor as a "nonpinch" does not merit such a thrashing. At that, the patient, who has been much involved in his directorial efforts, falls into a chair and describes an incident which, he acknowledges, has prompted his choice of skit and the inappropriate action he has outlined.

In childhood, he explains, he was the victim of a homosexual attack. Throughout the attack, the rapist exhorted him to "Be a man! Be a man!" Now he launches into a long monologue, questioning his understanding of what it is to be a man. As he speaks he slumps lower and lower in his chair. And as the monologue unfolds, two female patients enter the action without moving from the periphery of the room.

An older and rather maternal woman begins to question the patient's "ability to be a man." Another, a vibrant young woman in her twenties seated almost opposite the first urges the patient to "act right now and prove your masculinity." The atmosphere is highly charged, with the patient now weeping uncontrollably while the two opponent women continue to harass him.

The videotape replay of this scene brought the entire audience to a peak of involvement. The majority felt that the patient had forced this particular skit upon the group as a device for exposing his problems. He had not the courage to approach the two women directly and needed the screen of a performance to invite the judgment of society.

"War Games"

This skit consumed an entire 45-minute session.

The moderator chooses four male patients and outlines a situation: They are soldiers, relaxing for a moment in a battle-front canteen. Casual conversation has revealed that all four of them grew up in the same neighborhood.

The four patient/soldiers begin to reminisce about the old neighborhood.

The talk centers on their reasons for joining the army. They have fallen easily into the escape fantasy of the plot. One had to get away from his wife, a demanding, childish woman for whom the salary he brought home from two jobs was not enough. A second speaks of his disillusion with the Air Force, where he had hoped to become a helicopter engineer: "That's what I wanted to do but they wouldn't let me. I learned about them. You don't always get what they tell you you'll get." The third explains that he didn't get along with his parents; home was an unpleasant place to be, and so he joined the army. The fourth, Joe, is silent. His posture is rigid; his face immobile. Joe is in control of the situation.

The other three make rueful remarks about the army. They wish they were elsewhere and otherwise occupied. Joe speaks for the first time. "I like the small missiles," he says. "They're all right. I like the explosions; I like the noise."

The moderator introduces an element of danger, calling on the defenses of the players in terms of response to an anxiety provoking situation. At his instigation, a resident breaks into the scene. He is an enemy officer. His army has overrun the installation and the four soldiers are prisoners. The moderator joins him in the guise of an enemy colonel and instructs him to interrogate the prisoners without mercy. There is some mutual encouragement among the prisoners, who remind one another that only name, rank, and serial number need be supplied. The first three, despite the enemy officer's threats, reveal nothing. Only Joe is nonplussed. "I don't know the whereabouts of the other troops," he insists. "I really don't."

Joe is a patient with strong paranoid delusions of grandeur, feelings of omnipotence, a desire to control. The moderator/colonel singles him out, threatening to have him tortured if he fails to inform. "Get down on your knees," the colonel orders; and after some hesitancy, Joe complies.

Following the moderator's earlier instructions, a resident portraying a compatriot of the four prisoners joins the action. His army has recaptured the area, he says, and the tables are turned. The colonel and interrogation officer are now the captives of their own former prisoners. "What shall we do with them, men?" he asks the four patients. The consensus is that they should be put in a prisoner of war camp, but Joe demurs.

"Kill them, torture them," he says. "Do what they were going to do to us." And encouraged by several patients in the audience, he moves aggressively toward the moderator/colonel. "Down on your knees," Joe orders, his face expressionless. But the colonel refuses to obey. "Then I'll make you!" says Joe, and seems about to do so when the moderator hastily declares the scene concluded.

In the next scene, Joe is being welcomed back from the war. He is at home with his mother, who introduces a pretty young patient, a "neighbor," into the action. The "neighbor" adds several other patient/friends to the scene and a "Welcome Home" party is launched. Someone puts on a record, they pretend they are drinking champagne, and Joe's conversation becomes a trifle rakish. "I want some girls," he says. "One blond, one brunette." And when someone suggests dancing, he scoffs, "Dancing? We're already in bed."

But withal his face remains a mask, and the moderator challenges him: "Why don't you smile? Your face is stiff."

At once the partygoers become patients in a psychiatric ward, succoring and sympathizing with him. "That happened to me, too," one of them says. "You ask your doctor to give you less medication. That's what I did, and it worked."

"I don't mind being like this so much," says Joe. "I know it's helping. I'll be myself again later on. I really want that."

This is greeted by murmurs of assent. "You'll be okay, don't you worry." "Yah." "You'll be fine." At last Joe smiles.

In the first sequence of the skit, an anxiety-provoking situation with survival at stake brought to light the strong homosexual links that joined the four soldier/patients together. In the second sequence, Joe was unable to control the situation with females. His attitude of superiority was very flimsy, and the performance was filled throughout with flaws in what Joe imagined to be the approach of a veteran conqueror of women.

"Three Incidents"

The moderator has asked that a patient reenact three scenes from his life— one from childhood, one from adolescence, and one recent. Jennie volunteers. The first scene she will reenact occurred when she was 12—her memory goes back no further than this. It is a scene with a maid portrayed by Anne, a patient who is 34 to Jennie's 26.

Jennie says that her mother is leaving, and that she'll be just as glad to see her go—she's tired of being picked on and beaten. Anne asks if Jennie will not miss her mother. "A little," Jennie admits. But she's confident Anne will take good care of her and the other children who are left behind. Anne promises to try. But Jennie becomes petulant and whiny. "You don't feed us on time," she complains. "We're hungry, and you don't take good care of us, and you get mad all the time. I'm going to live with Grandma." Anne offers to make arrangements, but Jennie wants no interference from her. "You don't have to do anything," says Jennie. "I'll just go."

In the second scene Jennie is in her grandmother's house, with Anne portraying the grandmother. Jennie says that she doesn't like the maid and wants to stay with her grandmother instead. Anne assures her she may stay as long as she wishes. Jennie says that she misses her parents, that she has written to her mother, and that her mother has promised to send for her. "I'm going to America," Jennie declares. "I'm leaving Jamaica. I'm leaving Jamaica today." Anne questions the wisdom of the decision. "I'll miss you," Jennie replies. "I'll miss my boyfriend, too. Why you get so angry when I see him?" Anne says she considers the boyfriend an inappropriate associate for her granddaughter and, since wisdom comes with age, Jennie should listen to what she says.

For her third scene, Jennie projects her thoughts into the future when she will have left the hospital and, hopefully, returned to the daycare center where, before her breakdown, she worked as an assistant teacher. The scene takes place in a nursery classroom populated by the hospital community. Jennie wishes her class a good morning. She says she's been out sick, but now she's fine, and it's time to get down to work. She instructs her class to paint pictures. But two of the children (one medical student, one patient) decide they do not want to paint pictures; they want to eat cookies. "It isn't snack time yet," Jennie says. "First we work; then we have milk and cookies." But her charges are intractable. One (a resident) insists she has to go to the bathroom and can't go by herself. Subsequently she indicates, wailing loudly, that it's not really the bathroom she wants; it's home and Mommy. All of this Jennie copes with by smiling gently and uttering a few soft, soothing words.

The moderator, in the guise of director of the daycare center, informs Jennie by telephone that one of her pupils has told his parents that Jennie, his teacher, has struck him. She must speak to the child and get to the bottom of things or trouble will surely ensue. A medical student, Arthur, plays the child. Jennie asks him why he told his parents she had hit him. He replies that because she had in fact hit him. She says that that's not true. Arthur insists that it is so true. The yes-no volley continues fruitlessly for a few minutes. It remains unresolved, but Jennie's calm is unbroken.

This episode demonstrates how the patient dealt with her future life responsibilities. Her need to be supported and accepted in life and her response to therapy were visible in the last of her three incidents, the classroom scene. The effects of psychodrama played a decisive role in the evolution of the patient's future life plans.

"Pass the Secret"

The moderator invites eight patients and one medical student into the performing area, indicating that they are to arrange their chairs in a circle. When all the participants are seated, he tells them that he will relay a secret message to one player, who will whisper it to his neighbor, who will in turn pass the words along, until the last player announces what he has heard.

The moderator writes his message on a slip of paper: "The proper study of mankind is man." He hands it to the first player and the game begins. There is much giggling and grimacing as the message circles the group. In the final rendering it has become, "Poppa strut. Mine is mine." When the original and the final versions of the message are announced, the community roars with laughter.

Now the moderator turns the game over to the group and instructs the players to take turns inventing the message to be passed, and opening up game participation to include the entire community.

"No man is an island in his mind" becomes "No, I can't stand it this time." "One man's ceiling is another man's floor" quickly becomes "One man's feeling is another man's thought" but then deteriorates into "Pony dancing, another one's caught."

It is difficult to graphically reproduce the involvement and the depth of participation that "Pass the Secret" produced. If one envisages a cross-section schizophrenic population invited to relate in a skit of hide-and-seek words, where the fringe of each utterance lends itself to alterations and deviations in the individual's conceptualization, and if one pauses to think of pathological internalization, projective identification, the paleological thinking and primitive defense operations of a schizophrenic, then one will sense the validity of such a "game" of words.

"The Poem"

Annemarie was a longstanding withdrawn schizophrenic who was very resistant to psychodrama. She shunned exhibition in any guise, and her depleted narcissism found no source of nourishment in any form of therapy. She lived in the ward, participating without incentive or interest in different activities. When, after repeated attempts to persuade her, she finally agreed to act, it was on the condition that the sequence should involve only a father and a daughter, the father to be played by the moderator himself. During the course of the psychodrama, however, the moderator was able to shift the focus away from himself and mobilize outer stimuli by tapping the environment, the inner potentials of the patient and her desire to be recognized by the community.

MODERATOR: Annemarie and I will play a skit. We will be father and daughter. [To Annemarie] All the time I think about you. I'm so worried. You have no husband, no boyfriend. I don't know what will become of you if I die.

ANNEMARIE: I'll go to school.

MODERATOR: But what will happen afterwards? [No response] What do
you do in school?

ANNEMARIE: I write.

MODERATOR: What do you write?

ANNEMARIE: I write poetry.

In a very simple way they briefly discuss poetry. The moderator then
begins to introduce other men onto the scene—first a medical student, then
a patient, then a resident. Each time he brings one of his "friends" into the
scene he contrives an excuse to leave. Annemarie, distressed by his departures, attempts to preclude them or to join him wherever he claims he must
go. He is firm and reassuring, however, and she is left alone in psychodramatic conversation with three different men. Among the exchanges that
take place are the following.

STUDENT: What school do you go to?

ANNEMARIE: [To moderator] Can I make up an answer? [Upon affirmative
response, to student] The School of Medicine.

STUDENT: What do you study?

ANNEMARIE: Writing. Just poetry.

STUDENT: What do you write about? Forests? People?

ANNEMARIE: I write about people.

The following is excerpted from Annemarie's conversation with another
patient, Gary.

GARY: How do you like your dad? He's always trying to fix you up.

ANNEMARIE: He wants to get rid of me.

GARY: Naw. He's just worried about you in case he dies.

ANNEMARIE: I know.

GARY: He wouldn't have any trouble marrying you off. You're
pretty. [No response] I could come over to your house and
write some poems with you.

ANNEMARIE: No.

GARY: All right, I tried. I'd like to see some of your poetry, though.

ANNEMARIE: Why?

GARY: I like your father and you, too.

ANNEMARIE: That's no reason to show you my poetry.

The next exchange is from her dialogue with a resident.

RESIDENT: I'd like to take you to the movies tonight.
ANNEMARIE: No, I'm writing tonight.
RESIDENT: Would you let me read your poetry?
ANNEMARIE: I don't know; it depends.

At this point, the moderator returned to the scene, stepping out of his role.

MODERATOR: Why don't we play a game with poetry? I'll write the first line:
"In the midst of the night a door just opened."
[Handing paper to student] You next.

In turn, the medical student, the resident, and the patient, Gary, added a line to the poem, as follows.

STUDENT: "Though afraid to look there I couldn't help see. . . ."
RESIDENT: "A pair of young lovers wrapped arm in arm in the cool summer breeze."
GARY: "Though my thoughts were scrambled I had a sense of being which could help me to see."
MODERATOR: [To Annemarie] You finish the poem. [She writes and returns the paper to him. He reads:]
"From the bottom of my heart I was forced to see the truth about our lives."
[To Annemarie] Will you give a title to the poem?
ANNEMARIE: [After a lengthy pause] "The Misty Dawn of Truth."

After this psychodrama had taken place, the patient was able to participate in others, and the pattern of her sessions with her therapist improved considerably.

"The Minister"

The moderator outlines a situation: A young couple who are embroiled in marital difficulties have come to consult a minister because their marriage is foundering. He calls on two medical students, Larry and Rosalind, to play the couple, and a patient, Peter, to portray the minister.

Rosalind, the wife, states her case assertively. She is working, she says, in order to put her husband through medical school. She has no objection to this; however, her husband comes home from the hospital so exhausted each night that he can do no more than eat and fall into bed. Accordingly, her life consists of the drudgery of housework and the drudgery of a job with very little pleasure to compensate.

Peter, the minister, listens to her diatribe impassively. He mumbles a response in a voice too low to hear. The moderator asks him to speak up. In an only slightly louder voice he repeats his answer. "Pray to God. Put your faith in him. You do what I tell you. You pray."

Now Larry, the husband, offers his version. His wife had known before they married that she would be required to work while he finished his training. It's true he is tired when he comes home at night, but the situation will change once his education is complete. Rosalind cuts him short. "I know what's going to happen once you're through with school," she says. "You'll find someone else. You're just using me to pay for your education. You'll leave me the first chance you get. Well, I'm not going to be a sucker for you. I want out right now!"

They turn to Peter expectantly, and he mumbles his advice. "Pray. Pray for guidance. Pray for patience. Pray for love and understanding. Prayers are answered; I tell you so, and I know."

The students portraying the couple make an unsuccessful attempt to get Peter to address the situation with which they have presented him. Stubbornly, he continues to exhort them to pray. The moderator declares the skit concluded, but asks Peter to remain. The two students move back into the audience, and the moderator himself joins Peter in the center.

Peter is still the minister, he says, while he, the moderator, is another individual seeking help. The moderator leans toward Peter; his voice is loud, his manner aggressive. He presents himself to Peter as the lover of Rosalind. It is a relationship he enjoys very much, he says, and he will not consider ending it. But he is somewhat disturbed by the fact that his mistress is married to another man. What does Peter suggest he do? "Don't tell me to pray," he warns Peter. "I've tried that, and it doesn't help. Tell me what I should do."

Peter's rocklike composure is shaken. His hands tremble; his eyes dart. Once more he recommends prayer as the only solution to this problem and every problem, but his sermon is less facile and he stumbles over words. His discomfort electrifies the patients in the audience.

"I always thought prayer was silly myself," one female patient volunteers. "That was before I ended up in the hospital. Now I know better." But another disagrees: "Praying don't do no good. The minister talks to God on Sunday; then he fool around with women the rest of the week." A third patient, a man, challenges Peter on the minutiae of his faith. The seam that had momentarily opened in Peter's equanimity is now repaired. He answers every challenge with ease and assurance in the language of a religious tract.

Peter, a paranoid of long duration, had withdrawn into a religious sect and become a self-appointed minister following marital difficulties and abandonment by his wife. Decompensation occurred when a flood of paranoid thinking compelled the patient to seek help. During the course of his hospitalization he confessed a tremendous conflict between a very rigid superego and his inner strivings. The precipitating cause of hospitalization was an attempt to set fire to himself and reach God in a state of grace after punishment. Peter appears also in the following psychodrama.

"The Dance"

The moderator calls two patients into the center of the room. Pearl has proven in previous sessions that she can handle herself well under the stress of psychodrama. Julie, a recently admitted patient, looks much younger than her 24 years. She wears an expression of perpetual terror; her body is held rigidly erect, her hands never gesture, and her voice is so faint it can barely be heard.

Pearl tells Julie that she is leaving the hospital soon, and that her stay has helped her a great deal. Julie opens her mouth piteously, and Pearl interprets this to mean that she, too, would like to leave the hospital. "But you need more help," Pearl remonstrates. There is no response.

The moderator asks Julie if she cannot answer, and when she almost imperceptibly shakes her head no, he moves behind her chair to play her alter ego. "I'm so afraid," Julie's alter ego says. "I don't like it here, but I'm afraid to leave. I don't know what I'll find outside. I don't know why I'm here. I'm so little and helpless, and my voice is so small." Pearl urges Julie to talk to and relate with other people, to which Julie's alter ego replies, "I need support, I need people to tell me what to do. I'm so scared I can't even open my mouth to talk." Julie smiles gratefully, acknowledging the accuracy of the interpretation.

The moderator then attempts to help Julie vocalize. "Say your vowels; say AHHH," he instructs. She accedes as minimally as possible; a barely audible "ah" escapes her lips. Shifting to a different approach of body image utilization, he asks her if she likes to dance, and when she nods her head yes he dismisses Pearl and invites a patient named Peter into the center of the room to dance with Julie. A record is put on and they dance. Her eyes remain fixed on his feet and hers as they move. Only when the music is ending does she look up into his face and smile. Applause from the audience follows.

"What do you want to do now?" the moderator asks Peter. "What would you ordinarily do after a dance?"

"Go home," Peter replies roguishly.

"It's not that simple," says the moderator. "What comes after a dance?" Peter shrugs. "Conversation, I guess."

The center of the room then becomes a café where Peter and Julie have gone after the dance.

PETER: How'd you like the dance?

JULIE: Okay.

PETER: You think you dance nice?

JULIE: [with genuine concern] I don't know. Do I?

PETER: Yeah. Real nice.

JULIE: Do you want to dance some more?

PETER: I think the party's kind of far away. What do you like to do besides go to dances?

JULIE: Have some drinks maybe.

The moderator brings another patient, Carl, into the scene. He portrays an acquaintance of Peter's who has been drinking rather heavily in the café and decides to join Peter at his table. But Peter fails to acknowledge the presence of Carl, and continues to address only Julie.

PETER: Do you like to get drunk or do you just like to taste?

JULIE: To sip.

PETER: Yeah, that's good. So what else do you like—besides dancing and drinking?

CARL: Do you like to eat?

JULIE: Mashed potatoes. . . .

The moderator instructs Carl to try to take Julie away from Peter.

CARL: [To Julie] Is he your boyfriend? [She nods.] Oh, wow. Can I have you? [She shakes her head no.] Why not?

JULIE: [Indicating Peter] Ask him.

PETER: [To Carl] You're always getting drunk. Besides, she has kids.

CARL: [To Julie] You tell me why—why you like him? Could we make a date one day? Go out? Maybe take the kids? [At mention of the children, she smiles.] You have kids? How many?

JULIE: Two.

CARL: What are they?

JULIE: A boy and a girl.

PETER: [To Julie] So how're the kids doing? How big are they now? [She indicates the height of the children with her hand.]

CARL: [To Julie] How come you so quiet?

JULIE: I'm just quiet.

The moderator concludes the psychodrama and calls for commentary from the audience. The comments of the patients are unusually perceptive. One patient shrewdly points out that Julie's voice is tiniest of all when she is speaking of things that trouble her—her children, for example—but that it is considerably louder when she is talking of such neutral matters as dancing.

THE UTILIZATION OF POETRY AND PROVERBS

According to Arieti, "At times the poetry of an author involves a whole aspect of human existence." Poetry is employed in psychodrama because of its concretization and perceptualization. The use of metaphorical language, the phonetic value of rhyming sound, the symbolism of a passage that often leads to displacement in its interpretation, and the differentiation between metaphor and metamorphosis are factors that lead to the application of poetry as a powerful therapeutic vehicle to many pathological disturbances.

Following are two poems utilized in psychodrama sessions. The first, "My Ass", was selected for psychodramatization because of the double entendre of the word ass. It is mischievous in its concretization, and yet in an Aesopian sense lends itself to a great deal of participation from the audience.

1. "My Ass"

Supercilious
my ass
crossing
the bridge
and carrying
all my flour
to a near windmill
he knew
the road

but he shied
from the shadows
of the trees
    leery
of his goings.
At the border
he just halted
and in a deep grunt
mumbled
several names
meaning the trees
but a few humans
responded to invitation
and now
my ass
is gone
without me.

A paranoid patient with a long history of persecutory trends was able to give a "supercilious" look to the role of the ass carrying the flour to another patient who, investing all his immobility in the role of the windmill, crunched and devoured the imaginary flour with great gusto. The patient playing the ass selected members of the audience to play an alley of trees, sitting or leaning against them and enjoying his title role. The grunting and the selection of mumbled names provoked an outburst of rivalry, especially when the patients chosen to be "humans" realized the deceitful pitfall they were caught in.

At the end the "ass" strode away without anybody following him. "I'm going home," he yelled, halfway out the door. "I am discharged."

"Discharged, my ass," someone echoed.

The poem's concreteness, its surrealistic ending, and the participation required of the audience playing the chorus of trees all contributed to the popularity of this poem as a point of reference for psychodrama. Other favorable factors include the anthropomorphic expression of the patients' basic motivations, the pleasure of separation in the role of the animal (patient) from the bondage of authority (therapist), and the support of the community identifying with the star of the drama, reaching a peak of sublime and childlike delight in being "leery of his goings." It is worth mentioning that the most disturbed schizophrenic patient of the group was the one who contributed the "deep grunt" of the poem and was able to cooperate with the rest in crossing the bridge (which was enacted by a passive dependent patient who enthusiastically embraced his role).

Following is a second poem which was presented to the community for psychodramatization.

2. "Bondage"

I go blank
and then
the coffer of my mind
snatches . . .
and . . . purrs
surreptitiously
bounces
back and forth
the iridescence
of my heart
between its pillars
hide and seek
the politeness
of my beliefs
the tone
of my forceful
drive:
Toward him
I am bound!

This poem, quite abstract in its essence, was played by a pair of patients both of whom were paranoid schizophrenics—college graduates, articulate, emotionally labile and unpredictable in their behavior. In both cases the event precipitating hospitalization was loss of object relation with consequent deep disturbance in ego defenses and decompensation.

She begins: "I go blank," and she stares into space for several minutes.

He is next. "And then the coffer of my mind snatches." To the collective hilarity of the audience, he snaps his forehead and symbolically pours out imaginary things.

The next lines, "surreptitiously bounces," find both patients dancing up and down around their chairs with awkward and disorganized motions. "The iridescence of my heart between its pillars" is played by the female patient, who, at the suggestion of the moderator, uses the two chairs as pillars and pounds her chest repeatedly, while the male patient crouches on the floor enacting "hide and seek." "The tone of my forceful drive" is approached with reluctance. Neither patient is able to act the "forceful drive."

For both psychodramas the poem was inscribed on a board and kept in full view of the audience who participated with suggestions regarding interpretation of the words into physical actions and with expressions of emotional involvement—a synthesis and analysis of body language at a level of high abstraction.

Following the reading and acting out of the second poem, both patients had private therapeutic sessions with their respective therapists. The female was able to link memories of events laden with guilt and associated with early childhood frustrations. More aggressive, the male lashed out at his therapist for not being able to explain many of the dynamics that had led to the event precipitating hospitalization. In both cases a catharsis had taken place.

Concretization of the concept through imagery is found not only in poetry but also in many other forms of art. Parables and proverbs differ from poetry in form and aims. Their main purpose is to give a precept of good behavior or wisdom, whereas poetry aims to create an aesthetic expression. (Arieti)

In line with this concept, proverbs are used in psychodrama at Kings County. Proverbs used most commonly because of their multiple interpretations include:

1. Blood is thicker than water.
2. Matches are made in heaven.
3. People who live in glass houses shouldn't throw stones.
4. Fools make feasts and wise men eat them.

Space limitations preclude description at length of all the variations in interpretation that have emerged. As an illustration of the variety, however, one patient acted out the proverb "Matches are made in heaven" by portraying a rabbi in his synagogue, busily introducing male members of the community to female members in hopes of provoking a marriage. Another patient interpreted the same proverb homonymically, working away in heaven manufacturing safety matches.

Often patients approached the proverb "Fools make feasts while wise men eat them" very concretely, assuming that the food they foolishly prepared would be wisely consumed by the psychiatrists.

EVOLUTION OF A SESSION

The overall framework of the 45-minute psychodrama session within which the individual psychodramas fit is as follows.

Initial Stage.   A patient or several patients perform (either spontaneous or assigned topic).

Second Stage. The moderator introduces variations into the psychodrama or extends it with contributory material. Or the same plot is presented for enactment to a different set of patients.

Third Stage. Comment from the audience on the validity and significance of the performance just witnessed. Often the comments are extremely challenging. (One example, after "The Dance," was the patient who pointed out that Julie's voice was weakest when the subject was a sensitive one such as her children, but considerably louder when she spoke of neutral topics.)

Fourth Stage. The video receiver is turned toward the community so that the performance can be shown in instant replay.

Final Stage. Comment and therapeutic directives from moderator to staff after the patients have left the room. Critique of session, proposals for modification for future reference.

For the purpose of studying the mental and emotional productivity mobilized in the community soon after a session is ended, a questionnaire is given to each patient to be filled out and returned at the next session or discussed with his own therapist in private session.

Questionnaire

1. How did you feel at the beginining of the psychodrama session?
2. Which skit provoked you most? Why?
3. Why did you participate in the particular skit you were in?
4. If you did not participate today, will you tomorrow?
5. Did you feel different at the end of the session than you did at the beginning? If you can, explain the reason.
6. Do you discuss sessions with other patients?
7. Do you discuss sessions with your therapist?
8. Did the session help to bring out memories, emotions, forgotten events, or feelings that you had kept inside and tried to control?
9. Do you find any change in your personality since you started attending psychodrama sessions?
10. Do you prefer psychodrama to other forms of therapy? Why?

THE ROLE OF THE VIDEO APPARATUS

The video apparatus has marked clinical therapeutic value in the performance of psychodrama. When the video receiver is turned with its screen facing the players and audience, and the sequence is screened, the patients are transfixed:

The mirror image of their own past actions confronts them, eliminating any possible skepticism or dilution of impact that might greet a verbal description and analysis of what has just transpired.

The emotions have barely had time to cool when the revelation with all its implications is imposed.

Endoceptual experiences, body image expressions, mannerisms, stereotypes, verbalizations, hidden feelings, and fluctuating emotions in their wide gamut of variations—the whole world of inner and outer reality (intrapsychic and environmental) already fading and transformed in the recesses of memory—are brought again to the forefront of attention.

An evasion, denial, or resistance mechanism is pointed out to the audience as it is being replayed on the video screen. As a result, patients are sometimes able to achieve important insights that, until then, had eluded them.

The cathartic value of the performance is often enhanced or reinforced by instant replay.

Moreover, the video tape is a valuable point of reference for coordinating individual therapy following a session.

FACTORS INFLUENCING THE PERFORMANCE OF PSYCHODRAMA

1. Onset (selection of initial topic).
2. Aura preceding the opening of a session.
3. Prevailing mood of some patients and their interfering influence.
4. Exhibitionistic qualities of some patients and tendency to manipulate the milieu.
5. Upstaging occurring during performance.
6. Frequency of interruptions from audience (comments, resistance, aggressiveness, sudden exits, control of the floor, etc.)
7. Massive resistance to the authority of the moderator.
8. Too close identification with authority (staff, moderator, therapist).
9. Emotional involvement among different patients.
10. Total withdrawal (apathy, indifference, confusion, etc.)

The psychodrama performed at Kings County and described in this chapter is intrinsically unpredictable in its evolution. A session cannot be formally structured in advance because its development will be influenced by the numerous variables listed above. Furthermore, the homogeneity of the group, their cultural and social background, race, religion, age, intellectual endowment, type of psychosis, the general mood of the milieu, the traumatic events that have occurred previous to the session, all these are elements that influence the outcome. Other factors that play a role relate to the ability of the staff to intervene satisfactorily and with immediacy to maintain the empathy of the group toward the performers, especially when disruptive behavior among the onlookers is an unavoidable negative influence. The use of drug therapy or individual psychotherapeutic approach just prior to the session may establish an acceptable range of behavior or expression.

CONCLUSIONS

The socially controlled field (the hospital) in which a schizophrenic lives is very challenging to him. The more regressed he is, the more intensive are his experiences in a group situation where he is continuously tested as part of the milieu/therapeutic environment. Through the routine of everyday activity in this milieu, the psychotic individual learns again the concept of space-time boundaries and his gradual differentiation versus a new identity stemming at first from the environment and finally culminating in a partial or total rehabilitation of self.

Psychodrama of the kind performed at Kings County and described in this chapter plays an active role in that rehabilitation, either as a coadjutant to other formal therapies or as the sole emergency vehicle for breaking through the resistance, promoting within itself a cathartic strength when intellectualization and defense-resistances act as powerful barriers to desirable changes.

The method of approach in psychodrama affords different levels of intervention. It is my observation that if regression occurs it is controlled, repression is then eliminated, and acting out becomes modified, especially if it is utilized as a resolving factor. In the pathology of internalized object relations, psychodrama, then, serves a useful function because it succeeds in reestablishing safer boundaries between the intrapsychic world of the patient and his interpersonal one. The patient regains a new system of controls, more evident when the individual is supported by psychotherapy. In studying schizophrenic disorders that involve varying levels of disintegration, with mechanisms of arrest, regression, repression, withdrawal, and such, I have further observed that psychodrama has the following cumulative effects:

1. It increases the span of interpersonal relations.
2. Through interaction with the community, it increases the tolerance for stress.

3. Through critique of peers, therapists, videotape exposure, it increases the patient's comprehension of his own behavior.

4. It produces growing sociability and improved learning ability.

What is perhaps most outstanding in my findings is the impact that the patient's acting produces on the milieu and vice versa. This exchange of pathology, the individual versus the collective, can be utilized therapeutically in terms of the examination of the group processes between patients and their surroundings. Therefore, if a psychodrama therapist acquires skill in utilizing the awareness of the patient toward his needs and his frustrated wishes, he will have reached a definite road of approach that other avenues of therapy might fail to uncover.

This comparative use of experience, relived in acting out, establishes better relationships among the peers of the community and the therapist. The ultimate gratification that then comes from acting out a repressed conflict or an emotional catharsis might be reorganized on the basis of a concept framed long ago by Frieda Fromm-Reichmann.

She conceived the psychotherapeutic relationship as a joint enterprise between the capacity of the therapist and the potentiality of the patient. During the therapeutic process we attempt to fill the void that separates a human being from the others when we try to structure something, for example, a symbolic artifact that is placed in the hand of a person who has not yet learned the expression of communication. Psychodrama reestablishes that form of communication.

The drama of life lies in the strength of its psychic components, and the integration of one's ego occasionally puts forth a few newborn leaves: I am standing in a hospital corridor, I watch a patient in catatonic immobility, and I wave to her cheerfully. Her response is minimal: a very small, very timid lifting of the hand. But then I wave to her again, and this time she raises her arm with a bit more strength and self-confidence. I wave to her still again, and now my insistence perplexes her. She turns around to see if I am not after all waving to someone else behind her. I point my finger directly at her: "You!" my finger says. And she opens her eyes wide and points to herself: Me? When I nod confirmation she lifts her arm and waves to me with vigor and enthusiasm. I know then that I have established a basis for rapport and that eventually she will be able to dance. This elementary expression of human relations is the cradle of psychodrama.

In the final analysis, we must find ourselves ready to accept the words of the poet:

I am Nobody! Who are you?
Are you—Nobody—too?
Then there's a pair of us?

Don't tell! They'd advertise—you know!
How dreary—to be—Somebody!
How public—like a frog—
To tell one's name—the livelong June—
To an admiring bog!*

Success, after all, is not based essentially on achievement but on recognition of one's identity. Passengers we are on the highways of life, and if we pause from time to time to assess on the palette of our existence span the hues of our emotions and the colors of our thoughts we discover our similarities which are almost equal for each of us in Pirandellian fashion.

Eye meets eye, there, in the workshop of the artist as well as in the office of the therapist. The bridge that we cross is two-way. We encounter in order to relate, and we relate in order to feel.

A poet was once asked what would have been his greatest joy in life. "To receive a letter from someone," he answered, "asking me to explain one of my verses. I would know then that someone loves me in my creative effort; and poetry would then have acquired one more friend."

In my field, as a psychiatrist, I subscribe to the same experience.

REFERENCES

1. Arieti, S.: Schizophrenia: Other aspects; Psychotherapy. In *American Handbook of Psychiatry*, S. Arieti (Ed.), Basic Books, New York, 1959.

2. Arieti, S.: Schizophrenia: The manifest symptomatology, the psychodynamic and formal mechanisms. In *American Handbook of Psychiatry*, S. Arieti (Ed.), Basic Books, New York, 1959.

3. Arieti, S.: *The Intrapsychic Self*, Basic Books, New York, 1967.

4. Arieti, S.: Contribution to cognition from psychoanalytic theory. In *Communication and Community*, Jules Massermann, (Ed.), *Science and Psychoanalysis*, Vol. VIII, Grune and Stratton, New York, 1965.

5. Arieti, S.: *Interpretation of Schizophrenia*, Basic Books, New York, 1974.

6. Bour, Pierre: *Psicodramma E Vita*, Milano, Rizzoli, 1969.

7. Feldman, S. S.: *Mannerisms of Speech and Gestures in Everyday Life*, International Universities Press, New York, 1959.

8. Frankl, V. E.: Logotherapy and existential analysis; A review. *Amer. J. Psychother.*, 20:252–260, 1966.

9. Greenberg, I. A., (Ed.): *Psychodrama: Theory and Therapy*, Behavioral Publications, New York, 1974.

10. Kernberg, O. F.: Modern hospital milieu treatment of schizophrenia. In *New Dimensions in Psychiatry*, S. Arieti and G. Chrzanowski (Eds.), Wiley, New York, 1975.

* Emily Dickinson: *Collected Poems.*

11. Meerloo, J. A.: The universal language of rhythm. In *Poetry Therapy*, J. J. Leedy (Ed.), Lippincott, Philadelphia, 1969.

12. Moreno, J. L.: *Psychodrama*, Vol. 1 and 2, Beacon House, Beacon, NY, 1946, rev. 1964.

13. Moreno, J. L.: Psychodrama. In *American Handbook of Psychiatry*, S. Arieti (Ed.), Vol. II, Basic Books, New York, 1959, pp. 1374–1396.

14. Sechehaye, M.: *A New Psychotherapy in Schizophrenia*, Grune and Stratton, New York, 1956.

15. Spiegel, R.: Specific problems of communication in psychiatric conditions. In *American Handbook of Psychiatry*, S. Arieti, (Ed.), Vol. 1, Basic Books, New York, 1959, pp. 909–949.

16. Spiegel, R.: Creative process in the arts. *Communication and Community*, Jules Massermann (Ed.), *Science and Psychoanalysis*, Grune and Stratton, New York, 1965.

17. Yablonsky, L. and Enneis, J. M.: Psychodrama: Theory and Practice. In *Progress in Psychotherapy*, 1956, pp. 149–161.

PART THREE

BIOLOGICAL STUDIES

ON THE EVOLUTION OF THREE MENTALITIES

PATHOGENIC AND NEUROPATHOLOGIC ASPECTS OF SOME NEUROPSYCHOTROPIC
AGENTS

PHARMACOLOGY AND PSYCHOSOMATIC MEDICINE: THE EXPERIMENTAL AND CLINICAL
APPROACH TO A PSYCHOSOMATIC EVALUATION OF PSYCHOTROPIC DRUGS

THE PSYCHOPHYSIOLOGICAL BASIS OF THE PHARMACOTHERAPY OF ENDOGENOUS
PSYCHOTICS

CHAPTER FIFTEEN

ON THE EVOLUTION OF THREE MENTALITIES*

PAUL D. MACLEAN, M.D.

Herein too may be felt the powerlessness of mere Logic, the insufficiency of the profoundest knowledge of the laws of the understanding, to resolve these problems which lie nearer to our hearts, as progressive years strip away from our life the illusions of its golden dawn. (p. 416)

George Boole, *An Investigation of the Laws of Thought*

INTRODUCTION

Many people point out the apparent irony that the great strides in the natural sciences seem to be speeding us toward the Hill of Megiddo and the long-advertised final conflict between the forces of good and evil. Others, still blinded by the searing light of Hiroshima, are more introspective in expressing this concern: How, they ask, can we contain and harness the devastating powers of the atom before we have learned to understand and control the potentially catastrophic forces within ourselves?

In recent years anxiety about thermonuclear war has diminished somewhat in the light of warnings that the human race and many forms of life may be on the way to extinction because of scientific developments that have made possible overpopulation, pollution of the environment, and exhaustion of critical resources.

A curve showing the growth of the world's population[13] indicates that each successive doubling of people has taken place in half the time of the previous doubling.[6] At this rate the present population would be expected to double in 30 to 40 years. In 1969, U Thant, speaking as Secretary of the United Nations, made his famous pronouncement that there remained only 10 years to find solutions for the exploding population and related problems.

Warnings of this kind focus attention almost exclusively on the external environment. It is so easy to see the problems of meeting future demands for food, water, energy, and other basic requisites that planning experts seem to have overlooked the lessons of animal experimentation indicating that psychological "stresses" of crowding may bring about a collapse of social structure despite an ample provision of the necessities of life (e.g., Refs. 5 and 41). Systems analysts who have attempted to predict the limits of growth with the aid of computer technology[38] either admit to an inability to deal with psychological factors or neglect them altogether.

Michael Chance[7] has remarked that the parts of the universe that man first chose for study were those furthest removed from the self—meaning, of

---

* From the introduction of a book (in preparation) on the triune brain. Not subject to copyright, having been prepared by an officer of the U.S. Government.

course, the heavens and the science of astronomy. Later I mention a possible neurological explanation of why our sciences from the very beginning have focused on the external world. By contrast, and perhaps for similar reasons, there has been a retarded interest in turning the dissecting lamp of the scientific method onto the inner self and the psychological instrument by which we derive all scientific knowledge. It would almost seem that there had always been a supernatural injunction against doing so: "Of every tree of the garden thou mayest freely eat: But of the tree of the knowledge of good and evil, thou shalt not eat of it: for in the day that thou eatest thereof thou shalt surely die."

Until rather recent times religion and philosophy provided the principal spokesmen and interpreters in regard to psychological matters. Although having their modern origins in the 18th century, psychology and psychiatry could hardly be regarded as sciences until the latter half of the 19th century. The same would be true for neurophysiology and experimental psychology which encompass investigations on psychological functions of the brain. According to Kathleen Grange,[16] the term "psychology" was used in titles as early as 1703, while "psychiatry" first appeared on a title page in 1813. Psychiatry began to receive recognition as one of the medical sciences in 1854, when Griesinger at the University of Munich united for the first time the teaching of neurology and psychiatry. Meynert, Gudden, Forel, and others followed this practice and established it as a tradition in Europe. Since the middle of the present century, neurology has tended to follow an independent course, delving into psychological functions only insofar as particular disturbances in cerebration make it possible to diagnose the nature and location of brain disease. Psychoanalysis, which gave new conceptual and methodological dimensions to psychiatry, began to arouse public interest in 1900 with the publication of Freud's *The Interpretation of Dreams*.[14]

The late development of the psychological sciences is of itself of epistemological interest. This leads to the consideration that none of the psychological sciences devotes itself specifically to epistemological questions concerning the origin, nature, limits, and validity of knowledge. Except for sensation and perception, it is curious how little attention has been given by philosophers and others to the role of the brain in matters of epistemology.

Epistemology exists because of human societies, and human societies depend on the existence of individuals. I state these truisms to emphasize the incontrovertible centricity of the individual person with respect to public knowledge. In constitutional language, public knowledge, just as society itself, derives authority from individuals. In this sense, an individual is both supreme and indispensable.

Central to every individual is a subjective self—a self that Descartes[9] once referred to as "this me." A conceptual dissection of the subjective self requires that it be laid open not only in terms of its inner workings, but also in relationship to the societal and nonsocietal elements of the external environment. There are two sides to each of these relationships: the side that is intuitively and unsystematically experienced and the side that becomes known through the analytic and synthetic approaches of the various sciences. The animate relationships become systematically known through the social and life sciences, while formal knowledge of the inanimate derives from the natural sciences.

"Epistemics".   There is, however, no branch of science that deals specifically with an explanation of the subjective self and its relation to the internal and external environment. While such a study would draw on every field of knowledge reflecting on the human condition, it would build fundamentally on the psychological and brain-related sciences. In order to have a matching expression for epistemology, as well as an equivalent term for science, one might borrow a word directly from the Greek, and instead of speaking of a "science of the self," refer to an "episteme (ἐπιστημη) of the self." Then the body of knowledge or the collective disciplines dealing with this subject could be known as *epistemics.*

Let is be emphasized that the domains of epistemics and epistemology are the same. The difference is in the point of view. Epistemics represents the subjective view and epistemic approach from the inside-out, whereas epistemology represents the public view and scientific approach from the outside-in. The two are inseparable insofar as epistemics is nuclear to epistemology, and epistemology embraces epistemics. What is entailed is an obligatory relationship between a private, personal brain and a public, collective, societal brain.

Developments in the knowledge of the brain promise to have a profound influence on epistemology. In scientific and philosophic writings, it has been customary to regard the human brain as a global organ dominated by the cerebral cortex which serves as a *tabula rasa* for an everchanging translation of sensory and perceptive experience into symbolic language, and which has special capacities for learning, memory, problem solving, and transmission of culture from one generation to another. Such a view is blind to the consideration that in its evolution the human brain has expanded along the lines of three basic patterns which may be characterized as reptilian, paleomammalian, and neomammalian (see Figure 1).[25] Radically different in structure and chemistry and in an evolutionary sense countless generations apart, the three formations constitute, so-to-speak, three-brains-in-one, a *triune* brain.[28, 33] What this situation immediately implies is

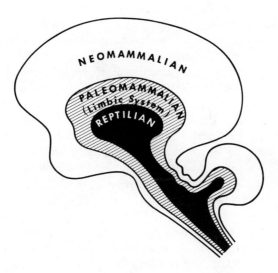

Figure 1. In its evolution, the human forebrain expands in hierarchic fashion along the lines of three basic patterns that may be characterized as reptilian, paleomammalian, and neomammalian. From Ref. 27.

that we are obliged to look at ourselves and the world through the eyes of three quite different mentalities. To complicate things further, two of the mentalities appear to lack the power of speech.

"Objectivity".* Achievements of the so-called hard or exact sciences have helped to promote the attitude that solutions to most problems can be found by learning to manipulate the external environment. It has been traditional to regard the exact sciences as completely objective. The self-conscious cultivation of the "objective" approach is illustrated in a statement by Einstein quoted by C. P. Snow[46]: "A perception of this world by thought, leaving out everything subjective became . . . my supreme aim." Monod, in a recent essay on the contributions of molecular biology[39], is equally insistent on applying the "principle of objectivity" in the life sciences. "The cornerstone of the scientific method," he writes, "is the postulate that nature is objective." Even in the world of fiction one finds a book reviewer saying, "Humanity is likely to be saved, if it is at all, by a search for an objective reality we can all share—for truths like those of science."[52]

Early in this century, John B. Watson and others of the behaviorist school, sought to revive the spirit of the Helmholz tradition and to establish

* The wording of this passage follows closely that of MacLean, 1970.

psychology as an exact science on an equal footing with physics and the other natural sciences.[45] In their study of animals and man they advocated a completely objective approach that dispensed with the consideration of consciousness, subjectivity, and introspection.[51] The irony of all such "objective" attitudes is that every behavior selected for study, every observation and interpretation, requires subjective processing by an introspective observer. Logically, there is no way of circumventing this or the more disturbing conclusion that the cold, hard facts of science, like the firm pavement underfoot, are all derivatives of a "soft" brain. No measurement or computation obtained by the hardware of the exact sciences enters our comprehension without undergoing subjective transformation by the "software" of the brain. The implication of Spencer's statement[47] that objective psychology owes its origins to subjective psychology could apply to the whole realm of science.

For such reasons it is important to consider how a fifth dimension, the subjective brain, affects our relative view of the world. In considering this problem, I do not intend to deal with the familiar Cartesian tropic of perceptual illusions. Rather, I focus on brain research concerned with the origins of other forms of experience and attitudes that may be of more basic significance for "epistemics" and epistemology, giving particular attention to forebrain mechanisms underlying "paleopsychic" processes and "prosematic" (nonverbal) behavior.

Subjective Experience.   For each one of us as individuals there is nothing so vital as our subjective experience. Without the essence of subjectivity, there would be no means of realizing our existence. Subjectivity represents a form of information. As Wiener stated more succinctly than Berkeley or Hume, "Information is information, not matter or energy."[53] At the same time, it is empirically evident that there can be no communication of information without the intermediary of what we recognize as physical behaving entities. This invariance might be considered a law of communication.

"Facts."   I should also mention at this point my conclusion that facts apply only to those things that can be agreed upon publicly as entities behaving in a certain way. The term validity does not apply to the facts themselves, which are neither true nor false *per se,* but rather to what is agreed upon as true by subjective individuals after a public assessment of the facts. What is agreed upon as true or false by one group may be quite contrary to the conclusions of another group.

Communicative Behavior

Next in importance to our subjective experience is the ability to share what we feel and think with other beings. Such communication must be accomplished through some form of behavior. Human communicative behavior can be broadly categorized as verbal and nonverbal. Like P. W. Bridgman, the physicist-philosopher, the great majority of people would probably conclude that "most communication is verbal."[3] Since we are so accustomed to think of ourselves as verbal beings, we have given less attention to the analysis of nonverbal behavior. This neglect is evidenced by our lack of a specific word for nonverbal behavior; we refer to it negatively by stating what it is not.

It is an everyday experience that in spite of all kinds of talk—no matter how well documented—we are never quite sure how we develop attitudes or reach decisions regarding all manner of human relationships. Who would feel confident in trying to identify the nonverbal factors affecting one's choice of spouse, friends, associates; a vote for a particular candidate; one's judgments as a member of a committee or jury? In an article on nonverbal communication in Japan, Morsbach[40] illustrates the bewilderment commonly felt in trying to reconstruct human decisions. In an anecdote conjuring a feeling of *déjà vu* he describes two professors who after a faculty meeting found themselves in agreement that everyone had spoken positively about a particular proposal that was subsequently voted down. "Don't you agree," one asked the other, "that everyone was in favor?" "Yes," was the reply, "but you did not hear the silences."

Contrary to the popular view, many behavioral scientists would be inclined to give greater importance to nonverbal than verbal behavior in day-to-day human activities. For example, when a psychologist, a behavioral ecologist, a specialist in environmental design, and an ethologist were asked to draw two squares representative of the weight that they would give verbal and nonverbal communication in everyday human activity, there was a striking similarity in their responses. In each case, the square for nonverbal behavior was about three times bigger than the one for verbal behavior. It must be admitted, however, that we are so ignorant of the hidden aspects of nonverbal behavior that it would be impossible to make quantitative assessments of their influence.

Nonverbal ("Prosematic") Behavior.   Nonverbal behavior mirrors in part what Freud (1900) called primary processes. In drawing a distinction between verbal and nonverbal behavior it is easier to see differences than similarities. But in a very real sense, nonverbal behavior like verbal behavior, has its semantics and syntax—in other words, *meaning* and *orderly arrangement* of specific acts.

It is nonverbal behavior that we possess in common with animals. Since it is hardly appropriate to refer to nonverbal behavior of animals,[19] it is desirable to use some other term for this kind of behavior. The Greek word "σημα" pertains to a sign, mark, or token. By adding the prefix "προ" in the particular sense of "rudimentary" one obtains the word "prosematic" which would be appropriate for referring to any kind of nonverbal signal— vocal, bodily, chemical.[34, 36]

It has been the special contribution of ethology to provide the first systematic insights into the semantics and syntax of animal behavior.[21, 48]

An analysis of prosematic behavior of animals reveals that somewhat parallel to words, sentences, and paragraphs, it becomes meaningful in terms of its components, constructs, and sequences of constructs. Since the patterns of behavior involved in self-preservation and survival of the species are generally similar in most terrestrial vertebrates, it is rather meaningless to speak, as in the past, of species-specific behavior. But since various species perform these behaviors in their own typical ways, it is both correct and useful to refer to species-typical behavior.

Introspectively, we recognize that prosematic communication may be either active or passive. When two or more individuals are within communicative distance, there is the possibility for either active ("intentional") or passive ("unintentional") communication to occur with respect to the "sender" or "receiver." Even when an individual is alone a sound, utterance, movement, or odor emanating from the self may have self-communicative value as it originates either actively or passively.

SYNOPSIS OF EXPERIMENTAL WORK

For the past 25 years, my research has been primarily concerned with identifying and analyzing forebrain mechanisms underlying prosematic forms of behavior which on phylogenetic and clinical grounds might be inferred to represent expressions of "paleopsychic" processes. In this work, I have taken a comparative evolutionary approach which has the advantage that it allows one to telescope millions of years into a span that can be seen all at once, and as in plotting a curve makes it possible to see trends that would not otherwise be apparent. It also shows the usefulness of research on animals for obtaining insights into brain mechanisms underlying human prosematic behavior.

Since animal experimentation provides us our only systematic knowledge of brain functions, I should comment briefly on the justification of using findings on animals for drawing inferences about the workings of the human brain. At the molecular or cellular levels, there is general enthusiasm for applying findings on animals to human biology. In the field of psychiatry, neurochemical and neuropharmacological discoveries in animals have radically changed the treatment of certain neuropsychiatric disorders. But many people believe that behavioral and neurological observations on animals have little or no human relevance.

Such a bias perhaps stems from a failure to realize that in its evolution, the human brain expands in hierarchic fashion along the lines of three basic patterns which were mentioned earlier and characterized (Figure 1) as reptilian, paleomammalian, and neomammalian. It deserves reemphasis that the three formations are markedly different in chemistry and structure and in an evolutionary sense eons apart. Extensively interconnected, the three basic formations represent an amalgamation of three-brains-in-one, or what may be appropriately called a *triune* brain.[28, 32, 33] The word triune also serves to imply that the "whole" is greater than the sum of its parts, because with the exchange of information among the three formations each derives a greater amount of information than if it were operating alone. Stated in popular terms, the amalgamation amounts to three interconnected biological computers, with each inferred to have its own special intelligence, its own subjectivity, its own sense of time and space, and its own memory, motor, and other functions.

This scheme for subdividing the brain may seem simplistic, but thanks to improved anatomical, physiological, and chemical techniques, the three basic formations stand out in clearer detail than ever before. Moreover, it should be emphasized that despite their extensive interconnections, there is evidence that each brain type is capable of operating somewhat independently. Most important in regard to the "verbal-nonverbal" question, there are clinical indications that the reptilian and paleomammalian formations lack the neural machinery for verbal communication. To say that they lack the power of speech, however, does not belittle their intelligence, nor does it relegate them subjectively to the realm of the "unconscious."

The basic neural machinery required for self-preservation and the preservation of the species is built into the neural chassis contained in the midbrain, pons, medulla, and spinal cord. As shown by the early experiments of Ferrier[12] and others, an animal with only its neural chassis is as motionless and aimless as an idling vehicle without a driver. But this analogy stops short because with the evolution of the forebrain, the neural chassis acquires three drivers, all of different minds and all vying for control.

The Reptilian-Type brain. Let us look first at the reptilian "driver." In mammals, the major counterpart of the reptilian forebrain is represented by a group of large ganglia including the olfactostriatum, corpus striatum (caudate nucleus and putamen), globus pallidus, and satellite gray matter. Since there is no name that applies to all of these structures, I shall refer to them in this synopsis as the R-complex. As shown in Figure 2, the stain for cholinesterase reveals a remarkable chemical contrast between the R-complex and the two other cerebrotypes. The shaded areas in Figure 3 show how this stain sharply demarcates the R-complex in animals ranging from reptiles to man. In using the fluorescent technique of Falck and Hillarp (1959), it is striking to see how the structures corresponding to those in the figure glow a bright green because of large amounts of dopamine.[20]

From an evolutionary standpoint it is curious that ethologists have paid little attention to reptiles, focusing instead on fishes and birds. Some authorities believe that of the existing reptiles, lizards would bear the closest resemblance to the mammal-like reptiles believed to be the forerunners of mammals. At all events, lizards and other reptiles provide illustrations of complex prototypical *patterns* of behavior commonly seen in mammals, including man. One can quickly list more than 20 such behaviors that may

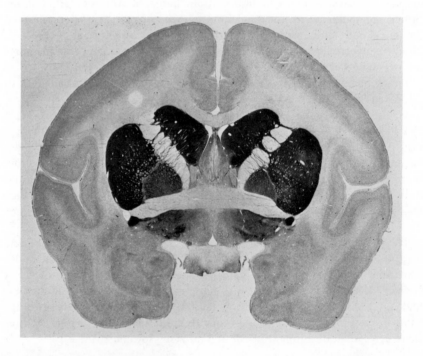

Figure 2.   This section from the brain of a squirrel monkey shows how the greater part of the R-complex is selectively colored (black areas) by a stain for cholinesterase. From Ref. 29.

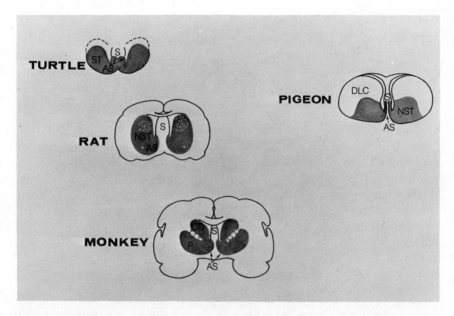

Figure 3. Shaded areas indicate how a stain for cholinesterase demarcates the greater part of the R-complex in animals ranging from reptiles to primates. With the fluorescent technique of Falck and Hillarp, the same areas shown above would glow a bright green because of the high content of dopamine. The pallidal part of the striatal complex does not fluoresce. No existing reptiles represent the forerunners of mammals. Birds are an offshoot from the *Archosauria* ("ruling reptiles"). Adapted from Ref. 42.

primarily involve self-preservation or the survival of the species[36]: (1) selection and preparation of homesite; (2) establishment of domain or territory; (3) trail making; (4) "marking" of domain or territory; (5) showing place-preferences; (6) ritualistic display in defense of territory, commonly involving the use of coloration and adornments; (7) formalized intraspecific fighting in defense of territory; (8) triumphal display in successful defense; (9) assumption of distinctive postures and coloration in signaling surrender; (10) routinization of daily activities; (11) foraging; (12) hunting; (13) homing; (14) hoarding; (15) use of defecation posts; (16) formation of social groups; (17) establishment of social hierarchy by ritualistic display and other means; (18) greeting; (19) "grooming"; (20) courtship, with displays using coloration and adornments; (21) mating; (22) breeding and, in isolated instances, attending offspring; (23) flocking; and (24) migration.

Five interoperative behaviors. There is an important *pentad* of prototypical forms of behavior of a general nature that may be variously operative in the activities above. In anticipation of some later comments, I name and briefly characterize them. They may be denoted as: (1) isopraxic, (2) perseverative, (3) reenactment, (4) tropistic, and (5) deceptive behavior. The word "isopraxic" will be used to refer to behaviors in which two or more individuals engage in the same kind of activity. Purely descriptive, it avoids preconceptions and prejudices commonly attached to such terms as social facilitation and imitation. Perseverative behavior applies to repetitious acts, such as occur in displays or in conflictive situations. Reenactment behavior refers to the repetition on different occasions of behaviors seeming to represent obeisance to precedent as, for example, following familiar trails or returning year-after-year to the same breeding grounds. Tropistic behavior is characterized by positive or negative responses to partial or complete representations of animate or inanimate objects and includes what ethologists refer to as "imprinting" and "fixed action patterns." Deceptive behavior involves the use of artifice and deceitful tactics such as are employed in stalking a prey or evading a predator. Except for altruistic behavior and most aspects of parental behavior, it is remarkable how many *patterns of behavior* seen in reptiles are also found in human beings.

As yet, hardly any investigations have been conducted on reptiles in an attempt to identify specific structures of the forebrain involved in the various behaviors listed above. All that is known thus far is that the neural guiding systems for species-typical complex forms of behavior lie forward of the neural chassis.

In contrast to reptiles, the R-complex of mammals has been subjected to extensive investigation. Curiously enough, however, 150 years of experimentation have revealed remarkably little about its functions. The finding that large destructions of the mammalian R-complex may result in no obvious impairment of movement speaks against the traditional clinical view that it subserves purely motor functions. At our Laboratory of Brain Evolution and Behavior, we are conducting comparative studies of reptiles, birds, and mammals in which we are testing the hypothesis that the R-complex plays a basic role in species-typical prosematic behavior.

In the work thus far, crucial findings relevant to prosematic behavior have developed from experiments on more than 100 squirrel monkeys (*Saimiri sciureus*). Animals of this species perform a characteristic display of the erect phallus in a show of aggression, in courtship, and as a form of greeting.[25, 44] Members of one subspecies consistently display to their reflections in a mirror, providing a means of systematically testing the effects of brain ablations on the incidence and manifestations of the display.[26] I have found that large bilateral lesions of the paleo- and neomammalian parts of the forebrain may have either no effect or only a transitory effect on the display. After bilateral lesions of the pallidal part of the R-complex,[29, 31] however, or interruption of its main pathways,[35] monkeys may no longer show an inclination to display. Without a test of the innate display behavior, one might conclude that they were unaffected by the loss of brain tissue.

These experiments provide the first evidence in mammals that the R-complex and its major pathways are basically involved in the performance of genetically constituted, species-typical, prosematic behavior. Such work represents a necessary first step for a more detailed analysis of forebrain mechanisms underlying "territorial" assertiveness, courtship, and social deportment. Since the mirror display also involves isopraxic factors, the experiments also indicate that the R-complex is implicated in *natural* forms of imitation.

The Paleomammalian Brain.   There are behavioral indications that the reptilian brain is poorly equipped for learning to cope with new situations. The reptilian brain has only a rudimentary cortex. In the lost transitional forms between reptiles and mammals—the so-called mammal-like reptiles—it is presumed that the primitive cortex underwent further elaboration and differentiation. The primitive cortex might be imagined as comparable to a crude radar screen, providing the animal a better means of viewing the environment and learning to survive. In all existing mammals the phylogenetically old cortex is found in a large convolution which the nineteenth century anatomist, Broca[4] called the great limbic lobe because it surrounds the brain stem. Limbic means "forming a border around." As illustrated in Figure 4, the limbic lobe forms a *common denominator* in the brains of *all mammals*. In 1952, I suggested the term limbic system as a designation for the limbic cortex and structures of the brain stem with which it has primary connections.[22]

The limbic cortex is structurally less complicated than the new cortex. Although it was once believed to receive information mainly from the olfactory and visceral systems, we have shown by recording from single nerve cells in awake, sitting monkeys that signals also reach it from the visual, auditory, and somatic senses.[33] There are clinical indications that the combined reception of information from the inside and outside worlds is essential for a feeling of individuality and personal identity.[30]

Also in contrast to the new cortex, the limbic cortex has large cablelike connections with the hypothalamus which has long been recognized to play a central role in integrating the performance of mechanisms involved in self-preservation and the procreation of the species.

Although the limbic system undergoes considerable expansion in the brains of higher mammals, the basic pattern of organization remains the same as in lower mammals. Electrophysiological studies have shown that

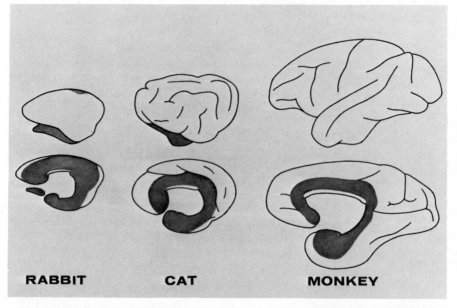

RABBIT   **CAT**   **MONKEY**

Figure 4.   The limbic lobe of Broca (shaded) is found as a common denominator in the brains of all mammals. It contains the greater part of the cortex representative of the paleomammalian brain. The cortex of the neomammalian brain (shown in white) mushrooms late in evolution. After Ref. 23.

this basically paleomammalian brain is functionally, as well as anatomically, an integrated system. In the past 40 years, clinical and experimental investigations have provided evidence that the limbic system derives information in terms of emotional feelings that guide behavior with respect to the two basic life principles of self-preservation and the preservation of the species.

Before further comment on limbic functions, it should be noted that many people maintain that it is inadmissible to make sharp distinction between "emotion" and "reason." Raphael Demos,[8] in an introduction to the dialogues of Plato, expresses a traditional philosophical view: ". . . we are apt to separate reason from emotion. Plato does not. Reason is not merely detached understanding; it is conviction, fired with enthusiasm." Piaget, the founder of the Center for Genetic Epistemology, is quite vehement, saying that "nothing could be more false or superficial" than to attempt "to dichotomize the life of the mind into emotion and thoughts." ". . . Affectivity and intelligence," he insists, "are indissociable and constitute the two complementary aspects of all human behavior" (p. 15).[43]

Granted the complementary aspects of "emotion" and "thought," we are faced with evidence from the study of "psychomotor" epilepsy that the two may occur independently because they are products of different cerebral mechanisms. Clinical observations provide the best evidence of the role of the limbic system in emotional behavior. Epileptic discharges in or near the limbic cortex result in a broad spectrum of vivid emotional feelings. It is one of the wonders of the brain that limbic discharges tend to spread in and be confined to the limbic system, not directly involving the neocortex. I have referred to this condition as a "schizophysiology"[23] and have suggested that the underlying factors may contribute to inexplicable conflicts between "what we feel" and "what we know."

In regard to structures possibly involved in mental illness, it is significant that limbic discharges may result in symptoms characteristic of the toxic and endogenous psychoses, such as feelings of depersonalization, distortions of perception, paranoid delusions, and hallucinations.[33] I referred earlier to the striking chemical differences of the three basic cerebrotypes. An accumulation of evidence indicates that many of the psychotherapeutic drugs owe their salutary effects to a selective action on the limbic system and the R-complex.

It is of special epistemological interest that at the beginning of a limbic discharge, a patient may have an intense free-floating feeling of what is real, true, and important or experience eureka-type feelings like those associated with discovery. There may be oceanic feelings such as occur in mystical revelation or under the influence of psychedelic drugs. Ironically, it seems that the ancient limbic system has the capacity to generate strong affective feelings of conviction that we attach to our beliefs, regardless of whether they are true or false!

Three Subdivisions of the Paleomammalian Brain.   The limbic system comprises three subdivisions.[24] The two older ones (see Figure 5) are closely related to the olfactory apparatus. Our experimental work has provided evidence that these two divisions are involved respectively in oral and genital functions. The findings are relevant to orosexual manifestations in feeding situations, in mating, and in aggressive behavior and violence. The close relationship between oral and genital functions seems to be due to the olfactory sense which, dating far back in evolution, is involved in both feeding and mating.

The main pathway to the third subdivision bypasses the olfactory apparatus. In evolution, this subdivision reaches its greatest development in the human brain. An assortment of evidence suggests that this remarkable expansion reflects a shift from olfactory to visual and other influences in sociosexual behavior. It is also possible that this subdivision, together with the prefrontal cortex of the neomammalian brain, has provided a neural substrate for the evolution of human empathy.

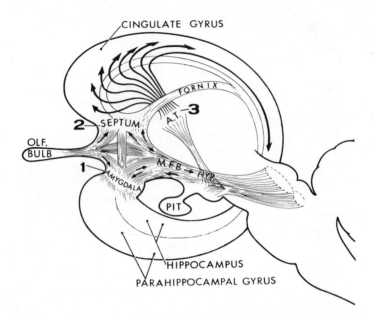

Figure 5. Diagram of three main subdivisions of the limbic system and their major pathways. See text for summary of their respective functions. Abbreviations: AT, anterior thalamic nuclei; HYP, hypothalamus; MFB, medial forebrain bundle; PIT, pituitary; OLF, olfactory. After Ref. 24.

Avenues to the Basic Personality. The major pathways to and from the reptilian-type and paleomammalian-type brains pass through the hypothalamus and subthalamic region. If the majority of these pathways are destroyed in monkeys, they are greatly incapacitated, but with careful nursing may recover the ability to feed themselves and move around. The most striking characteristic of these animals is that although they look like monkeys, they no longer behave like monkeys. Almost everything characteristic of species-typical simian behavior has disappeared. If one were to interpret these experimental findings in the light of certain clinical case material, one might say that these large connecting pathways between the reptilian and paleomammalian formations provide the avenues to the basic personality. Here, certainly, would seem to be the pathways to the expression of prosematic behavior.

The Neomammalian Brain. Compared with the limbic cortex, the neocortex (shown in white in Figure 4) is like an expanding numerator. As C. Judson Herrick has commented, "Its explosive growth late in phylogeny is one of the most dramatic cases of evolutionary transformations known to comparative anatomy."[18] The massive proportions achieved by the neo-cortex in higher mammals explains the designation of "neomammalian brain" applied to it and structures of the brain stem with which it is primarily connected. The neocortex culminates in the human brain, affording a vast neural screen for the portrayal of symbolic language and the associated functions of reading, writing, and arithmetic. Mother of invention and father of abstract thought, it promotes the preservation and procreation of ideas.[32] As opposed to the limbic cortex, the sensory systems projecting to the neocortex are primarily those giving information about the external environment—namely, the visual, auditory, and somatic systems. It therefore seems that the neocortex is primarily oriented toward the outside world. Here, perhaps, is a clue to what was mentioned earlier regarding the traditional emphasis of the sciences on the external environment.

Three Forms of Mentation

A brief discussion of questions relevant to brain research requires me to use the expressions protomentation, emotomentation, and ratiomentation. Protomentation applies to rudimentary mental processes underlying complex, prototypical forms of behavior mentioned above, as well as to propensions, a term used to cover mental states variously alluded to by such words as drives, impulses, compulsions, and obsessions. Emotomentation (emotional mentation) will refer to cerebral processes underlying what are popularly recognized as "emotions", ignoring at this time an important semantic distinction between "emotions" and "affects", as well as the classification of three species of affects that are subject to emotional expression.[28]. Paleopsychic processes are understood to cover those aspects of protomentation and emotomentation that are manifest by prosematic behavior. The meaning of ratiomentation (ratiocination) is assumed to be self-evident.

QUESTIONS RELEVANT TO BRAIN RESEARCH

In the past there has been the tendency to lump together many of the psychological processes that have just been alluded to in regard to proto-mentation and emotional mentation. Originally the German word "Trieb" which Freud (1900) used to refer to drive, impulse, or urge was inappropriately translated into English as "instinct." This twist apparently led to the commonly used expression "instinctual drives." Instincts were regarded as the biological driving forces that, analogous to the pressure head in a hydraulic system, impelled an individual to action. The pressure of the instinctive forces was believed to result in emotional feelings of an unpleasant sort, while the reduction of tension gave rise to pleasurable feelings. Freud used the impersonal word "id" (i.e., "it") to apply to the instinctual forces of the so-called "unconscious" part of the "mental personality." In 1933, at the age of 77, he stated in his *New Introductory Lectures,* "In popular language . . . we may say that the id stands for the untamed passions."[15]

Since the disposition to equate the "instincts" and "emotions" has continued to the present day, it is timely in this book to point out developments in the study of the brain and behavior that bring into better focus some distinctions between protomentation and emotional mentation. In addition to the role of protomentation in special prototypical behaviors such as are observed in the establishment of territory, we want to give consideration to the part it plays in the *pentad* of general prototypical behaviors as they become manifest in obsessive-compulsive behavior; day-to-day rituals of which we are hardly aware; the tendency to seek and give obeisance to precedent as in legal and other matters; superstitious actions; deceptive behavior; and "imitation" (isopraxis).

Because of their subjective obtrusiveness, perhaps a disproportionate emphasis has been given to the importance of "emotions" in influencing our day-to-day activities, but we should keep in mind the possibility that "emotions" may oftentimes be passive reflectors of psychic states rather than determinants of action, and that under many circumstances propense forms of protomentation may play a more basic role.

The world's literature provides abundant evidence that because of moral customs and society's numerous ways of meting out punishment for wrongdoing, we tend to give greater weight to the role of "emotions" in unpleasant affairs than in situations of joy and gratification. This biased attitude carries over into the scientific literature where one finds an authority on brain mechanisms of emotion referring to anger and fear as the "major emotions."[1]

Some Medical and Legal Aspects. The negative role assigned to the "emotions" in medical and legal matters has a long history. Miss Grange[16] points out that in the eighteenth century "moral" insanity was the equivalent of "emotional" insanity. In an article on Pinel, the well-known eighteenth-century psychiatrist, she explains how he helped to popularize the use of the word "moral" to describe emotional factors in mental experience. He believed that the chief cause of insanity was "moral," and his treatment of insanity was based on Aristotle's theory of "balancing the passions." Grange also describes how Pinel's writings inspired others to examine the emotions "in relation to health, to education, to politics, to crime, to urban and rural environments, to organic disease, and to the welfare of groups and individuals" (p. 452).[16] Today, just as two centuries ago, "emotions" are commonly believed to be the root of psychoneuroses, several forms of psychoses, "psychosomatic disease," alcoholism, narcotic addiction, implacable domestic situations, juvenile delinquency, and crime. But in all of these conditions, developing insights require that we keep in mind that protomentation may be more fundamentally involved than emotomentation, recalling, symbolically, that "the reptile does what it has to do."

There is another side of the "emotions" that has received less attention, possibly because it is considered an unalterable part of human nature. I refer now to the paradoxical capacity of emotional mentation to find support for opposite sides of any question. We take it for granted that the "emotions" will generate divisiveness in every field of discourse whether it is religious, ethical, artistic, sociological, legal, economic, political, educational, or scientific. However much this may be lamented, there is the potential benefit that argument and conflict may stir up the gene pool of ideas and lead to new and constructive concepts.

All such concerns about the "emotions" seem insignificant, however, compared with those deeply personalized feelings experienced when the utter isolation of death separates us from a loved one, or finally, after long prospect, forces itself upon each one of us.

Some Scientific Implications. After the presentation of behavioral and experimental data, it is of interest to consider how in scientific affairs protomentation and protoreptilian propensities may be influential in regard to the establishment of intellectual domain ("territory"), the idée fixe of such a scientist as Kepler, obeisance to precedent, adherence to doctrine, and intolerance of new ideas.

As regards emotional mentation, it seems a particular irony that in science, as in politics, the "emotions" make it possible to stand on any platform. How does it happen that different groups of reputable scientists presented with the same data often find themselves at opposite poles—and sometimes in bitter, acrimonious debate—because of diametric views of what is true? It is equally puzzling—and intellectually incongruous—that for years, and even centuries, the world order of science may emotionally cling to, and champion, "suspect" beliefs that are destined to crumble. What makes it psychologically possible for wise men to build higher and higher on foundations of such beliefs without fear of their sudden collapse? It is also curious that the emotional investment of some scientists is such that they remain convinced of the truth of a theory long after it has proven to be false. As the late E. G. Boring commented in paraphrasing a statement of Max Planck, "Important theories, marked for death by the discovery of contradictory evidence, seldom die before their authors."[2] In two recent essays Washburn[49] and Washburn and Ciochon[50] have made an instructive analysis of how emotional factors seem to have been instrumental in solidifying the thinking of proponents of divergent views of human evolution despite the admitted lack of sufficient data. They suggest some insightful correctives.

Why Brain Research? Why is it so necessary to investigate brain mechanisms to understand the various forms of paleopsychic processes under consideration? After all, the laws of formal thought have been derived without an understanding of the underlying machinery of the brain. It is the peculiarity of ratiomentation that it lends itself, as in the case of logic, to symbolic representation in the form of words or other signs which when semantically specified and syntactically related according to certain rules result in inevitable conclusions. A parallel situation applies to numerical procedures in which the steps of calculation can be so interlocked as to assure an outcome as predictable as the movements of a geartrain. Within a generation, we have seen the evolution from simple calculating machines to giant computers which, when programmed according to the laws of logic, can reach the solution of a problem in but a small fraction of the time formerly required.

In formal ratiomentation, we have the advantage of being able to specify the inputs into our own brains or the prosthetic brains of computers. But the situation is quite different in the case of protomentation and emotomentation. Here the known input is so obscured by an indefinable input from the person's ancestral past and personal life history that there is no means of ascertaining what the outcome will be. The successive mentational processes have neither been identified nor shown to obey laws that allow predictable conclusions.

Because of the inability to specify and control the internal input for paleopsychic processes, there is the hope that insights may be gained from an investigation of underlying mechanisms. Until the restrictions of the mechanisms are known, there can be as many explanations of paleopsychic processes as there are explicators.

Many learning theorists and behaviorists would take exception to this point of view, contending that the cranium and its contents may be regarded as a black box. Some adherents to operant conditioning claim that in utilizing the principle of reinforcement, any form of behavior can be shaped and predicted. Until it can be demonstrated, however, that neuroses in animals and human beings can be regularly induced and alleviated by operant techniques, one may reserve judgment about such claims.

Jeans has stated that "physics gives us exact knowledge because it is based on exact measurements." But if the ultimate scientific instrument, the human brain, is for one reason or another predisposed to artifactual interpretations, where does confidence lie in any field?

Time and Space. Although nuclear physicists are quick to point out the "evaporation" of the material world at the atomic level, many of them seem to retain an abiding faith in the existence of time and space. They would contend that if all particles were to disappear from the universe, space and time would still remain. There is an evident inconsistency in such an argument when we relook at what Kant said about the "transcendental aesthetic." In view of the tripartite division of the brain under consideration, we want to keep in mind the question whether there exist "reptilian time," "paleomammalian time," and "neomammalian time." A parallel question applies to space. Recently, students of environmental design have begun to consider the latter question in connection with urban planning and the desirable uses of space.[10, 17, 37]

CONCLUDING COMMENT

In these introductory remarks on the evolution of three mentalities, it has been the implication that the reptilian, paleomammalian, and neomammalian formations provide three underlying neural mechanisms for what have been provisionally referred to as protomentation, emotomentation, and ratiomentation. At the same time, I have used the expression *triune brain* to symbolize that no hard and fast boundaries exist between the three formations and their respective functions. With these provisions, I use a metaphor to summarize:

In the field of literature it is recognized that there is an irreducible number of basic plots and associated emotions. In describing the functions of the triune brain metaphorically, one might imagine that the reptilian brain provides the basic plots and actions; that the limbic brain influences emotionally the developments of the plots; while the neomammalian brain has the capacity to expound the plots and emotions in as many ways as there are authors.

With respect to epistemics, particular attention will be given to an analysis of clinical and experimental findings (some of which have been mentioned) that indicate that the two older evolutionary formations of the brain are fundamentally involved in the psychogenesis of propense and affective states and that their projecting pathways are essential for the prosematic expression of the basic personality.

Other problems to be considered include the major one concerning mechanisms of intercommunication of the three evolutionary formations which are so radically different in anatomy and chemistry. A discussion of this problem requires our delving not only into anatomical questions, but also into the nature of biochemical and bioelectrical signaling devices. Whatever these intersignaling devices are, it must be inferred that they involve nonverbal coding. Stated otherwise, there are indications that with the evolution of the forebrain structures underlying the three mentalities in question, no provision was made for intercommunication by the use of words. Expressed in phrases from the introductory quotation, this situation may help to explain "the insufficiency . . . of the laws of the understanding, to resolve these problems which lie nearer to our hearts. . . ."

REFERENCES

1. Bard, P.: A diencephalic mechanism for the expression of rage with special reference to the sympathetic nervous system. *Amer. J. Physiol.* **84**:490–513, 1928.

2. Boring, E. G.: Cognitive dissonance: Its use in science. *Science,* **145**:680–685, 1964.

3. Bridgman, P. W.: *The Way Things Are,* Harvard University Press, Cambridge, Mass., 1959, 333 pp.

4. Broca, P.: Anatomie comparée des circonvolutions cérébrales. Le grand lobe limbique et la scissure limbique dans la série des mammifères. *Rev. Anthropol.* **1**:385–498, 1878.

5. Calhoun, J. B.: Population density and social pathology. *Sci. Amer.* **206**:139–146, 1962.

6. Calhoun, J. B.: Space and the strategy of life. In *Behavior and Environment,* A. H. Esser, (Ed.), Plenum Press, New York, 1971, pp. 329–387.

7. Chance, M.: Towards the biological definition of ethics. In *Biology and Ethics,* J. Ebling, (Ed.), Academic Press, New York and London, 1969.

8. Demos, R.: Introduction. In *The Dialogues of Plato,* Transl. B Jowett, Random House, New York, 2 vols., 1937, 879 pp. and 939 pp.

9. Descartes, R.: *The Philosophical Works of Descartes,* Transl. E. S. Haldane and G. R. T. Ross, Cambridge University Press, Cambridge, Mass., 2 vols., 1967, 452 pp. and 380 pp.

10. Esser, A. H.: Environment and mental health. *Sci. Med. Man,* **1**:181–193, 1974.

11. Falck, B. and Hillarp, N. A.: On the cellular localization of catecholamines in the brain. *Acta Anat.,* **38**:277–279, 1959.

12. Ferrier, D.: *The Functions of the Brain,* Smith, Elder, and Company, London, 1876.

13. Foerster, H. von, Mora, P. M., and Amiot, L. W.: Doomsday: Friday, 13 November, A.D. 2026. *Science,* **132**:1291–1295, 1960.

14. Freud, S.: *The Interpretation of Dreams,* (1900) Standard Edition, Hogarth Press, London, 1953.

15. Freud, S.: *New Introductory Lectures on Psychoanalysis,* Transl. W. J. H. Sprott, The Hogarth Press and The Institute of Psycho-Analysis, London, 1949, 239 pp.

16. Grange, K. M., Pinel and eighteenth-century psychiatry. *Bull. Hist. Med.* **35**:442–453, 1961.

17. Greenbie, B.: *Design for Diversity,* Elsevier Scientific Publishing Company, Amsterdam, in press.

18. Herrick, C. J.: The functions of the olfactory parts of the cerebral cortex. *Proc. Nat. Acad. Sci. USA,* **19**:7–14, 1933.

19. Hinde, R. A.: *Non-Verbal Communication,* The University Press, Cambridge, Mass., 1972, 443 pp.

20. Juorio, A. V., and Vogt, M.: Monoamines and their metabolites in the avian brain. *J. Physiol.* **189**:489–518, 1967.

21. Lorenz, K. Z.: The companion in the bird's world. *Auk,* **54**:245–273, 1937.

22. MacLean, P. D.: Some psychiatric implications of physiological studies on frontotemporal portion of limbic system (visceral brain). *Electroenceph. Clin. Neurophysiol.* **4**:407–418, 1952.

23. MacLean, P. D.: The limbic system and its hippocampal formation. Studies in animals and their possible application to man. *J. Neurosurg.* **11**:29–44, 1954.

24. MacLean, P. D.: Contrasting functions of limbic and neocortical systems of the brain and their relevance to psychophysiological aspects of medicine. *Amer. J. Med.* **25**:611–626, 1958.

25. MacLean, P. D.: New findings relevant to the evolution of psychosexual functions of the brain. *J. Nerv. Ment. Dis.* **135**:289–301, 1962.

26. MacLean, P. D.: Mirror display in the squirrel monkey, Saimiri sciureus. *Science,* **146**:950–952, 1964.

27. MacLean, P. D.: The brain in relation to empathy and medical education. *J. Nerv. Ment. Dis.* **144**:374–382, 1967.

28. MacLean, P. D.: The triune brain, emotion, and scientific bias. In *The Neurosciences Second Study Program,* F. O. Schmitt (Ed.), The Rockefeller University Press, New York, 1970, pp. 336–349.

29. MacLean, P. D.: Cerebral evolution and emotional processes: New findings on the striatal complex. *Ann. N.Y. Acad. Sci.* **193**:137–149, 1972.

30. MacLean, P. D.: Implications of microelectrode findings on exteroceptive inputs to the limbic cortex. In *Limbic System Mechanisms and Autonomic Function,* C. H. Hockman, (Ed.), Charles C Thomas, Springfield, 1972, pp. 115–136.

31. MacLean, P. D.: Effects of pallidal lesions on species-typical display behavior of squirrel monkey. *Fed. Proc.* **32**:384, 1973.

32. MacLean, P. D.: The brain's generation gap: Some human implications. *Zygon J. Relig. Sci.,* **8**:113–127, 1973.

33. MacLean, P. D.: A triune concept of the brain and behavior, Lecture I. Man's reptilian and limbic inheritance; Lecture II. Man's limbic brain and the psychoses; Lecture III. New trends in man's evolution. In *The Hincks Memorial Lectures,* T. Boag, and D. Campbell, (Eds.), University of Toronto Press, Toronto, 1973, pp. 6–66.

34. MacLean, P. D.: The triune brain. In *Medical World News,* Special Supplement on "Psychiatry," New York, October, 1974a, Vol. 1, pp. 55–60.

35. MacLean, P. D.: Role of pallidal projections in species-typical behavior of squirrel monkey. *Trans. Amer. Neurol. Assoc.,* 100 1975, 110–113.

36. MacLean, P. D.: An evolutionary approach to brain research on "prosematic" (nonverbal) behavior. In *The Daniel S. Lehrman Memorial Symposium* on *Reproductive Behavior and Evolution,* Institute of Animal Behavior, Rutgers University, 1974, (to be published).

37. Mallows, E. W. N.: Urban planning and the systems approach. (I. B. M. System & Engineering Symposium, October, 1969) *Plan* (Successor to *S. A. Archit. Rec.*), **55**:11–24, 1970.

38. Meadows, D. H., Meadows, D. L., Randers, J., and Behrens, III, W. W.: *The Limits to Growth,* Universe Books, New York, 1972, 205 pp.

39. Monod, J.: *Chance and Necessity,* A. A. Knopf, New York, 1971.

40. Morsbach, H.: Aspects of nonverbal communication in Japan. *J. Nerv. Ment. Dis.* **157**:262–277, 1973.

41. Myers, K., Hale, C. S., Myktowycz, R., and Hughes, R. L.: The effects of varying density and space on sociality and health in animals. In *Behavior and Environment,* A. H. Esser, (Ed.), Plenum Press, New York, 1971, pp. 148–187.

42. Parent, A. and Olivier, A.: Comparative histochemical study of the corpus striatum. *J. Hirnforsch.* **12**:75–81, 1970.

43. Piaget, J.: *Six Psychological Studies,* Transl. A. Tenzer, Random House, New York, 1967, 169 pp.

44. Ploog, D. W., and MacLean, P. D.: Display of penile erection in squirrel monkey (Saimiri sciureus). *Anim. Behav.* **11**:32–39, 1963.

45. Shakow, D., and Rapaport, D.: The influence of Freud on American psychology. In *Psychological Issues,* International Universities Press, New York, 1964, Vol. 4, Monograph 13, 243 pp.

46. Snow, C. P.: *Variety of Men,* Charles Scribner's Sons, New York, 1967, 270 pp.

47. Spencer, H.: *Principles of Psychology,* D. Appleton and Company, New York, 2 vols., 1896.

48. Tinbergen, N.: *The Study of Instinct,* The Clarendon Press, Oxford, 1951, 228 pp.

49. Washburn, S. L.: The evolution game. *J. Hum. Evol.* **2**:557–561, 1973.

50. Washburn, S. L., and Ciochon, R. L.: Canine teeth: Notes on controversies in the study of human evolution. (in press)

51. Watson, J. B.: *Behaviorism,* The People's Institute Publishing Company, New York, 1924, 251 pp.

52. Weisberger, B. A.: *Book Review of "Black Mountain,"* The Washington Post, Washington, D.C., November 19, 1972.

53. Wiener, N.: *Cybernetics, or Control and Communication in the Animal and the Machine,* Wiley, New York, 1948, 194 pp.

CHAPTER SIXTEEN

PATHOGENIC AND NEUROPATHOLOGIC ASPECTS OF SOME NEUROPSYCHOTROPIC AGENTS

L. ROIZIN, M.D.

The "drug culture" and the "pill myth" have created conditions conducive to "drug abuse" and "drug dependence." Moreover, the increased and prolonged use of neuropsychotropic agents for the treatment of psychiatric and behavioral disorders frequently lead to multiple drug therapies. The latter, when further complicated by erratic consumption of alcohol[36] or by the occurrence of medical, psychiatric, and socioeconomical pathogenic cofactors, often induce multiple chemical-biological interactions that may potentiate, aggravate, or precipitate adverse or toxic reactions and even fatalities.

This chapter is limited to the salient pathogenic and neuropathologic aspects of the most commonly used neuropsychotropic agents for the treatment of various psychiatric disorders or hedonistic aims. The material used in the present study consisted of: (a) *Human* central nervous system and viscera of patients who developed adverse or toxic reactions, organic brain syndrome, and/or coma caused by accidental or intentional overdosage after having consumed: (1) tranquilizers; (2) opiates and narcotics; (3) amphetamines; (4) hallucinogens; and (5) lithium. The investigative and control material was obtained from various hospitals and institutions of the New York State Dept. of Mental Hygiene, through the Neuropathologic Registry at the New York State Psychiatric Institute and from the Chief Medical Examiner's Office of the Forensic Institute, New York City.[42-44] This material, combined with the review cases from the literature, amounted to a total of 1725 cases. (b) *Experimental*: up to the present time a total of 4033 animals were used for acute and chronic neurotoxicologic studies. This included mice, rats, and monkeys of both sexes and variable ages (from embryos to adults). (c) Spinal cord ganglia *tissue cultures*.

TRANQUILIZERS

The phenothiazines represent the most widely used drugs among tranquilizers.[14, 25] The adverse or toxic drug reactions involving the CNS and extraneural functions have been extensively reviewed by several authors.[12, 13, 23, 31, 37, 49] Most of these adverse or toxic effects are mild, transitory, and reversible in character[49] except the tardive dyskinesias.[12, 13, 37] However, some fatalities have been reported.[8, 13, 19, 22, 45, 49] Prenatal and teratogenic effects have also been observed by several investigators.[21, 24, 50]

Biochemical[17] studies of postmortem specimens of a patient treated for approximately 4 years with chlorpromazine, revealed the following drug concentrations (in descending order): lungs, liver, gallbladder (and bile), intestines, testis, hypophysis, adrenals, pancreas and in the CNS: thalamus and hypothalamus, temporal lobe and hippocampus, cerebellum, medulla, spinal cord (upper cervical), pons lenticular nucleus and corpus callosum. Tissue concentration of chlorpromazine in laboratory animals[5, 6, 11, 54] showed, with some individual variations, the following tissue distributions: lungs, liver, spleen, kidneys, intestine, and in the brain: cerebral cortex, basal ganglia, spinal cord, and cerebellum.

Histochemical studies[46] demonstrated distinct cytomorphologic patterns in different anatomotopographic regions of the CNS.

Histopathologic findings: biopsies of the liver, in patients with liver dysfunctions, showed various degrees of cholestasis associated, at times, with biliary thrombi in the central canaliculi and deposits of biliary pigment in the hepatic parenchymal and Kupffer cells and, at times, increased sudanophilia of hepatic parenchyma and occasional necrosis.[34, 4, 49] In human postmortem examinations, the most outstanding visceral pathology consisted of cholestasis and/or liver degeneration (at times with hepatitis), nephrosis (at times with biliary plugs), bronchopneumonia, petechial hemorrhages in the lungs, liver, myocardium, kidneys, and spleen.[30, 49]

The most significant neuropathologic findings were expressed by nonspecific variable chromatolysis and, at times, anoxic changes and various degrees of lipid degeneration, psuedo- or neuronophagia in various areas of the brain cortex, basal ganglia, hypothalamus and cerebellum, dystrophic alterations of the glia, and, at times, increased vascular permeability.[8, 13, 45, 49] In some instances paucity of neurons and depigmentation of substantia nigra in the mesencephalon were prominent.[46] Laboratory animals, in different experimental conditions, mainly after high and toxic dosages, presented a variety of histopathologic changes of the liver and CNS.[33, 45, 49]

Ultrastructural[46, 47] changes, particularly of the organelles, endoplasmic reticulum, qualitative, and quantitative variations of ribosomes, and some membrane systems, were also observed in the liver and CNS cellular constituents (including synapses and their content) *in vivo* and *in vitro*.

OPIATES AND NARCOTICS

The most prominent neuropathological findings, in chronic opiate addiction, consisted of fibrous proliferation of the leptomeninges, edema of the brain, degenerative changes of the cerebral neurons and Purkinje cells, lipid infiltration, pyknosis, satellitosis, and progressive degeneration leading to patchy neuronal loss. Symmetrical softening of the globus pallidus and early softening of the cerebral cortex, including laminary necrosis of

Ammon's horn similar to cerebral anoxia, were observed in cases who survived larger doses.[43]

Cocaine and derivatives can produce lesions similar to opiates. Injection for spinal anesthesia have caused, in individual cases, regional degeneration of the anterior horn cells with some demylination.[55] In fatalities following injections, nuclear chromatolysis and dissolution of Nissl substance in neurons of the CNS[32] and perivascular ring hemorrhages[3] were seen. In chronic cocaine addiction, mild neuronal degeneration with lipid infiltration resembling those in morphinism (see below) were detected.

Morphine:[43] Acute morphine toxicity is associated with congestion of blood vessels (particularly larger veins) with diapedesis of erythrocytes, perivascular hemorrhages, and cerebral edema. In some cases, the white matter of the brain appears studded with hemorrhagic petechiae.[10]

In chronic morphine addicts fibrous thickening of the leptomeninges, degenerative changes of the cortical nerve cells (particularly pyramidal) with patchy loss of neurons, nonspecific lipid degeneration of the nerve cells, microglia, and endothelial cells, and thickening of the blood vessel walls were encountered.[10] In experimental animals (surviving up to 20 days) pyknosis of small and medium size pyramidal cells, loss of tigroid material, swelling, homogenization or vesicle formation in the cytoplasm of neurons, clumping of nuclear chromatin, beadlike swelling of dendrites, and focal hemorrhages in the CNS were detected. In more chronic conditions, morphologic alterations with fatty degeneration were prominent, particularly in the cerebral cortex, corpus striatum, and Ammon's horn. It is not certain whether such changes are the intercurrent effects (depression) on the respiratory and cardiac centers with the resulting anoxic effects or whether they may be related to secondary vasomotor reactions.

Heroin and current clinical-pathological aspects of this drug dependence has been discussed in an exuberant number of papers. The neurotoxicologic and particularly the neuropathologic features have been summarized in the following recent publications.[42-44] The fatality rate among heroin addicts (between the ages 15 and 35) undergoing methadone-maintenance treatment ranges between 1 and 1.3%. This percentage appears to rise to 10% among drug abuse patients who have been discharged or who have voluntarily discontinued the detoxification or withdrawal treatment. Alcohol, multiple drug intake, medical and behavioral, or psychiatric cofactors represent the most common potentiating and aggravating elements.

The most common anatomopathological findings in heroin addicts are represented by: pulmonary edema (may also result from hypoxia due to respiratory depression or failure) and pulmonary complications, liver pathology (hepatitis, liver degeneration, and postnecrotic cirrhosis), secondary infections (viral, bacterial, mycotic), trauma (violent deaths, accidents, etc.), cardiovascular, and, in some instances, renal insufficiency, chondroosteomyelitis, transverse myelitis, anaphylactic, or allergic mechanisms.

The neuropathologic findings include a variety of mild to prominent nonspecific neuronal degeneration in various anatomotopographic regions of the CNS, some of which recall the microscopic features of an anoxic process.

The histopathologic changes of the liver were expressed principally by hepatitis (Figure 1*a* and *b*) and lipid degeneration of the hepatic cells (Figure 1*c* and *d*).

Moderate to prominent degrees of alterations in distribution and concentration of enzyme reaction products of TPP,* G-6-P,** and AcP† occurred in various cytoarchitectural and anatomotopographical regions of the CNS. In addition, perivascular glial (principally astrocytic) reactions were more prominent in TPP preparations which, at times, showed also increased vascular permeability as illustrated in Figure 2*a–c*.

The most pronounced electron microscope changes in the CNS were related to the ultrastructure and distribution of the endoplasmic reticulum (particularly Golgi complex) (Figure 3*a* and *b*), mitochondrial pleomorphism, ribosomes, synaptic complex, and their subunits, degenerative products in the cellular cytoplasm, vascular walls, and perivascular regions. Of particular significance is also the presence of axonal degeneration and dystrophies as well as some senile plaquelike formations.[43] In the liver alterations and, at times, the disorganization of the endoplasmic reticulum and related subunits of mitochondria, multivesicular bodies, heterogenous and membranous structures, and abnormal amounts of lipid products (Figure 4*a*), glycogen granules (Figure 4*b*) as well as necrobiotic material (Figure 4*c*) were prominent. Additional research is required to determine the specificity of the pathological processes related to the interaction or combined action of multiple biodynamic factors (see pathogenesis), heroin and methadone, particularly in long-term consumption. In relation with the latter, one should be aware of (*a*) severe toxic effects and fatalities occurring in children following accidental ingestion of concentrated doses of methadone; (*b*) variable enzyme reaction patterns; and (*c*) presence of ultrastructural changes in the CNS and liver in rats following the administration of concentrated doses of methadone.

* Thiamine pyrophosphatase.
** Glucose-6-phosphatase.
† Acid phosphatase.

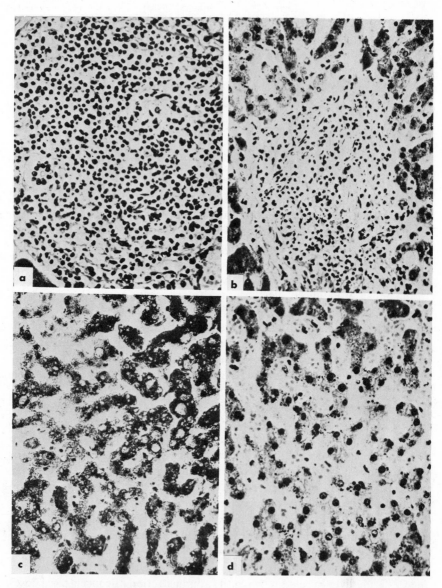

Figure 1.   Human liver: *a* and *b*: hepatitis; the inflammatory exudate is composed principally of mononuclear cells. Hematoxylin and Eosin stain; magnifications *a*: 416× and *b*: 312×; *c* and *d*: various degrees of degenerative changes involving, in particular, the hepatic cells; *c*: Sudan III stain, magnification: 260×; and *d*: Hematoxylin and Eosin stain, magnification: 640×. 416×

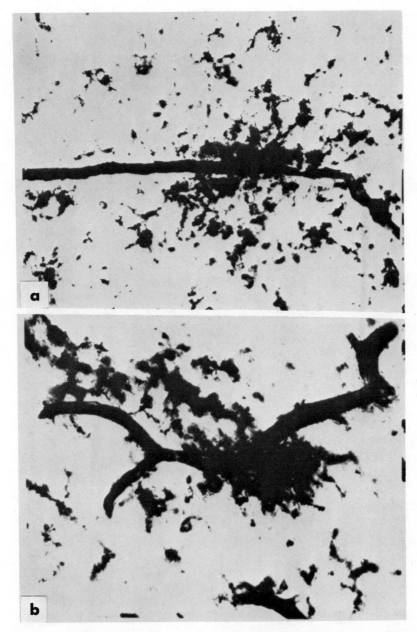

Figure 2.   Rat CNS: frontal cortex (*a* and *b*) showing various degrees of perivascular glial reactions associated with increased vascular permeability. Thiamine pyrophosphatase method, magnifications: *a*: 360× and *b*: 540×.

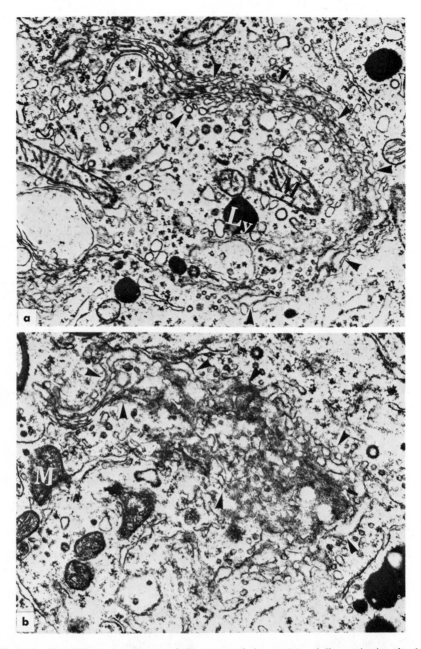

Figure 3. Rat CNS: various degrees of ultrastructural changes (*a*) and disorganization (*b*) of the endoplasmic reticulum, especially of the Golgi complex (arrows); Uranyl acetate and lead citrate counterstains. RCA,EMU-3G electron microscope, magnifications: *a*: 20,280× and *b*: 26,364×; M = mitochondria, Ly = lysosomes.

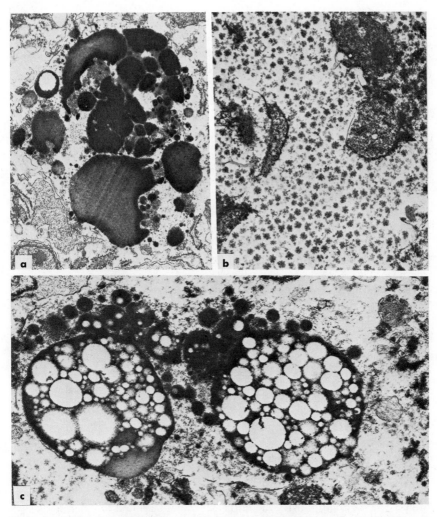

Figure 4. Human liver: abnormal presence of lipid products (*a*), glycogen granules (*b*), and necrobiotic material undergoing various degrees of metabolization or digestion (*c*). Uranyl acetate and lead citrate counterstains. RCA,EMU-3G, magnification: 16,900×.

STIMULANTS OF THE CNS

Amphetamines

Toxic reactions and "amphetamine psychosis" (chronic course and dementia) with reversible and irreversible organic changes of the brain are well known.[51-53] Lesions of vascular character expressed by congestion and subdural and subarachnoid petechiae, flat gyri, neuronal swelling, and tigrolysis, occasional neuroglial degeneration, and scattered pericapillary hemorrhages have been reported in some amphetamine fatalities.[9] Cortical neuronal degeneration was found in long-term users of amphetamines with clinical evidence of organic brain syndrome.[20, 51] Biochemical studies detected a decrease of aerobic lactic acid formation in the brains of patients and experimental animals with chronic amphetamine intoxication. More recent biochemical and metabolic investigations support the view that the central stimulatory action of the amphetamine and its peripheral sympathomimetic effects are mediated through the release of catecholamines. It has been suggested that the adrenergic receptor could be a component of the adenyl cyclase system. As far as the brain tissue is concerned, subcellular distribution studies of adenyl cyclase are compatible with synaptic localization and extrapolation from studies with pineal gland homogenates suggests a postsynaptic localization. Furthermore, electron microscope examinations of the CNS affected by experimental chronic methamphetamine intoxication[28] disclosed coalescence of membranes between axons at the nerve endings and between axons and dendrites, and hypertrophy as well as hyperplasia of the endoplasmic reticulum within the cytoplasm of neurons. Some of these ultrastructural findings may be indicative of possible disturbance of neural conduction and transmission mechanisms in the CNS.

Hallucinogens

LSD-25 (lysergic acid diethylamide-25) is, among a variety of hallucinogens (mescaline), DOM (2.5-dimetoxy-4-methyl-amphetamine hydrochloride), DMT, and DET (dimethyl and diethyltryptamine, respectively), psilocybin, different species of morning glory, one of the most commonly used and abused.[43, 48] Special attention has been recently focused upon its behavioral and interaction with narcotics and alcohol[44] as well as possible teratogenic effects.[24, 48] In relation with the latter, it should be noted that solutions with molecular weight below 500 pass through the placenta[26] and accumulate in the fetal blood. The blood brain barrier is more permeable in the fetus and newborn than in the adult. Fetal vulnerability to noxious agents and anoxia is particularly more prominent in the first trimester of gestation. Also children are more vulnerable than adults, while elderly people, undernourished, infirm, and under stress, have decreased tolerance to toxicity.[2, 56] The very rare cases of lethal overdose die in a short period of time without revealing remarkable CNS changes except "cardiac collapse." Neuropathologic observations, thus far, are forthcoming from experimental investigations.[7, 27, 48] Nuclear vacuolization associated with disappearance of nuclear chromatin and intranuclear Nissl staining granules, cytoplasmic chromatolysis, as well as depletion of Nissl substance and neuronal degeneration in cerebral cortex were detected following the use of variable doses in acute and chronic studies. Some hepatic cells also displayed nuclear vacuolization. Acid and alkaline phosphatases[7] in the CNS of LSD-25 treated animals disclosed some qualitative changes including liver and kidneys. Reversible changes and decrease of Nissl substance with concomitant alterations of the nucleus and nucleolus, contraction of oligodendroglia and, at times, increased number of glia were also observed in CNS cultures after administration of LSD-25.

Electron microscope examinations of neurons of spinal cord ganglia tissue cultures revealed alterations of the fine structure of the nucleoli, and endoplasmic reticulum, qualitative and quantitative variations of lysosomes, mitochondria, multivesicular bodies, as well as prominent pleomorphism, and proliferation of some organelle membranes. In this relation it is of interest to note the binding of LSD to subcellular fraction from brain[16] and brain membranes.[4]

Lithium[39]

The administration of lithium salts has been revived recently particularly in the treatment of protracted or recurrent manic phases of manic depressive psychosis. The mechanisms of lithium toxicity and its residual effects is still obscure with the exception of renal involvement. In addition, a slight effect or toxic reaction involving the central nervous system has been observed even during therapeutic doses.

To examine the neurotoxicological effects, short- and long-term experiments with variable routes of administration and doses of lithium carbonate or lithium chloride were carried out in different strains of animals maintained on special low sodium diets. Only the studies on the acute phase in rats have been reported. The drug was administered by: (a) intravenous infusion (I.V.) and (b) intraperitoneal injection (I.P.).

Dosage. (a) I.V.: Varied between 0 to 11.7 meq/kg of lithium administered as the chloride salt. (b) I.P.: 11.5 to 35.4 meq/kg. The animals were frequently examined and after lithium administration were under constant observation. Physiological parameters were examined by the E&M Physiograph which recorded pulse, blood pressure, and respiration. Prior to and following lithium administration, blood samples were taken for lithium estimation.

Results. Some of the earliest clinical responses noted (2 to 5 minutes after initiation of I.V. infusion) on qualitative observations were changes in the pulse rhythm and rate of respiration. In one of the animals, which

TABLE 1. LITHIUM LEVELS IN BLOOD SAMPLES TAKEN AT DIFFERENT INTERVALS FOLLOWING ADMINISTRATION[a]

| Male Rat No. | Lithium Administered (meq/kg) | Time of Sample[a] (minutes) | Concentration in Blood | |
			Hemoglobin (mols/liter)	Lithium (meq/liter)
7138	11.8	—	8.3	15.8
7157	17.7	9	4.9[c]	37.2[d]
7167	17.7	15	9.7	23.5
7193	17.7	20	8.6[b]	23.0[d]
7185	17.7	26	8.2[b]	20.3[d]
7178	17.7	30	12.4[b]	15.2[d]
7160	17.7	30	9.2	13.9
7163	35.4	>30	—	24.5[d]

[a] Time interval from beginning of infusion to collection of sample.
[b] Samples collected before infusion, average 8.6 mols/liter.
[c] Samples collected before infusion, 6.9 mols/liter.
[d] Samples collected before lithium infusion were below the level of sensitivity of 1.5 meq/liter.

received 150 mg/100 g body weight, the Physiograph recordings demonstrated an approximate 25% increase in pulse rate and about 70% increase in respiration rate with an associated decrease in depth. The animal died within 30 minutes after injection. It is of interest to note that the enhancement of the pulse and respiratory rate diminished gradually during this time. In some other animals irregularities in pulse and respiration rates were also observed. Animals that survived for 24 hours presented various degrees of a tendency to sleepiness, reduced spontaneous activity, awkwardness, hunched posture, an inclination to retreat into a corner of the cage, and intermittent tremors of the whole body. At times the body tremors were activated or enhanced by stimulation. On some occasions, mechanical stimuli or noises caused the animals either to jump or leap in the air like a kangaroo or to run for a short distance with a wobbling or ataxic gait of the posterior extremities. In addition, the majority of the animals were affected by diarrhea and polyuria followed by anuria. In these instances some animals became lethargic and semicomatose which was followed by coma and eventually death by failure of blood pressure and respiratory functions.

The majority of the animals tolerated well the low sodium diet. All the animals gained weight for the duration of the current experiments which lasted up to 40 days.

Lithium levels. At various time intervals following lithium injections blood samples were collected and analyzed. The lithium levels in blood are summarized in Table 1. As can be seen, the concentration in blood reflects the dose levels. In addition, the concentration in blood decreased with time. For instance, after administration of 17.7 meq/kg the blood level at 9 minutes is 37.2 meq/liter, at 20 minutes is 23.0 meq/liter and at 30 minutes is 15.2 meq/liter. In most samples the hemoglobin levels were approximately normal. However, in one animal the level was below normal

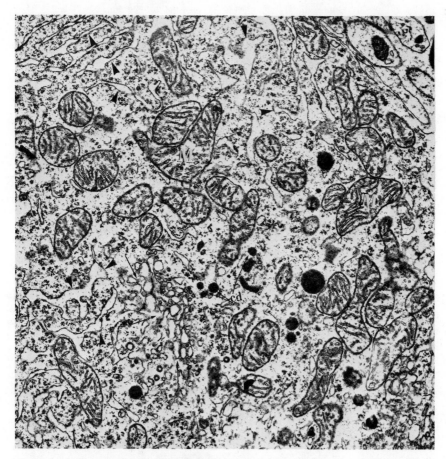

Figure 5. Rat hypothalamus: demonstrating in particular increased number of mitochondria or polymorphometabolosomes (M): Uranyl acetate and lead citrate, RCA,EMU-3G, magnification: 16,820×. Long arrows: Golgi complex, short arrows: rough endoplasmic reticulum; D.C. = dense core vesicles.

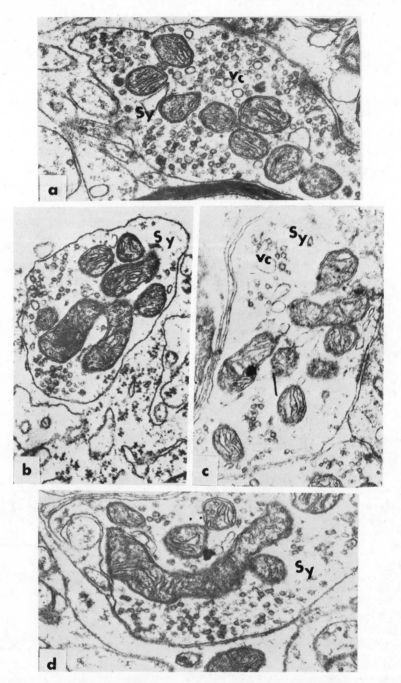

Figure 6. Rat hypothalamus: increase in number of PMS in synaptic (Sy) terminals and quantitative variations of synaptic vesicles. RCA,EMU-3G. Uranyl acetate and lead citrate, magnification: 29,000×. C.V. = synaptic vesicles.

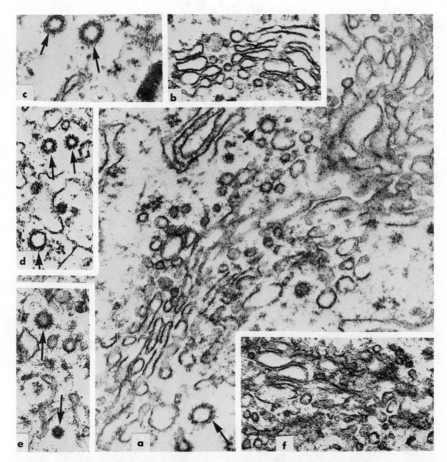

Figure 7.   Rat CNS: variations in distribution, structural patterns and osmiophilia of the Golgi complex (canaliculi and subunits). The arrows indicate: thickening, coating or incrustation-like features of the limiting membranes. Uranyl acetate and lead citrate. RCA,EMU-3G. *a*: pons, *b*: pons, *c*: hypothalamus, d–f: pons; magnification: 33,930×.

before the lithium infusion and it decreased following the infusion. In another animal, there was a marked increase in the hemoglobin level indicating a possible loss in fluid.

The animals were sacrificed at different time intervals from 30 minutes to 24 hours after the administration of the drug. To date, the most outstanding electron microscopic findings consisted of: (1) variable increases in the number of mitochondria or pleomorphometabolosomes (PMS) in the cytoplasm of the nerve cells (Figure 5), their processes, and some synapses (Figure 6*a–d*). (2) Changes in the fine structure, patterns, and osmiophilia

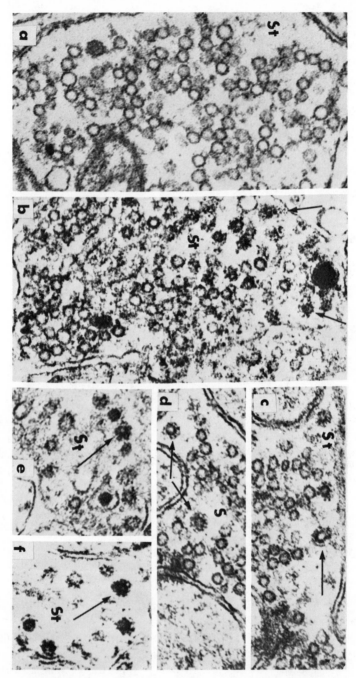

Figure 8.   Rat hypothalamus: various presynaptic terminals (*t*) revealing average fairly well preserved synaptic vesicles (*a*) to be compared with synaptic vesicles (S.V.) displaying modifications and spike-like features or incrustations of their limiting membranes (arrows). Uranyl acetate and lead citrate. RCA,EMU-3G, magnification: 31,842×.

of the PMS membranes and matrix. (3) Variations in the pattern of distribution and osmiophilia of the Golgi canaliculi, vesicles, or vacuoles, and particularly their limiting membranes (Figure 7a–f). (4) Increased osmiophilic density, coating, granularity, or incrustationlike phenomena displayed also, in many instances, by the synaptic vesicles (Figure 8a–f).

It would be premature to make definite conclusive remarks concerning the relationship between the shown ultracellular changes and particularly the membrane alterations and the lithium effects. However, in considering the possible pathogenic mechanisms it should be noted that: (a) the membrane unit systems compartmentalize the structural organization of the organelles, which are endowed with characteristic functional and metabolic properties; (b) they maintain an orderly arrangement of some of the enzyme assemblies; (c) they channel the intermediary metabolites or histometabolic processes and (d) they regulate the ionic flux (active and passive transport).

REFERENCES

1. Adams, R. and Foley, J.: The neurological disorder associated with liver disease. *Assoc. Res. Nerv. Ment. Dis.* **32**:198–237, 1952.

2. Adelson, L.: Pathologic findings in patients dead of common poisons. *Amer. J. Clin. Pathol.* **22**:509–519, 1952.

3. Barros, E.: Über die sogenannte spezfische Wirkung der Krampf gifte, ins besondere des Tetanus giftes auf die motorischen Ganglien-Zellen des Rückenmarks. *Z. Gesamte Neurol. Psychiat. Orig.* **93**:720–749, 1924.

4. Bennett, J. P. and Snyder, S. H.: Stereospecific binding of LSD to brain membranes: Relationship to serotonin receptors. *Brain Res.* **94**:523–544, 1975.

5. Bollard, B. M., Roizin, L., and Robinson, E. H.: Tissue distribution and metabolic effects of compazine (prochlorperazine). *Fed. Proc.* **21**:80, 1962.

6. Bollard, B., Roizin, L., Sabbia, R., and Horwitz, W. A.: Distribution of free and S^{35} labeled prochlorperazine (compazine) in mammalian tissues. *Fed. Proc.* **22**:317, 1963.

7. Buscaino, G. A. and Frongia, N.: Modificazioni biochimiche, electroencephalografiche istochimiche ed istologiche in cani, durante l'intossicazione sperimentale acuta e cronica da dietilamide dell' acido lisergico. *Acta Neurol.* **8**:641–695, 1953.

8. Cares, R. M.: Tranquilizers, sedatives and hypnotics. In *Pathology of the Nervous System,* Vol. 2, J. Minckler, (Ed.), McGraw-Hill, New York, 1971a, pp. 1682–1685.

9. Cares, R. M.: Alkaloids, antipyretics, analgesics, and other pharmaceuticals. In *Pathology of the Nervous System,* Vol. 2, J. Minckler (Ed.), McGraw-Hill, New York, 1971b, pp. 1685–1691.

10. Courville, C. B.: Forensic Neuropathology. VIII. The mechanism and structural effects of poisons upon the brain. *J. Forensic Sci.* **8**:179–199, 1963.

11. Cuatico, W., Roizin, L., Sabbia, R., Horwitz, W. A. and Wodraska, G.: S^{35} prochlorperazine autoradiography of the central nervous system. *Int. J. Neuropsychiat.* **1**:364–370, 1965.

12. Crane, G. E.: Tardive dyskinesias in patients treated with major neuroleptics: a review of the literature. *Amer. J. Psychiat.* **124**(Suppl.):40–48, 1968.

13. Cristensen, E., Möller, J. E., and Faurbye, A.: Neuropathological investigations of 28 brains from patients with dyskinesia. *Acta Psychiat. Scand.* **46**:14–23, 1970.

14. Delay, J. and Deniker, P.: Drug-induced extrapyramidal syndromes. In *Handbook of Clinical Neurology,* Vol. 6, P. J. Vinken and G. W. Bruyn (Eds.), North Holland, Amsterdam, 1968, pp. 248–267.

15. Ehrenpreis, S. and Teller, D. N.: Interaction of drugs of dependence with receptors. In *Chemical and Biochemical Aspects of Drug Dependence,* S. J. Mulé and H. Brill (Eds.), CRC Press, Cleveland, 1972, pp. 177–217.

16. Farrow, J. T. and Van Vunakis, H.: Binding of d-lysergic acid diethylamide to subcellular fractions from rat brain. *Nature* **237**:164–165, 1972.

17. Forrest, F. M., Forrest, I. S., and Roizin, L.: Clinical, biochemical and postmortem studies on a patient treated with chlorpromazine. *Agressologie,* **4**:259–265, 1963.

18. Greiner, A. C. and Berry, K.: Skin pigmentation and corneal and lens opacities with prolonged chlorpromazine therapy. *Can. Med. Assoc. J.* **90**:663–665, 1964.

19. Greiner, A. C. and Nicolson, G. A.: Pigment deposition in viscera associated with prolonged chlorpromazine therapy. *Can. Med. Assoc. J.* **91**:627–635, 1964.

20. Greenwood, R. and Peachey, R. S.: Acute amphetamine poisoning; an account of 3 cases. *Brit. Med. J.* **1**:742–744, 1957.

21. Hoffeld, D. R., Webster, R. L., and McNew, J.: Adverse effects on offspring of tranquilizing drugs during pregnancy. *Nature,* **215**:182–183, 1967.

22. Hollister, L. E. and Kosek, J. C.: Sudden death during treatment with phenothiazine derivatives. *J. Amer. Med. Assoc.* **192**:1035–1038, 1965.

23. Jellinger, K.: Neuroaxonal dystrophy: Its natural history and related disorders. In *Progress in Neuropathology,* Vol. 2, H. M. Zimmerman (Ed.), Grune and Stratton, New York, 1973, pp. 129–180.

24. Kalter, H.: Teratogenicity, embryolethality and mutagenicity of drugs of dependence. In *Chemical and Biological Aspects of Drug Dependence,* S. J. Mulé and H. Brill (Eds.), CRC Press, Cleveland, 1972, pp. 413–463.

25. Malitz, S. and Hoch, P. H.: Drug therapy: Neuroleptics and Tranquilizers. In *American Handbook of Psychiatry,* Vol. 3, S. Arieti (Ed.), Basic Books, New York, 1959, pp. 458–476.

26. Martland, H. and Martland, H., Jr.: Placental barrier in carbon monoxide, barbiturate and radium poisoning. *Amer. J. Surg.* **50**:270–279, 1950.

27. Matveev, V. F.: Pathomorphological alterations in the brains of experimental animals under chronic lysergic acid intoxication. *Sov. Neurol. Psychiat.* **5**:129–138, 1972.

28. Miyakawa, T., Sumiyoski, S., Deshimaru, M., Murayama, E. and Tatetsu, S.: Electron microscopic studies concerning the structural mechanisms of the development of mental disturbance in experimental chronic methamphetamine poisoning. *Acta Neuropathol.* **14**:215–225, 1969.

29. Mulé, S. J.: Phospholipid metabolism. In *Narcotic Drugs, Biochemical Pharmacology,* D. H. Clouet (Ed.), Plenum Press, New York, 1971, pp. 190–215.

30. Olchanskii, Y. O. and Morozov, B. V.: Death due to necrotizing nephrosis following aminozine. *Zh. Nevropatol. Psikhiat. Imeni Korsakoff,* **62**:762–764, 1962.

31. Quismorio, F. P., Bjarnason, D. F., Kiely, W. F., Dubois, E. L., and Friou, J.: Antinuclear antibodies in chronic psychotic patients treated with chlorpromazine. *Amer. J. Psychiat.* **132**:1204–1206, 1975.

32. Peters, G.: *Spiezielle Pathologic der Krankheiten des Zentralen und Peripheren Nervensystems,* Thieme Verlag, K. G., Stuttgart, 1954, pp. 339.

33. Popova, E. N. and Krivitskaya, G. N.: The influence of some psychotropic drugs on brain structures. *Z. Nevropathol. Psikhiat. Imeni Korsakoff,* 75:1064–1069, 1975.

34. Popper, H., Rubin, E., Gardio, D., Schaffner, F., and Paronetto, F.: Drug-induced liver disease. A penalty for progress. *Arch. Intern. Med.* 115:128–136, 1965.

35. Porter, C. C.: *Chemical Mechanisms of Drug Action,* Charles C Thomas, Springfield, Illinois, 1970, p. 165.

36. Rankin, J. G., (Ed.): Alcohol, drugs and brain damage. In *International Symposium on Alcohol and Drug Problems,* Alcoholism and Drug Addiction Research Foundation of Ontario, Toronto, Canada, 1975, p. 98.

37. Rodova, A. and Nahunck, K.: Persistent dyskinesias after phenofluazines. *Cesk. Psychiat.* 60:250–254, 1964.

38. Roizin, L.: Evolution of fundamental CNS pathogenic concepts. In *The World Biennial of Psychiatry and Psychotherapy,* S. Arieti (Ed.), Basic Books, New York, 1970, pp. 560–602.

39. Roizin, L., Akai, K., Lawler, H. C. and Liu, J. C.: Lithium neurotoxicologic effects. I Acute phase (preliminary observations). *Dis. Nerv. Syst.* 31:38–44, 1970.

40. Roizin, L., Gold, G., Alexander, G., Miles, B., Kaufman, M. A., Lawler, H. C., and Akai, K.: Prenatal effects of hallucinogens. In *Drug Abuse-Current Concepts and Research,* W. Keup (Ed.), Charles C Thomas, Springfield, Illinois, 1972, pp. 123–127.

41. Roizin, L., Gold, G., Kaufman, M. A., Fieve, R., Alexander, G., and Ueno, Y.: Experimental potentiation of phenothiazine toxicology. 1. Effects of liver disorders. *Int. Symp. Action Mech. Metabol. Psychoactive Drugs, Agressologie,* 9:379–381, 1968.

42. Roizin, L., Helpern, M., Baden, M., Kaufman, M. A., and Akai, K.: Toxosynpathies (a multifactor pathogenic concept). In *Drug Abuse-Current Concepts and Research,* W. Keup (Ed.) Charles C Thomas, Springfield, Illinois, 1972, pp. 97–116.

43. Roizin, L., Helpern, M., Baden, M., Kaufman, M. A., Hashimoto, S., Liu, J. C., and Eisenberg, B.: Neuropathology of drug dependence. In *Chemical and Biological Aspects of Drug Dependence,* S. J. Mulé and H. Brill (Eds.). CRC Press, Cleveland, 1972, pp. 389–411.

44. Roizin, L., Helpern, M., Baden, M., Kaufman, M. A., Hashimoto, S., Liu, J. C., and Eisenberg, B.: Methadone fatalities in heroin addicts. *Psychiat. Quart.* 46:393–410, 1972.

45. Roizin, L., Kaufman, M. A., and Casselman, B.: Structural changes induced by neuroleptics. *Rev. Can. Biol.* 20:221–229, 1961.

46. Roizin, L., Kaufman, M. A., Gold, G., Iyengar, V. K. S., Liu, J. C., and Keoseian, S.: A multidisciplinary investigation of the phenothiazines. *Ment. Hyg.* 50:574–579, 1966.

47. Roizin, L., Liu, J. C., and Akai, K.: Electron microscopy of basal ganglia in chronic prochlorperazine administration. *Fed. Proc., Fed. Amer. Soc. Exp. Biol.* 34:849, 1975.

48. Roizin, L., Schneider, J., Willson, N., Liu, J. C., and Mullen, C.: Effects of prolonged LSD-25 administration upon neurons of cord ganglia tissue cultures. *J. Neuropathology and Exp. Neurol.,* 33:212–225, 1974.

49. Roizin, L., True, C., and Knight, M.: Structural effects of tranquilizers. *Proc. Assoc. Nerv. Ment. Dis.* 37:285–329, 1959.

50. Roux, C.: Action teratogene de la prochlorperazine. *Arch. Fr. Pediat.* 16:968–971, 1959.

51. Sano, I. and Nagasaka, G.: Ueber chronische Weckaminsucht in Japan. *Fortschsitte Neurol. Psychiat. Ihrer Grenzgebiete*, 391–394, 1956.

52. Tatetsu, S.: Methamphetamine psychosis. *Folia Psychiat. Neurol. Jap., Suppl.* **7**:377–380, 1963.

53. Van Praag, H. M.: Abuse of dependence on and psychoses from anorexigenic drugs. In *Drug Induced Diseases*, L. Meyler and H. M. Peck (Eds.), Excerpta Medical Foundation, Amsterdam, 1968, 281–294.

54. Wechsler-Berger, M. and Roizin, L.: Tissue levels of chlorpromazine in experimental animals. *J. Ment. Sci.* **106**:1501–1505, 1960.

55. Weil, A.: *A Textbook of Neuropathology*, 2nd ed. Grune and Stratton, New York, 1945, p. 191.

56. Wintrobe, M.: The problem of adverse drug reactions. In *Symposium: Adverse Drug Reactions, JAMA*, 404–405, 1966.

CHAPTER SEVENTEEN

PHARMACOLOGY AND PSYCHOSOMATIC MEDICINE: THE EXPERIMENTAL AND CLINICAL APPROACH TO A PSYCHOSOMATIC EVALUATION OF PSYCHOTROPIC DRUGS

ADRIANO MARINO

The main aspects of the topic under discussion may be summarized as follows: (1) experimental approach to psychosomatic medicine; (2) psychosomatic approach to pharmacology; (3) pharmacological application in psychosomatic medicine. Although the work of our particular group is concerned mainly with experimental methods in applied pharmacology, some clinical applications of our results and ideas have also been carried out. This chapter outlines the theoretical, experimental, and clinical basis for a rational application of psychopharmacotherapy in internal medicine. For this purpose, a preliminary differentiation of somatic, somatopsychic, and psychosomatic effects of psychotropic drugs is attempted. Accurate choice of drug is then oriented toward corresponding manifestations of the disease.

In cardioangiology these kinds of effects have been described[19-21] as follows:

Somatic effects. Side effects independent of psychotropic activity result from direct action on heart and blood vessels or are mediated through cardiovascular neuroregulation. Somatic effects may influence both psychogenic and non psychogenic cardiovascular diseases.

Somatopsychic effects. Result from action on the psychic repercussions of psychogenic and non psychogenic cardiovascular diseases.

Psychosomatic effects. Result from action on the psychogenic factor which determines, precipitates, or contributes to the development of cardiovascular diseases.

This classification is applicable to any branch of internal and general medicine.

SOMATIC EFFECTS

The choice between drugs with the same psychotropic activity may depend exclusively on their somatic effects. For instance, reserpine and chlorpromazine are both psychodepressants and tranquilizers, but with respect to the heart, the former induces bradycardia, the latter, tachycardia; with respect of gastric function, reserpine causes increased HCl secretion, while chlorpromazine may cause a slight decrease. Therefore, in the case of anxiety reactions with tachycardia reserpine is indicated while chlorpromazine is preferred if there is bradycardia. In the management of anxiety reactions with gastric hypersecretion, chlorpromazine is indicated and reserpine contraindicated. However, the latter may be used in the presence of hyposecretion. Yet in the management of spastic gastrointestinal diseases with a depressive reaction or substrate, among the various antidepressants, drugs like amitriptyline with a high anticholinergic activity are preferable. The somatic effects of psychotropic drugs may provide indications or contraindications for their use apart from psychological or psychosomatic indications. One example is the high antiemetic efficacy of the phenothiazine neuroleptics which control several somatogenic types of vomit (anesthesia, surgery, pregnancy, alcoholism, uremia, toxic or infectious gastroenteritis, carcinomatosis, irradiation, digitalis, morphine, antibiotics, stilbestrol, and nitrogen mustard). Apart from motion sickness vomiting (in which they are ineffective) and psychogenic vomiting (in which their psychotropic activity also plays an important role), the phenothiazines are effective in relieving the foregoing kinds of vomit through mechanisms which are mainly somatic and almost independent of their psychotropic activity.

Among somatic contraindications, the following can be listed: reserpine for peptic ulcer (because it is an ulcerogenic agent), iproniazid for liver disease (hepatotoxic), and chlorpromazine for leukopenia (because it may induce agranulocytosis).

These somatic effects contribute towards differentiating the various groups of psychotropic drugs. For instance, psychostimulants like amphetamine and thymeretics like iproniazid may be differentiated on the basis of their somatic effects (apart from their behavioral and biochemical differences): the former raises blood pressure, decreases appetite, and shows no specific liver toxicity; conversely, the latter reduces blood pressure, increases appetite, and has potential hepatotoxicity.

As another example, I show the classification of psychotropic drugs in respect of their somatic effects on blood pressure. (see Table I)

From the experimental point of view, the investigation of somatic effects is conducted by standard pharmacological methods supplemented by particular devices to rule out interference from psychological factors in the experimental situation. For instance, in the search for a somatogenic bradycardia induced in vivo by a tranquilizer, the animal should be relaxed to prevent emotional tachycardia. Otherwise, the somatic cardiac effect of the drug could not be detected, because of masking by the psychic effect.

As another example, I quote our research on the somatic effects of amitriptyline on the heart *in vivo* in normal or emetinized rabbits. No severe EKG changes were observed in normal rabbits after hypotensive doses of amitriptyline (0.3 to 3.3 mg/kg, I.V., I.P., per os). On the other hand, the drug (6.66 mg/(kg) (die), I.P. per 7 days) provided protection against lethal and EKG alterations induced by acute (0.35 mg/(kg) (min), I.V.) poisoning in the rabbit. The animal lethal dose of emetine was 9 ± 2.7 in the control group (only emetine), 23 ± 2.4 in the group treated with amitriptyline, and then emetinized ($+155\%$ with respect to the control group).

The experimental data mentioned above, especially relating to protection

TABLE 1.   CLASSIFICATION AND SOMATIC PRESSOR EFFECTS OF PSYCHOTROPIC DRUGS[a]

   I.   *Nonspecific psychodepressant drugs.* sedatives, hypnotics, general anesthetics, narcotics (−).
  II.   *Specific psychodepressant drugs*
        A.   Major tranquilizers (phenothiazines, thiaxanthene, Rauwolfia, benzoquinolizine, and butyrophenone derivatives) (− − −).
        B.   Minor tranquilizers (glycol, benzodiazepine, dibenzazepine, diphenylmethane, and various derivatives) (no effect, apart from mebutamate and diphenylmethane derivatives) (− −).
 III.   *Nonspecific psychostimulant drugs.* convulsant drugs (+ +).
  IV.   *Specific psychostimulant drugs*
        A.   Nonantidepressant psychoanaleptics: (*a*) with low psychoselectivity (caffeine ±, nicotine ±, cocaine ±, ACTH and cortisone +, salicylates); (*b*) with major psychoselectivity and cholinergic activity (DMAE, centrophenoxine); (*c*) with major psychoselectivity and adrenergic activity (amphetamines, metamphetamine, methylphenidate, pipradol, Deltamine, ethylaminophenylnorcamphane, phenylpyrrolidine-pentane, etc. (+ +).
        B.   Antidepressant thymoleptics (dibenzazepine iminodibenzyl derivatives or imipramine group and analogous derivatives; dibenzocycloheptadiene derivatives or amitriptyline group and analogous derivatives; dibenzoxepinone derivatives; dibenzothioepinone derivatives; various (− −).
        C.   Antidepressant thymeretics MAO-inhibitors (hydrazides, hydrazines, amines) (− − −).

---

[a] Hypotensive effect (−); hypertensive effect (+).

against the specific cardiotoxicity of emetine, may contribute towards excluding a somatic cardiogenic mechanism underlying the antihypertensive efficacy of amitriptyline in man (see later).

SOMATOPSYCHIC EFFECTS

These effects are observed in the psychic repercussion of psychogenic and non psychogenic somatopathies. Since in the latter there are no psychosomatic components, the use of psychotropic drugs is relatively simple. The patient presents anxiety or depression secondary to organic disease without psychogenic component (megacolon, rheumatic endocarditis, congenital heart disease); the internist should prescribe psychodepressants or psychostimulants in addition to the specific somatic therapy, taking into account their respective somatic effects.

But the somatopsychic repercussion and the psychosomatic component may coexist. This is the case in many psychosomatic diseases, such as peptic ulcer, ulcerative colitis, thyrotoxicosis, essential hypertension, peripheral arteriopathies, coronary insufficiency, and cardiac arrhythmia.

It becomes apparent that the internist must attempt to differentiate these two components. Close contact between the internist and the psychiatrist is mandatory under these circumstances. The problem is not only of theoretical but also of practical interest for therapy.

Psychic repercussion and substrate may be of the same type, both being sensitive to the same psychodrug: or conversely, they may be different or opposite, as in the case of psychogenic hypertension in which a somatopsychic repercussion of anxiety and agitation may be combined with a psychic substrate of depression and hostility.[1, 3, 35] Under these circumstances, the choice of psychodrug is quite difficult and its use may be dangerous, as outlined in Table 2.

TABLE 2. SOMATIC, SOMATOPSYCHIC AND PSYCHOSOMATIC EFFECTS OF PSYCHOTROPIC DRUGS ON ESSENTIAL HYPERTENSION[a]

| | Action of the Drug on the Pathogenic Component | | | |
| | Psychosomatic | | Somatopsychic | Somatic |
Drug	Hostility	Depression	Anxiety	Hypertension
Chlorpromazine	−	++	− − − −	− − −
Reserpine	−	+++ +	− − −	− − −
Mebutamate	−	+	−	−
Benactyzine	+++	+	−	−
Chlordiazepoxide	− − −	±	− −	no
Amphetamine	+	− +	++	++
Iproniazid	++	− − −	++	− −
Pargyline	+	− −	+	− −
Imipramine	−	− − −	+	− −
Amitriptyline	−	− − −	− −	− −
Amitriptyline + chlordiazepoxide	− − − −	− − − −	− − − −	− −

[a] The drug acts in the same way as the pathogenic component of the disease (+). The drug antagonizes the pathogenic component of the disease (−).

For instance, among tranquilizers, benactyzine should be contraindicated in the treatment of psychogenic essential hypertension (PH), because of its potential for increasing or precipitating hostility (the psychic substrate of the disease); this is despite its fairly hypotensive and tranquilizing effects which would antagonize, respectively, the somatic and somatopsychic components of the disease. In our opinion, even reserpine, the well-known hypotensive and tranquilizing agent, may be contraindicated in PH, because of its specific psychodepressant effect that may aggravate the psychic substrate of the disease. This might explain the higher incidence of depression and suicide under reserpine treatment in hypertensive patients compared with schizophrenics. Among psychostimulants, amphetamine increases vasoconstriction and anxiety, producing a slight antidepressant effect. Therefore, this drug is contraindicated in the treatment of PH. Conversely, among antidepressant drugs, amitriptyline may be very useful especially in the early treatment of PH. Indeed, it is a drug with hypotensive, tranquilizing, and antidepressant effects, which may antagonize, respectively, the somatic, somatopsychic, and psychosomatic components of the disease.

Adopting this criterion, 29 patients with essential hypertension and depressive-anxiety syndrome, have been treated with amitriptyline (25 to 60 mg orally per day, for between 2 and 6 months) in a double blind crossover experiment. In the cases of severe anxiety, amitriptyline has been combined with chlordiazepoxide (10 to 20 mg orally per day). All the treated patients improved significantly after the treatment, from both the psychological and cardioangiologic points of view. Before treatment the mean values of blood pressure were as follows: maximum 209 ± 3.75; minimum 109 ± 2.98; differential 100 ± 2.77. After treatment we found the following values: maximum 157 ± 2.4; minimum 88 ± 1.9; differential 69 ± 2.19. Therefore the treatment reduced the control values respectively by 25% to 20% to 31% ($p < 0.01$). A neurophysiologic interpretation of the mechanisms underlying these clinical results may be found in report by Schmitt and Schmitt[36] who discovered an inhibitory effect of amitriptyline (and related drugs) on the vasomotor centers.

In another clinical investigation,[29] amitriptyline and chlordiazepoxide were administered to 11 patients with anorexia nervosa, that is, another psychosomatic syndrome in which anxiety and depression are often simultaneously present. In all these patients, in whom previous pharmacological and psychotherapeutic treatments had proved uneffective, a dramatic improvement in their psychological and somatic states (anorexia, body weight) was observed after amitriptyline + chlordiazepoxide.

Finally, the anticholinergic somatic effect of amitriptyline combined with its antidepressant and tranquilizing effects have been shown to be useful in the treatment of spastic gastrointestinal disease, especially when the thymoleptic was associated with chlordiazepoxide.[22]

The experimental study of the somatopsychic effects of psychodrugs belongs to general psychopharmacology. Just as the internist must differentiate the somatopsychic repercussion from the psychosomatic component of a disease, the pharmacologist should differentiate, in the early stages of experimental evaluation of a drug-inducing behavioral changes, the psychic or somatic origin of the corresponding effects. For instance, at first glance the depression induced by a cardiotoxic drug such as emetine is no different from that induced by a psychotropic drug like reserpine. However, posology and certain behavioral techniques allowed us to differentiate between the depressive effects of the two drugs. Indeed, depression appeared only after cardiotoxic doses of emetine, while reserpine depressed spontaneous behavior at doses without somatic interference. Moreover, at doses which do not influence spontaneous behavior, reserpine blocked the formation of, and inhibited, avoidance conditioned responses, while emetine showed no effect on the latter. Only at the terminal stage of emetine poisoning, when the animals were almost completely incapable of moving or crossing the barrier to avoid the shock was there a marked reduction of conditioned avoidance.[17, 20]

PSYCHOSOMATIC EFFECTS

Whereas conventional pharmacological and psychopharmacological methods can be applied to investigate the somatic and somatopsychic effects of psychodrugs, specialized technical training and psychosomatic initiation are required to investigate the psychosomatic effects. Appropriate methods are necessary to evaluate the activity of a drug from the psychosomatic point of view. Neurophysiology and experimental psychology provide such methods although they are not often used by pharmacologists. For instance, among the neurophysiological methods, it is possible to record the cardiovascular or gastrointestinal changes produced by stimulation or ablation of certain structures within the central nervous system which play a role in the genesis and regulation of emotions.[6-8, 12, 13, 34] The interference of psychodrugs with these neurogenic visceral changes could be investigated. Actually something has already been done by pharmacologists in this regard. For instance, Berger's group[2] investigated the depressor effects of meprobamate, mebutamate, reserpine, and Luminal on arterial hypertension induced by electrical stimulation of medullary and hypothalamic pressor areas; Dasgupta and Werner[5] investigated the effects of chlorpromazine on pressor responses to hypothalamic and spinal stimulation;

Schmitt and Schmitt[36] discovered a selective depressor effect of amitriptyline and related drugs on the vasomotor centers.

From a psychosomatic point of view criticism of this type of method may
be summarized as follows: (1) there is contamination from the various
technical artifacts present in acute experiments; (2) the evocative factors are
neurological, lacking any psychogenic component; (3) the resulting cardiovascular responses are too elementary lacking the usual pathogenic complexity.

Therefore, the experimental situation is too far removed from clinical
reality and from basic psychosomatic assumptions. It is more suitable for
the investigation of sites of action of psychodrugs than for their psychosomatic evaluation. For this purpose, psychological methods are more useful.
These include: recordings of motor and autonomic components of the
orienting reflex, motor and autonomic conditioned reflexes bearing in mind
the concepts of autokinesis and schizokinesis proposed by Gantt[10]; visceral
and vegetative changes following conflict situations, experimental neurosis,
and various kinds of psychic stress exemplified by the "fighting" rats or
mice[26]; audiogenic or vibratory stress inducing hypertension[33]; and the
examples of "executive monkeys" developing peptic ulcer,[4] and the "jealous
hypertensive baboons."[14] Concerning the latter, it has been observed that
patients with essential hypertension are psychologically oriented for
combat, but their aggressive action is unconsciously and powerfully
restrained. An ingenious experimental situation was devised along these
lines by Russian investigators at the primate station in Sukhumi. Baboons
who had become self-selected mates were separated. The female was placed
in a large cage with a strange male. Her mate was placed alone in a smaller
cage alongside. The authors observed that the cuckolded mate regularly
developed sustained hypertension.[14, 37, 38]

It would be very interesting to study the psychosomatic action of
psychotropic drugs on these complex somatic reactions produced by specific
psychological stresses. More often such action has been evaluated on more
elementary reactions. According to Gantt's group,[10, 11] curare and decame-
thonium do block the motor orienting and conditioned responses without
affecting the cardiac responses, while meprobamate abolishes the cardiac
conditioned or emotional responses, having only a slight effect on the motor
conditioned responses, reserpine and chlorpromazine block orienting
tachycardia in dogs. Thus in the case of chlorpromazine, the psychotropic
action is dominant with respect to the somatic effect (the drug often induces
tachycardia to compensate for hypotension).

Another method[15, 16, 18, 22, 23] used by our group is based on a combination
of psychological and pharmacological techniques aimed at bringing the
experimental approach closer to clinical observation. An experimental

"organ situation" which could be compared to the "organ inferiority" of psychosomatic medicine is experimentally evoked by means of pharmacologic treatment specifically toxic for that organ. On the other hand, psychological stress is induced by a conflict situation in animals previously conditioned to an avoidance situation. In this way, the influence of psychological stress on the target organ is evaluated.

Furthermore, the protective action of psychotropic and somatotropic drugs, acting either on the psychogenic (psychological stress), or somatic (organ inferiority) factors can be investigated with respect to the resulting somatopathy.

The results of our experiments are summarized in Tables 3 and 4.

The material I have presented refers to research performed or about to be performed in psychosomatic pharmacology. The practitioner faces a still more complicated problem. He should reach the diagnosis of the disease and then differentiate between the symptoms directly related to organic disease, those related to anxiety or depression secondary to the organic disease, and those having a primary functional psychogenic origin. The latter may in turn develop into an organic disease. Again, all the symptoms may be present simultaneously. In other words, the internist, should define the somatic somatopsychic and psychosomatic components of the disease. Finally, to achieve correct and rational pharmacotherapy, the practitioner should be familiar with the somatic, somatopsychic and psychosomatic effects of drugs. As this is a major task for one person alone, it should be undertaken by a team of experts in these respective fields (general practitioner, internist, and psychiatrist trained in psychosomatics, psychotherapy, and psychopharmacotherapy).

At the present time, it is difficult to conceive of such a multidisciplinary approach because it is hard to bring together a team of experts for each single patient. However, this difficulty could be overcome by mutual contact and shared information among the experts in preference to continuing polemics between organicists and psychogeneticists. In my opinion, the pharmacologist might prove to be an appropriate pacifying mediator. From the ideas presented in this chapter, the following practical conclusions may be drawn:

1. Psychotropic drugs have already shown a high and undoubted efficacy in mental diseases. Since in mental disease, the relevant psychodynamics may be as complicated as in psychosomatic diseases, there is no reason to preclude the application of psychotropic drugs from the management of the psychic component in psychosomatic diseases.

2. Recently, it has become apparent that some psychoanalytically oriented schools do not deny the validity of psychopharmacoterapy, at least as an adjunct to dynamic psychotherapy.

TABLE 3. EXPERIMENTAL PSYCHOSOMATIC DISEASE INDUCED BY STRESS + ORGAN INFERIORITY

Organotoxic Drugs—Doses mg/kg—Route and Type of Administration—Animal [b]	S.	Potentiation	O.I.
Adrenaline: 1–2–5–10, I.P.—single—G. (Ref. 21)	CF	+++	CV
[b] Nor-adrenaline: 10–15–20–25, I.P.—sequential—G.	CF	+++	CV
[b] Isoproterenol: 200–400–600, I.P.—sequential—G.[c]	CF	No	CV
[b] Isoproterenol: 400 to 2800, I.P.—sequential—M.[c]	CF	No	CV
[b] Isoproterenol: 400, I.P.—single (100 × 4)—M.	FT	No	CV
[b] Isoproterenol: 400; 400 to 2800, I.P.—single; sequential—M.	IC	No	CV
Emetine: 5, S.C.—daily—G. (Ref. 16)	CD	No	MY
Emetine: 5, S.C.—daily—G. (Ref. 16)	CF	++	MY
Emetine: 5, S.C.—daily—G. (Ref. 15)	SW	+++	MY
Strophanthin: 0.3–0.6–0.9–1.2, S.C.—sequential—G. (Ref. 31)	CF	+++	MY
[b] Thyroxine: 0.1–0.5–1–3, I.P.—sequential—G.	CF	+	CR
Pitressin: 60 U.tannate in oil, i.m.—single—G. (Ref. 24)	CF	++++	COR
Hypertensin: 0.1–1–4, I.P., 0.05–0.5–1, I.V.—sequential—G. (Ref. 28)	CF	+++	CV
[b] Pentylenetetrazole: 50 to 200, I.P.—sequential—G.	CF	±	CNS
Pentylenetetrazole: 50 to 500, I.P.—sequential—M. (Ref. 26)	FT	No	CNS
Streptomycin: 100, I.P.—daily—G. (Ref. 32)	CF	No[d]	CNS
Adrenaline: 0.05 + Ergotamine: 3, S.C.—sequential—G. (Ref. 30)	CF	+++	PA
[b] Oil + chloroform: 0.2–0.4, S.C., intratympanic—single—G.	CF	++	L

[a] G. = guinea pigs; M. = mice.
[b] Unpublished data.
[c] In four equal doses.
[d] Decreased toxicity.
S. = stress (CF = conflict; CD = avoidance conditioning; FT = fighting; IC = isolation confinement; SW = swimming exercise).
O.I. = organ inferiority (CV = cardiovascular; MY = myocardium; CR = cardiorespiratory; COR = coronary; CNS = central nervous system; PA = peripheral arteriae; L = labyrinth).

TABLE 4. PSYCHOSOMATIC EXPERIMENTAL EVALUATION OF PSYCHOTROPIC AND SOMATOTROPIC DRUGS

Protective drugs	Doses		Toxic	Stressor	Protection	
	Route	mg/kg			Normal Animals	Stressed Animals
1. Chlordiazepoxide (Ref. 27)	I.M.	10	Adrenaline	Conflict	+	+++
2. Chlordiazepoxide[b]	I.M.	10	Labyrinthitis	Conflict	No	++
3. Diazepam[b]	I.P.	1		Conflict		[a] b.c.+++ [a] decond. no
4. Glutamine[b]	I.M.	150		Conflict		b.c. no decond. +
5. Mogadon[b]	I.M.	10	Cardiazol	Conflict	+++	++++
6. Mogadon (Ref. 26)	I.M.	10	Cardiazol	Fighting	++++	++++
7. Mebutamate (Ref. 31)	I.M.	20	Strophanthin	Conflict	++	++
8. Mebutamate (Ref. 28)	I.M.	20	Hypertensin	Conflict	+	+++
9. Chlorpromazine[b]	I.M.	5	Isoproterenol	Isolation	–No	
10. Methiomeprazine[b]	I.M.	5	Isopreterenol	Isolation	–No	
11. Methiomeprazine[b]	I.M.	5	Nor-adrenaline	Conflict	++	+++
12. Promazine (Ref. 24)	I.P.	4	Pitressin	Conflict	++	+++
13. Pentaerythritoltetranitrate (Ref. 27)	O.S.	5–25	Adrenaline	Conflict	No	No
14. 1 + 13 (Ref. 27)			Adrenaline	Conflict	+	+++
15. Dipyridamol (Ref. 24)	I.P.	4	Pitressin	Conflict		+++
16. 12 + 15 (Ref. 24)			Pitressin	Conflict		+++

[a] b.c. = behavioral changes;/decond. = deconditioning.
[b] unpublished data.

359

3. Because of economic, logistic, and scholastic difficulties, routine psychoterapy has not yet been established in many countries. Therefore, it might seem advisable for the internist to use psychodrugs together with "petite psychothérapie." However, it is indisputable that practitioners should become more familiar with the pharmacology of psychotropic drugs to avoid the combination of "petite psychotérapie" with a psychopharmacoterapy as "petite" as "psychotérapie" but much more dangerous. Empiric psychopharmacoterapy of internal diseases holds many more actual disadvantages than potential advantages.

4. To make this therapy rational and scientific, the data of experimental pharmacology should be applied to psychosomatic pathology and medicine. For further researches and details the reader may consult my textbooks.[39,40,41]

REFERENCES

1. Alexander, F.: *Medicina Psicosomatica,* Editrice Universitaria, Firenze, 1956, pp. 128–137.

2. Berger, F. M., Douglas, J. F., Kletzkin, M., Ludwig, B. J., and Margolin, S.: The pharmacological properties of 2-methyl-2-secbutyl-1,3-propaniedol dicarbamate (mebutamate, W-583), a new centrally acting blood pressure lowering agent. *J. Pharmacol. Exp. Ther.* **134**:356, 1961.

3. Boss, M.: "Petite" psychothérapie et "grande" psychothérapie des hypertendus essentiels. *Acta Psychosom.* **3**:1, 1959.

4. Brady, J. V.: Ulcers in executive monkeys. *Sci. Amer.* **199**:95, 1958.

5. Dasgupta, S. R. and Werner, G.: Inhibition of hypothalamic, medullary and reflex vasomotor responses by chlorpromazine. *Brit. J. Pharmacol.* **9**:389, 1954.

6. Delgado, J. M. R.: Circulatory effects of cortical stimulation. *Physiol. Rev.,* 40/suppl., 4, 146, 1960.

7. French, J. D.: Brain physiology and modern medicine. *Postgrad. Med.* **27**:559, 1960.

8. Fuster, J. M. and Weinberg, S. J.: Bioelectrical changes of the heart cycle induced by stimulation of diencephalic regions. *Exp. Neurol.* **2**:26, 1960.

9. Gantt, W. H.: Factors involved in the development of pathological behavior: schizokinesis and autokinesis. *Perspect. Biol. Med.* **5**:473, 1962.

10. Gantt, W. H. and Newton, J. E. O.: Meprobamate on acquired cardiovascular responses and experimental catatonia. *Pharmacologist,* **2**:63, 1960.

11. Gliedman, L. H. and Gantt, W. H.: The effects of reserpine and chlorpromazine on orienting behavior and retention of conditioned reflexes. *Sth. Med. J. (Birmingham, Ala.)* **49**:880, 1956.

12. Hess, W. R.: *Arch. Psychiat.* **88**, 813, 1929: quoted in French, J. D.: The reticular formation. In *Handbook of Physiology-Neurophysiology,* vol. 2, Chap. 52, pp. 1281–1305.

13. Keller, A. D.: Ablation and stimulation of the hypothalamus: circulatory effects. *Physiol. Rev.* **40**:116, 1960.

14. Lapin, J. P.: see in UTKIN, I. A. (1961) and WOLF, S. (1960).

15. Marino, A.: Factor increasing emetine cardiotoxicity. *Pharmacologist* **2**:73, 1960.

16. Marino, A.: Psychological stress and emetine cardioxicity. *Experientia (Basel)* **17**:117, 1961.

17. Marino, A.: Electrocardiographic and behavioral effects of emetine. *Science,* **113**:385, 1961.

18. Marino, A.: Influence of psychological stress on the specific cardiotoxicity of drugs. *Nature (Lond.)*, **203**:1289, 1964.

19. Marino, A.: Gli psicotropi in cardiologia. *Relaz. Clin. Sci.* **16**(87):22–27 (1st part); **16**(88):13–17 (2nd part), 1964.

20. Marino, A.: La farmacologia sperimentale e clinica degli alcaloidi e derivati della Rauwolfia e dei derivati benzochinolizinici con particolare riferimento ai loro effetti cardiovascolari. *Clin. Ter.* **31**:230, 1964.

21. Marino, A.: Gli psicolettici fenotiazinici in cardioangiologia. *Recent Progr. Med.* **38**:150, 1965.

22. Marino, A.: Psychopharmacology and psychosomatic medicine. *Sett. Psicosom. Int.* Roma, September 11–16, 1967; *Med. Psicosom. (Roma)* **237**:1968.

23. Marino, A. and Bianchi, A.: Une mèthode mixte, psychologique et pharmacologique pour l'étude expérimentale de la pathogenèse des affections psychosomatiques et l'évaluation des médicaments psychotropes et somatotropes. *Arch. Int. Pharmacodyn.* **140**:143, 1962.

24. Marino, A., Bianchi, A. Giaquinto, S., and Casola, L.: Induzione e trattamento della cardiopatia sperimentale da stress psicologico e pitressina. *Arch. Int. Pharmacodyn.* **141**:377, 1963.

25. Marino, A., Colucci D'Amato, F., Miracco, A., and De Marino, V.: Psicodinamica e psicofarmacoterapia della ipertensione essenziale. *Clin. Ter.* **41**:219, 1967.

26. Marino, A. and Cosimo, W.: Attività protettrice di un nuovo tranquillante, 10 1,3-diidro-7-nitro-5-fenil-2H-1,4-benzodiazepina 2-one (Mogadon), sulla letalità e convulsività da Cardiazol nel topo normale o combattente. *Rass. Med. Sper.* **12**:121, 1965.

27. Marino, A., De Marino, V., Mastursi, M. and Salvatore, D.: Interferenze dello stress psicologico, del Pentaeritrolo-Tetranitrato e del Clordiazepossido con gli effetti tossici ed ecgrafici dell'adrenalina nella cavia. *Rass. Med. Sper.* **12**:45, 1965.

28. Marino, A., Galdi, R. and Parise, A.: Azioni ed interferenze della ipertensina, dello stress psicologico e del mebutamato sull'elettrocardiogramma della cavia. *Arch. Ital. Sci. Farmacol.* **12**:276, 1962.

29. Marino, A. and Gambardella, A.: Ricerche preliminarri sulla psicofarmacoterapia delle anoressie psicogene. *Clin. Ter.* **41**:51, 1967.

30. Marino, A., Mazzeo, F., di Mezza, F., and Bracale, G.: Arteropatia periferica da adrenalina + ergotamina + psicostress nella cavia. *Arch. Int. Pharmacodyn.* **156**:455, 1965.

31. Marino, A., Parise, A., and Galdi, R.: Protective effect of mebutamate in the experimental cardiopathy induced by strophantin and psychological stress. *Arch. Int. Pharmacodyn.* **145**:276, 1963.

32. Marino, A., Tortora, R., Robertaccio, A., and Sallusto, L.: Effetti della streptomicina sul comportamento spontaneo e condizionato. Interferenze fra tossicità streptomicinica e stress psicologico. *Rass. Med. Sper.* **11**:173, 1964.

33. Rosecrans, J. A., Watzman, N., and Buckley, J. P.: The production of hypertension in male albino rats subjected to experimental stress. *Biochem. Pharmacol.* **15**:1707, 1966.

34. Rushmer, R. F.: Regulation of the heart's functions. *Circulation,* **21**:744, 1960.

35. Saul, L. J.: Physiological effects of emotional tension. In *Personality and the Behavior Disorders,* Vol. 1, J. McV. Hunt, (Ed.), Ronald Press Co., New York, 1944, pp. 269–305.

36. Schmitt, H. and Schmitt, H.: Actions modératrices des antidépresseurs du groupe de l'imipramine, amitriptyline sur les centres cardiovasculaires. *Arch. Int. Pharmacodyn.* **165**:276, 1967.

37. Utkin, I. A.: Theoretical and practical questions of experimental medicine and biology in monkeys. Transl. under grant by Russian Scientific Translation Program of N.I.H., Pergamon Institute, 1961.

38. Wolf, S.: Stress and heart disease. *Mod. Conc. Cardiov. Dis.* **29**:599, 1960.

39. Marino, A.: Farmacologia Clinica e Farmacoterapia, Idelson (Ed), 1973.

40. Marino, A.: Psiconeurofarmacologia e Farmacologia Psicosomatica, Vallardi (Ed), Milan, 1974.

41. Marino, A.: Cardioangiofarmacologia, Vallardi (Ed), Milan, 1976.

CHAPTER EIGHTEEN

THE PSYCHOPHYSIOLOGICAL BASIS
OF THE PHARMACOTHERAPY
OF ENDOGENOUS PSYCHOTICS

HANS HEIMANN, MAGDALENA SCHMOCKER,
AND ECKART STRAUBE

In the last several decades, the experimental investigations of the psychophysiology of endogenous psychoses have concentrated mainly on information processing, covering such areas as attention, anticipation, perception, cognitive processes, memory, and decision-making. Because the numerous findings concerning the component parts of these functional pathways are often contradictory, it is impossible to summarize the findings.

On the other hand, psychophysiologically oriented investigations into the effectiveness of psychotropic drugs on endogenous psychoses are rare. They are often unsuited to give the clinician simple, theoretically based insights into the effectiveness of psychotropic drugs. A further problem is created by specialization. The clinician who deals only with patients in everyday life, with their histories and psychic disturbances of an individual nature, has difficulty relating his problems to the theoretical models of the psychophysiologists. Even the highly praised teamwork, which often only consists of each specialist doing his part of the work on his own, cannot solve this problem, because the specialists often lack a thorough knowledge of and practical experience in the related fields. In this chapter, we comment on the psychophysiological processes in question and their significance for our understanding of the effectiveness of psychotropic drugs. We restrict the discussion to the depressive syndromes and schizophrenic disturbances, and try to elucidate the problem from the point of view of the clinician looking for a method enabling him to go beyond the limitations of the descriptive psychopathological syndromes. A few preliminary remarks are necessary to clarify the association between clinical symptoms and syndromes on the one hand, and psychophysiological measurements on the other.

PRELIMINARY REMARKS

1. The functional levels that are investigated when we introduce physiological variables (e.g., heart rate, pulse amplitude, skin resistance, or EEG), that is to say the autonomic functions and arousal, are often directly related by clinicians to symptoms of pathological behavior and experience. This is an oversimplification. The clinician expects that the results of these investigations will give him simple explanations of the symptomatology of a clinical observation or will objectively verify his patients' statements. This may be true for the correlation of the quantitative measurement of salivation and the feeling of a dry mouth, but otherwise polygraphic measurements of psychiatric patients correlate with nosological or syndromatic clinical data only to a very limited degree.

The incongruity of clinical and physiological data is, in our opinion, due to our incomplete knowledge of the psychophysiological systems (which may only be assessed at the periphery) and also to the well-known difficulties of clinical description. With our present knowledge, it is advisable to treat syndromatically the physiological data of both the depressive and schizophrenic psychosis as *additional,* but not *explanatory* information about the clinical state.

Psychophysiologic experiments furnish otherwise unattainable additional information about psychopathological states. This can be explained by the differences in the investigation strategies of the clinician and the psychophysiologist. Whereas the clinician tries to understand his patient's condition through subjective explorations (i.e., patient's history, interview, etc.), the psychophysiologist subjects his patient to different experimental conditions that will enable him to make statements about the psychophysiological responsiveness of this patient. In this respect, his methods are similar to those of the psychologist.

2. Psychophysiological basal levels and responsiveness are at present most often interpreted in terms of a general activation theory. Activation means the state of readiness of the organism to process information and to act. According to Haider,[8] the activation system of the organism is organized in a hierarchical way, ranging from the basal long-term mechanisms of circadian vigilance changes, through the tonic and phasic activation responses to specific stimulus constellations of the environment, to the highly differentiated selective mechanisms of attention and expectation. Those processes, which can be grouped under the headings Orientation Reaction, Habituation, and Conditioning, are relevant for the clinical assessment of psychophysiological responsiveness.

The Orientation Reaction is an instantaneous state of readiness of the organism evoked by a novel stimulus. This reaction enhances reception of additional information, promotes coping behavior, and is comprised of a set of physiological changes (orienting responses).

Habituation is a decrement in the orienting responses when the same stimulus is repeated; that is, the stimulus becomes familiar and unproblematic for the organism.

Conditioning means reinstating an orienting response and/or a reaction to a habituated stimulus, by coupling it with an unconditional stimulus, which always provokes a reaction.

Sokolow[15] has developed a neural model of orienting responses and their habituation, which is shown in Figure 1.

According to Sokolow,[15] habituation, that is, the decrement of orienting responses when stimuli are familiar, is initiated by the matching of old information to the incoming information. This process occurs in the model-

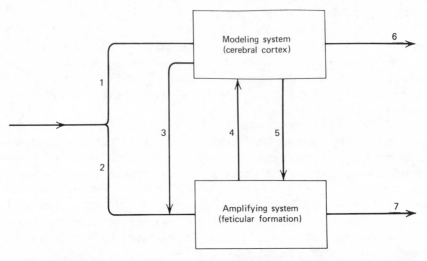

Figure 1. 1. Specific information transmission from the receptors to CNS. 2. Unspecific collateral pathway to reticular formation. 3. Feedback, if model is already existing (blocking the reception of the stimulus, that is, disactivation of the reticular formation). 4. Activating pathway to cortex and 5. back again to reticular formation, if a model of the situation does not exist. 6. Output after elaboration of an internal model. 7. Influences on vegetative functions by the activation level of the reticular formation.

ing system of the cortex and the thalamocortical functional circuits. The tonic and phasic orienting responses are initiated in the amplifying system, that is, in the unspecific reticular system of the brain stem and parts of the limbic system.

As a result of psychophysiological investigations with schizophrenic patients, one supposes that schizophrenic disturbances are primarily located in the modeling system (information processing), whereas such investigations with depressive patients tend to locate the disturbance in the amplifying (activation) system.

Both of Sokolow's systems,[15] the modeling system and the amplifying system are closely connected with each other, disturbances in one system having an effect also on the other system. The deficiency in cognitive filtering of relevant information in schizophrenics can be interpreted as either the cause or the result of a general overactivation of the organism; on the other hand, in the case of retarded depressive syndromes, the fact that the activation is inadequate for the stimulus, means that the intake of information is limited to a narrowly confined range. However, many experimental results lead us to believe that in the case of schizophrenic functional disturbances, it is *primarily* the selective functions of attention that are affected, and in depressive syndromes, *primarily* those activation processes that are coupled with the emotions.

DEPRESSIVE SYNDROMES

Already Gellhorn,[4] Alexander,[1] Selbach,[13] and others have considered depression to be an inactivated state, characterized by an increase in trophotropic tone and a decrease in sympathetic tone. More differentiating, Lader[12] and Kelly[11] found that inhibited and agitated depressive patients differed in their activation reactions as measured by forearm bloodflow and the skin conductance reaction.

In our own investigations, matters looked even more complicated. Ninety-five patients (in- and outpatients) diagnosed as depressed and/or anxious (schizophrenic and organically impaired patients excluded) were tested with regard to their psychophysiological reactivity to different stimuli. The parameters measured were EEG, finger pulse amplitude, respiration, and skin resistance. The stimuli consisted of tones of different intensities, a conditioning setting in which a habituated tone was coupled with a strong noise, simple tasks (arithmetic, motor reaction, etc.), and a part of JUNG's verbal association test.

Looking only at the reactivity in the skin resistance, we can distinguish four types of reactivity that differ from the normal range of reactivity.

In agreement with Claridge,[3] we assume that a tonic and a modulating activation system exists. Shifts in the basal level of skin resistance supposedly are controlled by the tonic system. Lability of the tonic system is defined as excessive shifts in skin resistance (measured as the difference between minimal and maximal values of skin resistance obtained during the entire experiment). Brief changes in skin resistance, which persist not longer than some seconds, are under the control of the modulating system. Spontaneous fluctuations and the orienting responses to discrete stimuli are generally this type of brief phasic reaction.

Further criteria of a more complex nature are the habituation rate and the strength of conditioning.

With these criteria, the four aforementioned types of depressive and depressive-anxious syndromes can be distinguished, as shown in Figure 2.

The Inhibited Type

The tonic system of this patient is stable. The difference between the maximum and minimum skin resistance is small. On the other hand, the modulation system is badly disturbed, for the patients in this group do not

Type	Tonic System	Modulation System				
	Difference between Max. and Min. Skin Resistences	Reaction to Intensive Stimuli	Reaction to Minor Stimuli	Spontaneous Fluctuations	Habituation	Conditioning
Inhibited	Small	Small	None	Rare	Rapid	Weak
Activated	Small	Normal	Present	Frequent	Slow	Strong
Labile—inhibited	Large	Large	None	Rare	Rapid	Weak
Labile—activated	Large	Large	Present	Frequent	Slow	Strong

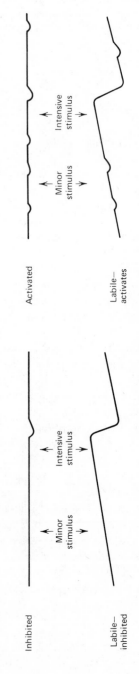

Figure 2. Types of reactivity (skin resistance) in depressive/anxious syndromes.

respond at all to tones; response to intensive stimuli is minor and spontaneous fluctuations are seldom observed. Habituation is rapid, and conditioning poor.

The Activated Type

The tonic system is again stable. The difference between the maximum and minimum skin resistance is small. The modulation system, however, is activated. The patients respond distinctly to minor stimuli. Many spontaneous fluctuations can be observed. Habituation is slowed down and conditioning strong.

The Labile and Inhibited Type

Here, the tonic, as well as the modulation systems are affected. The differences between the maximum and minimum skin resistance levels is large. In addition, very strong tonic reactions to intensive stimuli can be observed with these patients, as these lead to a breakdown of the tonic system. The modulation system is inhibited, as with the first type.

The Labile and Activated Type

The tonic modulation system corresponds to that of the labile type, the phasic modulation system, however, to that of the activated type.

Given complex stimulus situations, that is, Jung's association experiment, the patients do not always behave conformably to this classification. For example, there are depressive patients of the activated type who respond to minor tones but not to verbal stimuli, and conversely, patients of the inhibited type who show frequent and distinct reactions to verbal stimuli but none to tones.

This illustrates again the complexity of human information processing, which may be entirely different for neutral and emotional stimuli.

Figure 3 illustrates the *frequency distribution of the 4 types* of our 95 patients. The two labile types are less frequent than those with a stable tonic system. According to our experience, the treatment with psychotropic drugs is particularly difficult with the labile-activated type. This type shows in the self-rating scale of V. Zerssen the lowest frequency of negative and the highest number of positive answers. This shows that patients of this type suppress disorders when rating their own state of health.

Figure 4 shows the frequency distribution of diagnoses of the four types. One should note that endogenous depressions can be found in all four types, while the neurotic and reactive depressions occur more frequently with the activated type and less often with the inhibited type.

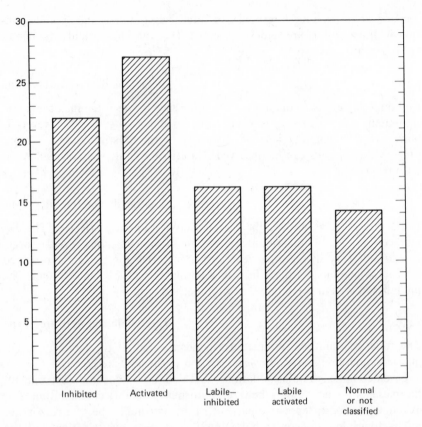

Figure 3. **Frequency distribution of the four types of reactivity (skin resistance) with depressive/anxious patients (N = 95).**

This means that, from a psychophysiological point of view, specificity exists only in a syndromatological, rather than a nosological, sense.

According to investigations by other authors, most anxious patients would belong to the activated type, as well as one group of schizophrenic patients ("responders" of Gruzelier[6, 7]). However, there exist nonresponders among chronic schizophrenic patients who would probably be classified as inhibited types in our experimental setting.

One can only speculate that in all patients who show the inhibited type of reactivity, the capability of orienting and reacting to changes in the environment is deficient, and therefore, adaptation is impeded.

In our opinion, any successful therapy should restore the basic processes of Orientation Reaction, Habituation, and Conditioning. For this reason, we plan in the future to measure the effects of a psychotropic drug in a given patient by looking at changes in psychophysiological reactivity under the influence of a single dose. From these measurements, we can then make suggestions for treatment.

SCHIZOPHRENIC FUNCTIONAL DISTURBANCES

The numerous investigations of disturbances in selective thinking, intake, and information processing of schizophrenics show that the problem is much more complex than in the case of depressive illness. Generalizations are therefore much more problematic. For example, assertions that phenothiazine reduces psychophysiological activity and responsiveness in schizophrenics, or that it normalizes the either too-high or too-low psychophysical activity in schizophrenics[18] are too vague to allow us to make a reliable hypothesis in clinical pharmacology. At the risk of oversimplifying, we would like to concern ourselves with at least one psychophysiological

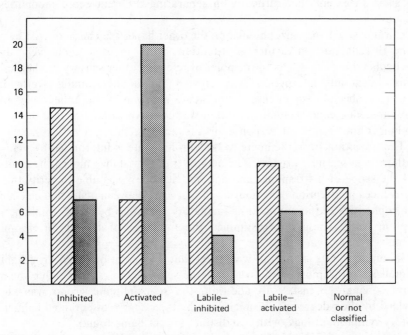

Figure 4. Frequency distribution of diagnoses of the four types of reactivity (skin resistance) ($N = 95$). ▨: endogenous and involutive depressions. ■: neurotic and reactive depressions.

aspect of schizophrenic functional disturbances that seem to us to be central to our understanding of the effectiveness of phenothiazines.

It has been shown repeatedly that schizophrenic functional disturbances are characterized by a pronounced response lability, if the environmental conditions are controlled. This can be seen by a large variance in the physiological values and in the lack of consistency when measurements are repeated. The statement that both chronic and acute schizophrenic states show an excessive general activation which can be normalized by giving major tranquilizers does not coincide with experimental findings.

In his neuronal model of attention functions, Sokolow[15] states that a central inhibitory mechanism must exist, which allows one to choose between relevant and irrelevant perceptual objects (see Figure 1). Similarly, Broadbent[2] speaks of a filter function necessary for selective perception. In acute schizophrenia, this filter is porous, and a stimulus overload occurs at the information processing centers.[14] The patients ability to structure his environment in such a way as to be able to cope with a particular situation is reduced, and his sensitivity to random, irrelevant stimuli is increased. The result is that the acute schizophrenic is more easily distracted; that is, his ability to sustain his attention and to structure his environment is reduced to such an extent that difficulty in separating different sense modalities occurs.

Chronic states of schizophrenia, on the other hand, are characterized by a general reduction in scanning, attention being focused exclusively on particular things or events to the point of rejecting other sensory modalities. This is generally interpreted as a screening-out of the stimulus overload, which has become so intense in the acute phase as to be unbearable. In these patients, conditionability is often slowed down or lacking and there is no longer any orientation response, or it is inconsistent.

The transition from the acute to the chronic state is interpreted by many authors as a learning process. The patient tries to stabilize himself by limiting the scope of his response and actions. Straube[17] was able to verify that differences in attention behaviour do in fact exist between acute and chronic schizophrenics of the paranoid-hallucinatory subgroup by using simple perception tests. These tests examined the influence of random irrelevant stimuli.

In another test series, it was seen that the emotion-laden irrelevant stimuli were the most attractive for some schizophrenics, preventing them from solving the task.[16] In addition, the schizophrenic group was not divided by their degree of chronicity but by their degree of paranoid hallucinatory symptomatology, with two distinct groups being found.

Gruzelier and Venables[6] were able to verify with psychophysiological investigations (GSR) the existence of two extreme groups in a heterogenous sample of schizophrenics: so-called responders and nonresponders.

The responders did not habituate to criteria (three successive failures to respond). However, using this criteria, there was no fixed relationship to chronicity. These investigations illustrate the psychological and physiological multidimensionality of the schizophrenic illness, which must be remembered if one considers the effect of psychopharmaca.

If one considers acute schizophrenia, as we have done, to be a disturbance of an inhibitory mechanism during stimulus processing, it is relatively easy to understand the effectiveness of major tranquilizers, in that major tranquilizers create a chemical safety valve filter. The association between chronic schizophrenia and major tranquilizers is much more complex. In this case, the drugs also have the effect of reducing the potential stimulus overloading, and one would imagine that the defense mechanism which chronic schizophrenics have learned should no longer be necessary. However, the changes that these patients show when major tranquilizers are given are generally unspectacular. This is because they must first of all learn to give up the defense mechanism of limiting the field of attention. This is often impossible without a long, consistent rehabilitation, which, in order to be successful, needs the protective function of a stable human relationship.

For the further development of clinical pharmacology of schizophrenia, it will be necessary to examine *together* psychological (clinical behavior, cognitive disturbances, etc.) and psychophysiological aspects of the disturbance and to examine the interaction between the modelling system and the amplifying system in the sense of Sokolow,[15] under various drug conditions. Until this is done, it will not be possible to make differential statements about the effectiveness of medications. In the future, it will be psychophysiological investigations into disturbances of the filter mechanism in schizophrenics and, as we showed in the second part of this paper, the investigations of the activation systems that will bridge the gap between the fundamental biochemical hypotheses and the clinical reality which the psychiatrist has to deal with in everyday life.

SUMMARY

Sokolow's[15] model of information processing is presented as a theoretical framework for psychophysiological investigations. Psychophysiological findings in depressive and schizophrenic disturbances are discussed within this framework as providing additional information about psychopathology.

Psychophysiological measurements are proposed as helpful in determining treatment as well as evaluating new psychotropic drugs.

REFERENCES

1. Alexander, L.: *Objective Approaches to Treatment in Psychiatry,* Thomas, Springfield, 1958.

2. Broadbent, D. E.: *Decision and Stress,* Academic Press, London, 1971.

3. Claridge, G. S.: Personality and arousal. A psychophysiological study of psychiatric disorder. *International Ser. Monogram Experimental Psychology,* Vol. IV, Pergamon Press, Oxford, 1967.

4. Gellhorn, E. and Kiely, W. F.: Autonomic nervous system in psychiatric disorder. In *Biological Psychiatry,* J. Mendels (Ed.), Wiley, New York, 1973, pp. 235–261.

5. Gottlieb, G. and Paulson, G.: Salivation in depressed patients. *Arch. Gen. Psychiat.* **5**:468, 1961.

6. Gruzelier, J. H. and Venables, P. H.: Skin conductance orienting activity in heterogenous sample of schizophrenics. *J. Nerv. Ment. Dis.* **155**:277–287, 1972.

7. Gruzelier, J. H. and Venables, P. H.: Skin conductance responses to tones with and without attentional significance in schizophrenic and non-schizophrenic psychiatric patients. *Neuropsychologia,* **11**:221–230, 1973.

8. Haider, M.: Neuropsychology of attention, expectation, and vigilance. In *Attention, Contemporary Theory and Analysis,* D. I. Mostofsky (Ed.), Appleton-Century-Crofts, New York, 1970, pp. 419–432.

9. Heimann, H.: Methodologische Probleme bei der Effizienzprüfung von Psychopharmaka. *Arch. Psychiat. Nervenkr.* **220**:255–268, 1975.

10. Heimann, H.: Psychobiological aspects of depression. In *Masked Depression,* P. Kielholz (Ed.), Hans Huber, Bern, 1973, pp. 32–60.

11. Kelly, D. and Walter, C. J. S.: A clinical and physiological relationship between anxiety and depression. *Brit. J. Psychiat.* **115**:401, 1969.

12. Lader, M. H. and Wing, L.: Physiological measures in agitated and retarded depressed patients. *J. Psychiat. Res.* **7**:89, 1969.

13. Selbach, H.: Die endogene Depression als Regulationskrankheit. In *Das depressive Syndrom,* H. Hippius and H. Selbach (Eds.), Urban & Schwarzenberg, Munich, 1969.

14. Silvermann, J.: Stimulus intensity modulation and psychological disease. *Psychopharmacologia, Berlin,* **24**:42–80, 1972.

15. Sokolow, Y. N.: Neuronal models and the orienting reflex. In *The Central Nervous System and Behavior,* M. A. Drazier (Ed.), J. Macey Foundation, New York, 1960.

16. Straube, E. and Klemm, W.: Sprachverhalten Schizophrener. *Arch. Psychiat. Nervenkr.* **221**:67–85, 1975.

17. Straube, E.: Experimente zur Wahrnehmung Schizophrener. *Arch. Psychiat. Nervenkr.* **220**:139–158, 1975.

18. Tecce, J. J. and Cole, J. D.: Psychophysiologic responses of schizophrenics to drugs. *Psychopharmacologia, Berlin,* **24**:159–200, 1972.

CLINICAL CONTRIBUTIONS

CHAPTER NINETEEN

SIMPLE FORM OF SCHIZOPHRENIA: WHAT DID IT TURN OUT TO BE?

VLADIMIR G. LEVIT, M.D., DR. MED. SCI.

D espite the numerous studies of the Simple form of schizophrenia and the frequent reference to it in the medical literature, this common type of schizophrenic illness still remains inadequately investigated. In discussions of the variants and types of schizophrenia, the question of the Simple form continues to be actively debated. It has been pointed out by W. Mayer-Gross[54] that the most difficult type to identify is the Simple form of schizophrenia. A follow-up study carried out recently in St. Louis[64] resulted in the conclusion that the Simple form does not exist at all, while a group of Harvard psychiatrists[83] presented their findings under the suggestive title "Simple Schizophrenia: Syndrome or Shibboleth?". Nevertheless, this diagnostic group continues to occupy a prominent place in daily clinical practice. It has been included in all psychiatric classification for at least three quarters of a century and may currently be found in the *International Classification of Diseases,*[32] and in the *Diagnostic and Statistical Manual of Mental Disorders*[15] approved by the APA.

To merely negate a diagnostic entity of this importance is not sufficient. Such a negation must be substantiated by the most extensive evidence. Moreover, one must be prepared to explain the persistence of the diagnosis among practicing psychiatrists and to suggest a more accurate and useful way of viewing the phenomena in question. The following data, presented as a contribution toward the resolution of this issue, are the results of a detailed study conducted by the author over the course of 11 years, 1962–1973, during the period of his association with the Institute of Psychiatry of the Academy of Medical Sciences U.S.S.R., Moscow.

HISTORICAL SURVEY

To understand the current debate about the Simple form, it is helpful to review rapidly the work that helped establish it as a diagnostic category. Brief descriptions of a clinical state, later to be referred to as Simple schizophrenia, are to be found in the works of the earliest psychiatrists, T. Willis,[91] Ph. Pinel,[69] and others, but astonishingly clear description may be attributed in 1798 to John Haslam of Bethlehem Hospital, London (cited by A. Pick[68] and J. Zelmanovitz[95]). The features observed among Haslam's patients, progressive increase in severity of dementia with dominance of apathy and abulia, were later interpreted with reference to several different psychoses: Demence Precoce,[62] Primäre Verrücktheit,[73, 68] Hebephrenia,[23, 27, 34] Hereditäre Neurosen,[76] and so on. The diagnoses were quite different, but so far as can be judged by the actual description, the clinical pictures were very similar.

J. Haslam described cases in which the course of illness led to severe dementia. Significantly, the psychiatrists who followed him tended to depict cases with a less serious course of development.[20, 28, 61, 73] These cases were also referred to as the Simple schizophrenia several decades later.

E. Kraepelin, in the fifth edition of his *Textbook on Psychiatry,*[42] defined the special nosological entity "Dementia Praecox," giving detailed attention to the form described by Haslam, Morel, and others. "Simple Dementia," as he called it, was distinctly characterized by the gradual development of dementia accompanied by apathy and abulia, and by the absence or mildness of other psychopathological signs. The onset of the illness was insidious, almost unremarkable; the course—slow but steady. This concept of the Simple schizophrenia, passing unchallenged, acquired a universal and almost canonical status. It was reproduced in numerous handbooks and guides, and may still be found, essentially unmodified, in the latest American textbooks. The following are some examples:

In this type the most marked disturbances are of emotion, interest and activity. If hallucinations occur, they are rare and fleeting, and delusions never play an important role.[39]

Insidious reduction of external attachments and interests, apathy, impoverishment of interpersonal relations, poverty of thought, and an absence of florid schizophrenic symptoms.[5]

The Simple schizophrenia's principal disorder is a gradual, insidious loss of drive, interest, ambition and initiative. He is usually not hallucinated or delusional.[45]

The Simple form of Dementia Praecox became an independent clinical entity—"Dementia Simplex"—as a result of the work of O. Diem in 1903,[16] who again focused on comparatively mild cases, in which the schizoid changes in personality observed by Haslam, Kraepelin, and others were less marked. Likewise, E. Bleuler,[6] in his efforts to define the boundaries of the illness that he had named "schizophrenia," classified the Simple form as an independent and basic one.

Thus we observe almost from the start the same division of opinion concerning (1) the course of the Simple schizophrenia, and (2) its nosological independence, that characterizes current debate. As a rule, one describes the Simple form as an independent form of schizophrenia. It usually develops soon after puberty and expresses itself through the slow, progressive worsening of schizophrenic symptoms, accompanied by distortion or exaggeration of features associated with adolescent change. "Positive disturbances," such as hallucinations and systematized delusions, are not characteristic. One generally notes two variants. The first, with gradual deterioration and progression toward global dementia of an apathoabulic type, is that described by Haslam and Kraepelin. The second, described by Diem, is characterized by a less severe psychosis, absence of apathy and abulia, slow development of schizoid or pseudopsychopathic disturbances or excited type (heboid),[35] schizophrenic changes in personality, and acute positive disturbances of pseudoneurotic type: asthenia, obsessions, hypochondria, and such. According to some authorities, the Simple form would cover both these variants; others admit only the first; and a third group, only the second—in which case, the first variant is described as Hebephrenia.

The willingness to include under a single heading cases that differ from each other so markedly in their severity can perhaps be related to the well-established idea that the development of Dementia praecox as a whole, as well as its Simple form, can be arrested at any stage, depending on various external factors. The differences between variants, however, cannot be ignored. They appear from the very onset of the illness, being evident in the particular clinical manifestations of the initial syndrome. Moreover, in addition to the continuous course, cases of the Simple schizophrenia with undulating ("shiftlike"), and even recurrent, courses have been described. In fact, given the wide range of possible courses the disease may follow, some psychiatrists have preferred to speak about the *group* of the Simple schizophrenias, or of the Simple form in the plural.[11, 19, 57, 94]

Whatever one says, there can be no doubt that in the process of its evolution as a diagnostic entity, the concept of the Simple schizophrenia gradually lost its specificity. One result of the lack of unanimity is a marked variability in the relative frequency of this diagnosis. The discrepancy factor was about 1400 (see Table 1). In one sample 55.3% of all cases classified as schizophrenia were considered to be the Simple form, while at the other extreme, a second sample yielded a frequency of only 0.04%. It would be interesting to note the complete absence of the diagnosis Simple schizophrenia in the very last edition of *A Psychiatric Glossary* published by the APA.[71]

The reasons for the differences in understanding the Simple schizophrenia are several. First and foremost is the diversity of the clinical variants to which the same term is applied. Second is the fact that the definition of the Simple schizophrenia has depended from the beginning more on "negative" than on "positive" statements: *absence* of florid delusions, hallucinations, catatonic symptoms, and so on—and is obviously inadequate. Terminological inexactitudes constitute a third factor. For example, Kraepelin and others, who considered the Simple dementia to be relatively independent form of schizophrenia, made the mistake of including within this category the residual apathoabulic states that followed acute attacks. And

TABLE 1. TABULATED SUMMARY OF RELATIVE FREQUENCIES OF DIAGNOSIS OF SIMPLE SCHIZOPHRENIA WITHIN WHOLE GROUP OF SCHIZOPHRENICS

Ref.	Investigator	Year	No. of Patients	Contigent	Prevalence of Simple Schizophrenia
37	E. Kasanskaya	1934	106	Inpatients	29.2
19	A. Edelstein	1945	365	Outpatients	46.7
36	O. Kant	1948	741	Male schizophrenics	49.6
36	O. Kant	1948	679	Female schizophrenics	3.3
12	R. Counts	1954	94	Men called up for military service	55.3
89	H. Weiner	1958		Review	0.3–55.0
2	A. Ambrumova	1962	1000	Follow-up of inpatients	9.0
7	V. Borinevitch et al.	1964	1240	All the schizophrenics from two regions of Moscow	1.7
96	N. Zharikov et al.	1966	1429	Epidemiological study	1.5
83	A. Stone et al.	1968	Approx. 4500	Inpatients during 1960–1963	0.24
83	A. Stone et al.	1968	Approx. 4560	Inpatients during 1963–1965	0.18
83	A. Stone et al.	1968	Approx. 4080	Inpatients during 1965–1967	0.04

last, but not least, is the fact that O. Diem and E. Bleuler included under the label, the Simple schizophrenia, cases that came to be regarded several decades later as "sluggish" pseudoneurotic, or pseudopsychopathic schizophrenia.[17, 84, 29] These forms, like the Simple form with which they were confused, are currently classified as independent entities both in the APA Classification,[15] and in the International Classification of Diseases.[32]

Psychiatrists commonly try to resolve such vague issues by appealing to longitudinal observations on the course of the disease over long duration. Only an analysis of the total longitudinal history of a psychosis can possibly lead to conclusions convincing enough to support a diagnostic contention, as has been argued by S. Korsakov,[41] E. Kraepelin,[44] A. Meyer,[58] and others. This approach is particularly relevant to the controversial question of the Simple schizophrenia and its nosological independence. Unfortunately, although the clinical features associated with the Simple form in its initial and manifest stages have been fully described,[1, 65b, 67, 70, 99] the "terminal states" (outcome) of this form have not been adequately investigated. Only a few studies address themselves to this aspect of the problem,[11, 40, 94] among them two studies by American psychiatrists.

Starting with the data from frequency studies and a review of the classic descriptions of the Simple schizophrenia in American textbooks, A. Stone and colleagues[83] set out to show that this category is not applicable to a coherent group of patients and is therefore no longer a viable psychiatric diagnosis. They stated, "It is a vague and inherently unreliable diagnosis without foundation in psychological theory or psychiatric practice; we believe it should be discarded." Their conclusion was substantiated by clinical reexamination of eight patients so diagnosed many years before.

A. Munoz and colleagues[64] arrived at the same conclusion through a somewhat different approach. Upon conducting follow-up studies in cases of the Simple and the Hebephrenic schizophrenia, these authors found that the clinical pictures characteristic of the former did not remain stable. Viewed over the course of the years, the symptoms were seen the change, and new clinical pictures arose: paranoid with predominantly affective disorders, and so on. The authors presented their paper at a conference "Life History Research in Psychopathology," where several psychiatrists[26, 92, 93] supported their conclusion that Simple schizophrenia was not a viable diagnostic entity and called for the revision of the diagnostic manuals.

Follow-up studies of this sort are very difficult to carry out; that is why they are rare and the number of cases investigated is typically not large. Our own discussion is based on the detailed, phenomenological investigation of 200 cases, all of which were followed up. It is our intention to provide the reader with objective information which will allow him to form his own conclusions. We will therefore withhold our own opinions until the discussion section that follows the presentation of the data. Although it has sometimes been necessary to define the observed symptoms categorically, we have tried for the most part to restrict ourselves to descriptive language.

METHOD OF INVESTIGATION

The main object of our investigation was to determine what had happened to those patients who at the time of hospitalization (first hospitalization in the majority of cases) had presented the symptoms considered characteristic of the Simple form. In other words, we wanted to see how schizophrenia would appear when studied after many years' duration. In selecting our patients, we disregarded the diagnostic label although the majority of the patients were in fact diagnosed as Simple schizophrenics. The main criterion for selection was the clinical picture; in particular we looked for evidence and predominance of sluggishness, apathy, and passivity. These symptoms were presumed to have emerged during the predominantly continuous course of the disease, rather than as the outcome of an acute psychotic attack. Patients exhibiting a pronounced pseudoneurotic or hypochondriacal symptomatology were not considered in the sample, even though they had been diagnosed in the hospitals or dispensaries as Simple schizophrenic.

At the beginning of our work the patients for this study were selected from among those who had been observed by the Frunze Psychiatric Dispensary (outpatient clinic) which was the clinical base of the Department of Catamnestic Study of the Institute of Psychiatry AMS, U.S.S.R.

This dispensary was chosen for the following reasons. The Frunze administrative region was one of the oldest districts of Moscow and had a relatively stable population. All case histories had been kept in the archives of this dispensary for the last 15 years. In contrast to other dispensaries, a single register for all psychiatrists was maintained and kept in excellent order.

Using this source of information we observed a remarkable fact. Only a relatively short duration of the Simple schizophrenia was recorded. In addition, most of the patients were fairly young and had been hospitalized once or twice. Following their release they tended to disappear from the dispensary. At the same time in this clinic, other forms of schizophrenia (Paranoid, Schizoaffective, "Sluggish-course" or pseudoneurotic) were followed up and relatively large numbers of patients both with short and long duration of illness were found.

Four possible explanations of this situation occurred to us. First, the course of the Simple schizophrenia became progressively worse so that patients were directed to suburban hospitals for chronic cases, thereby removing contacts with the outpatient clinic. But this supposition was controversial to the published data. A very serious study headed by V. Favorina[22] was devoted to the investigation of the population of such hospitals and no Simple schizophrenics were found. Second, the Simple schizophrenia might have resulted in the death of young patients, thus eliminating them from the group of chronic schizophrenics. However, such a supposition could only be hypothetical and was in fact contradicted by clinical evidence: schizophrenic patients can die because of the illness itself, but only in cases of the Hypertoxic Catatonia (so called Stauder's Tödliche Katatonia[81, 85]).The third possibility was that the clinical phenomena changed in such a way that after the manifest stage it became impossible to classify the illness as the Simple form. In other words, the schizophrenia could no longer be considered as the Simple form. This explanation seemed plausible. The fourth and last explanation was that the so-called old Simple schizophrenics were not under the control of the outpatient clinic because the illness became less severe: the symptoms became less disruptive; then the patients were able to adapt themselves socially without the help of the psychiatrist. Neither the patients nor their relatives would thus need to appeal to the dispensary. This explanation likewise seemed plausible.

As a result of our initial observations we defined our problem as twofold: to find out—what had become of those patients, originally diagnosed as Simple schizophrenics, and to determine—what is finally understood as the Simple schizophrenia.

To obtain observations on patients with long duration of illness, we extended the field of our investigations to include the archives of the Gannushkin Clinical Hospital. This institution, in which the patients of Frunze region were generally hospitalized, is one of the oldest psychiatric facilities in Moscow, famous for the high quality of its charts. Both these sources were searched, and these cases were studied that met the criteria described above. There were 162 patients, 15 of them had never been hospitalized, 25 patients were added from Kashchenko Psychiatric Hospital (the clinic of the Institute of Psychiatry, AMS, U.S.S.R.) and 13 from other psychiatric hospitals where the author was a consultant. The criteria for inclusion were the same.

Before the interview of each investigated patient, all data available to us from hospitals, outpatient clinics, and other institutions were carefully analyzed. All record data were checked, and if they were not sufficiently complete they were marked for supplementation by information to be secured in the course of the interview. We then proceeded to personally interview and evaluate the patients. Attention was given to the full history of the illness (anamnesis), complete phenomenological picture to the patient's present problems, and his social adaptation. As a rule, these interviews were conducted using the facilities of the Frunze Dispensary, other outpatient clinics, and hospitals depending on the patient's condition. All interviews were conducted by the author, a trained physician and practicing psychiatrist.

In 30 cases out of the 200, we were unable to secure an interview—19 patients refused to be examined; 6 had left Moscow; and 5 had died at the time of the study. In these cases, we consulted relatives, physicians, and the records of medical institutions, and evaluated the consensus of opinion. By means of this approach, it was possible to reconstruct in considerable detail the entire medical history of the 200 patients in the sample. The results of the catamnestic studies enabled us to formulate initial hypotheses,[47] which were then tested in an epidemiological study of the total population of patients registered as schizophrenic in Kiev district of Moscow (1429 cases).[50]

DESCRIPTION OF THE STUDY SAMPLE

Of the 200 patients in the total sample, 76% were male (3.2:1 ratio). Mean duration of illness was 20.5 years. The first hospitalization in the majority of cases occurred between 1948 and 1957. The follow-up examination was conducted between 1962 and 1965.

Sixteen patients were ill less than 10 years; 87 were ill from 11 to 20 years; the remaining 97 had been ill for more than 20 years at the time of the interview. Distribution according to the age of onset of illness was as follows: 10 patients at age 3; 9 patients from 4 to 7; 24 patients from 8 to 11; 116 patients from 12 to 15; 25 patients from 16 to 19; 15 patients from 20 to 23; in a single case, illness developed at age 26 (see Figure 1).

The sample was divided into five groups, according to the course of the schizophrenic process which was found during the follow-up. The first three groups illustrate the slow and relatively favorable course. We considered it to exhibit three conditional stages: initial, manifest, and terminal or final. In terms of this division the patients of *group one* (81 patients, mean duration of illness 19.5 years) showed complete development of symptoms mentioned above over several years. Thus we referred to the manifest stage of the Simple schizophrenia in these cases. In *group two* (22 patients, the mean duration of illness was 19.8 years) an atypically protracted and veiled attack (shift or der Schub-*Germ.*) was followed by remission with a high degree of resocialization, so that it was possible to speak of "social recovery." The clinical picture of the manifest stage showed evidence of sluggishness, but this symptomatology was accompanied by atypical or "masked" adynamic

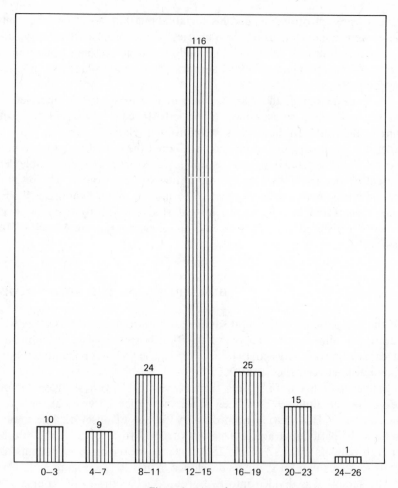

Figure 1.   Age of onset.

depression with another pseudoneurotic and pseudopsychopathic symptoms. *Group three* (26 patients) showed the longest duration of illness, 28.1 years. As in group one, the process showed itself to be "sluggish" throughout its continuous course. For the purposes of this discussion this group is the most interesting and is analyzed in detail below.

A malignant course, typical for Hebephrenia and other so-called "nuclear" forms, was observed in *group four* (34 patients), where the mean duration of illness was 18.5 years. Symptoms characteristic of the Simple form were soon complemented by florid positive symptoms: paranoid delusions, hallucinations, lucid catatonia (as opposed to oneiroid catatonic symptoms), hebephrenic features, and such. *Group five* (37 patients), with average duration of illness 19.2 years, differed from the rest of the sample. The disorders in these patients had taken the form of well-defined psychotic exacerbations. This became evident only as a result of the follow-up studies. The clinical pictures during the initial stage of the disease resembled pictures of Simple schizophrenia, but during the following attacks one could see acute schizoaffective symptoms. In other words, in groups four and five we observed the metamorphosis of the of the disease: clinical pictures corresponding to the description of the Simple schizophrenia gave way to manifest symptoms of florid psychosis.

Thus follow-up of the various cases revealed diverse developments. Schizophrenia originating as the Simple form had assumed the characteristics typical of other forms—"nuclear forms," such as Lucid Catatonia, Hebephrenia, and Juvenile paranoia, in group four; or shiftlike forms, as observed in groups two and five. It would be well to mention that the same type of phenomena has been noted by other investigators, and some psychiatrists have begun in recent years to speak conditionally of the "transformation" of the Simple form into other forms. For example, one encounters references not only to the independent Simple schizophrenia, but also to the "Simple schizophrenic picture,"[63] "the Simplex-syndrome,"[47] and "the Simplex-stage" in the development of the schizophrenic process.[100]

In our sample, the psychopathological disturbances that had become manifest over the course of illness in groups four and five made it clearly impossible to continue speaking of the Simple form, while with regard to patients in the second group, the degree of apparent remission enabled us to speak of it only conditionally. Only among patients of the first and third groups, where the process had remained "sluggish" and continuous throughout the follow-up period, were the clinical pictures still in accord with the standards for the Simple schizophrenia as outlined by O. Diem.[16] Since however the process in group one patients had not exceeded the terminal, last stage, complete description of the full course of illness was only possible for those cases labelled as group three. The rest of our discussion is restricted to the patients in this group.

CHARACTERISTICS OF THE SELECTED GROUP

Preliminary note may be made of the fact that of the 26 patients under consideration, 23 were male. Distribution of patients according to sex differed statistically from the distribution in the other four groups: 88.5% against 73% ($t = 2.18$). In 84.6% of the group, family histories revealed a genetic overloading, although this figure was commensurate with figures for the rest of the total sample. Also 38.4% had relatives who had suffered from different variants of the "sluggish course" of schizophrenia, and 23.1% had relatives who had suffered from acute psychotic forms, while 15.4% had relatives who had psychopathic personalities, were chronic alcoholics, or had suicidal tendencies; relatives of the remaining 7.7% were unidentified.

Clinical Picture During Initial Stage

In the majority of cases (65%), the first signs of schizophrenia appeared between 10 and 16 years of age and included autistic tendencies and the weakening of attachments. Interest in studies declined, and progress in school became poorer, especially in exact sciences. Students missed classes, fell behind, and were often forced to repeat the term. They confessed to feelings of laziness, to an inability to concentrate, to absentmindedness; poverty of thought[3] was noticeable. At the same time, they showed an inclination for pursuits not generally shared by their peers, as for example, the study of philosophy, yoga, or ancient religions. Such preoccupations, which we may call "overvalued ideas," suggested a symptom of "metaphysical intoxication."[52, 98] Compared to the interests common to normal adolescents, they appeared one-sided, unproductive, and autistic. The patients became stubborn, disobedient, and rude; some of them showed additional symptoms, including sloppiness, mendacity, and a preoccupation with instinctive drives.

Clinical Picture at Manifest Stage

After a period varying from 2 to 6 years from the onset of illness, the process reached the manifest stage. Autism and emotional impoverishment became more severe. The patients became more distant from their families. They refused to participate in household chores or to acknowledge responsibilities. They became increasingly impractical and incompetent. At work or in school, their productivity dropped and they were fired or expelled. In the absence of abstract preoccupations, they became totally idle, passive, and sluggish. In short, they failed to live up to the expectations they had aroused.

Against this background of gradual changes in personality, pseudoneurotic disturbances became manifest or more pronounced, although they never reached such intensity and variety as usually characterize pure, genuine pseudoneurotic forms. There were symptoms of asthenia, and such obsessive phenomena as irrational fear, compulsive counting and obsessive recall. Hypochondriacal apprehensions that were vaguely expressed during the initial stage were supplanted by a definite, fixed idea that there was "something wrong" with the patient's health. Carefully dissimulated dismorphophobic preoccupations were sometimes observed. The patient's aversion for his immediate surroundings increased, and he began to imagine that his closest friends and relatives were hostile toward him. Rudimentary auditory hallucinations, such as calls and mocking or accusing voices, were noted, as well as occasional and transient unpleasant feelings of indefinite nature, generally localized within the head. The overvalued ideas characteristic of the initial stage became increasingly prominent. All these symptoms were accompanied by superficial affective fluctuations of the cyclothymic type.

Clinical Picture During Follow-Up

Our most important initial observation concerned the relatively favorable condition of the patients, given the prolonged course of the illness. More than 80% of the group had been living regularly at home; only 5 of the 26 patients had been continuously (or almost continuously) confined to psychiatric hospitals. The majority had been hospitalized only once or twice for short periods, at the earlier stages, as a rule. Two persons had never been hospitalized. Six persons held steady jobs of a simple kind, and one other was a teacher of mathematics, though frequently changing his places of employment. The rest seemed to lack the initiative necessary to look for work, even in those cases where obvious financial difficulties might have encouraged them to do so. Some declared that they were "not against it in principle" or were "planning to look into it," while others rejected the whole idea of work, explaining that no job could be found that suited them. In response to specific proposals, they claimed that the job did not correspond to their temperament, was uninteresting, or did not pay enough.

Their interests appeared to be extremely limited. They passed their time leafing through books and magazines, or skimming over textbooks related to some specialized field which they never managed to master. They usually had no friends or acquaintances and did not feel the need of any company. Their activities were generally of a solitary nature. Although some patients evinced a special sensitivity to nature, to animals, or to a few works of art, such feelings were exceptions to their normal state of emotional impassivity. The patients seemed oblivious to the difficulties involved in running a household. They never offered to help with chores, even when their assistance was obviously needed. If they did do anything, they were absentminded, slow, and disorganized. Relatives commented that the patients were "heartless" and insensitive and affected great superiority. Patients who lived alone proved incapable of caring for themselves and became fully dependent on relatives, acquaintances, or neighbors. Such phenomena as extreme excitability or rudeness became even weaker with the course of time.

The appearance and behavior of the patients were unusual enough to arouse attention. Facial expressions and bodily postures were extremely mannered and affected. Dress was for the most part slovenly, more rarely smart though old fashioned—never natural and correct. Their speech was filled with platitudes, hackneyed expressions, and inappropriate of thought. Interrogated directly, their answers were frequently evasive or indefinite. They would speak for a long time, apparently without any real concern for the interlocutor. No real signs of monologue with schizophasia[87] were observed however. Certain properties of their behavior suggested psychic infantilism. Their future plans were totally unrealistic. Incapable of anything practical, they expressed their intention to create monumental works, appear at the Bolshoi Theatre, become celebrated mathematicians, or publish a scientific article a day. They made no attempt to realize their plans. They showed naive judgment, proposing, for example, to solve financial difficulties by marriage or enlistment in the army. They would discuss intimate matters with unseemly boldness and demonstrated a marked dependence on and attachment to their relatives.

The clinical pictures revealed by this follow-up study were not limited to the personality changes described above. All the previously manifested clinical symptoms were retained or developed. Vague hypochondriacal symptoms were observed in 12 cases, but were, as a rule, rudimental in nature. Only two patients evinced a profoundly dissimulated conviction of their personal ugliness. Symptoms of asthenia were also observed. Eight patients complained of rapid fatigue, auditory hyperesthesia, and headache, and in three cases there were additional suggestions of depersonalization. Eight patients showed obsessive features including phobias, recollections— sometimes unpleasant, sometimes of an abstract nature—and an obsessive need on the part of the patient to analyze his own behavior. These disorders appeared in waves and were accompanied by feelings of external influence; that is they became fragments of Kandinsky-Clerambaut syndrome. Division, confusion, or interruption of thought would sometimes supervene in a similar manner.

Pronounced fluctuations of mood were observed in 15 cases, with changes in affective intensity apparent over the course of a 24-hour period. As before, episodes of mild depression, expressed as gloominess and dissatisfaction, were dominant. While maintaining an appearance of outward indifference, one patient confessed to feeling sick, old, unwanted, incapable, lonely, and miserable. Some patients sank into a state of prolonged mental torpor in which they would analyze their own faults and reproach themselves. Thoughts of suicide did not occur. In a few cases, short alternate episodes of euphoria, signified by tomfoolery, forwardness, excitability, and fussiness were observed.

The preoccupation with overvalued ideas (most prominent in the case histories of six patients) led, in the late stage of illness, to increasingly absurd and unproductive fantasies. The patients spent their days drawing schemes for urban transport routes, attempting to design television sets of extraordinary power, or inventing an engine on "ion-molecular principles" so as to facilitate the tourist excursions that were never undertaken. They continued their ineffective preparations for a career as a concert musician or their work on a thesis, the purpose of which they could not even formulate.

Delusional and hallucinatory symptoms were characterized by poverty and monotonousness. Nine patients thought they detected signs of malevolence in the people about them, but we observed no steady delusions of persecution. (This accords with the observations of Diem[16]). Only two persons believed their relatives were capable of poisoning or infecting them intentionally. Hallucinatory symptoms included rare calls, a ringing in the head, and a feeling of cephalic overrepletion.

In summary, the gradual aggravation of personality disturbances observed in the late stage was, as a rule, accompanied by the gradual weakening of the emotional component. In some cases too, affective fluctuations became shorter and less intensive.

One final symptom, rudimentary catatonia deserves to be mentioned. It has been described by Scholz,[75] Kraepelin,[43] Diem,[16] and Arieti.[4] It appeared in the clinical picture after the other disturbances, almost always at the last stage, and was usually indicated by motor signs. Facial expression and body posture of effected patients became hardened in such a way as to suggest the appearance of a mannequin. Movements were characterized by extreme sluggishness and slowness, which sometimes degenerated into episodes of substupor. Incidental features manifested by some patients included facial grimaces, staring, grotesquely mannered or awkward and abrupt movements, stereotype, and impulsive, aggressive outbursts. Monotonous swinging of the arms, incessant stamping, and screaming (stereotype of movement and speech) appeared more rarely.

A quarter of the patients studied were found to be susceptible to brief exacerbations, which lasted from several hours to several days. Direct fear and anxiety were absent, but some patients were effected in insomnia, accompanied by a vaguely expressed hallucinations, psychic automatism, and feelings of mistrust. During these episodes, patients stopped going out, imagining that plots were being laid against them. A few who had shown signs of dissimulated hypochondria began sleeping on the floor, washing their head daily, cooking strange meals, and so on. The exacerbation could be displaced by reinforcement of the symptoms of catatonia—substupor, negativism, or chaotic excitement with confusion and derealization.

Social Adaptation: Quantitative Evaluation

Here we must make a short digression. Estimations of the clinical status of the investigated patients included not only a detailed description but also a quantitative evaluation of the level of social adaptation (SAL).[47] We used a five-grade scale based on such criteria as activity—employment, studies, housework, and such—productivity, and social involvement. A middle index of social adaptation level (MISAL) was computed for groups of patients at each year of their illness. Plotting this index figure against duration of illness, we obtained curves showing the dynamic change in level of social adaptation with reference to time. These permitted us to form a single visual picture of the diverse phenomena previously described. For the patients in group three, the curves took the characteristic form shown in Figure 2.

We observed an almost continuous decline in social adaptation to MISAL = 2.5, with the most prominent changes occurring in the first years of illness. Rate of decline was significantly reduced in the second decade, and a clear though slow tendency toward social recovery was observed after the 19th year. This tendency also appeared in the graph of SAL for group one and produced a U-like curve for group two of the sample.

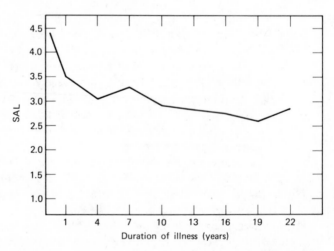

Figure 2.   Level of social adaptation (average for patients in group 3).

Treatment

An attempt was made to evaluate the effect of active therapy on the course of the disease. The data studied were extracted from the case histories. An evaluation of the methods used was beyond the scope and possibilities of our follow-up. Within the small group of 26 patients, the distribution of treatment was as follows: 11 patients received multiple courses of various types of active therapy (neuroleptics, insulin coma treatment, and others); 4 patients received only a single course of insulin coma treatment; 3 patients were treated with drug induced seizures and ECT; 5 patients were not treated at all; we were unable to obtain any information on the remaining 3 patients. It was impossible to draw any firm conclusions from the study of this group, but our general impression was that the fate of each patient depended primarily on the peculiarities of the ongoing psychosis and was not substantially altered by the type of therapy.

This impression was supported by observations extended to the total sample. The patients were grouped according to the treatment they had received and their latest SALs compared. As may be seen from Table 2, the highest levels of adaptation were observed among the patients who had not been treated at all. Those who had been treated actively continued to show low levels of adaptation despite the treatment.

ANALYSIS AND SUMMARY OF DESCRIPTIVE DATA

The clinical picture revealed during this follow-up analysis turned out to be complex. In the course of the prolonged development of the disease, a gradual accretion of new symptoms, none of which reached its full development, was observed instead of the transformation of one syndrome into another which is characteristic of other forms. Acute psychotic states failed to develop, and weak exacerbations were present in only a few cases and were of short duration. The initial syndrome, as noted, became increasingly polymorphic. Changes in personality were joined first by pseudoneurotic symptoms of an asthenic, obsessive kind, then by rudimentary psychic automatism, and last by vaguely expressed catatonic symptoms. This characteristic order of succession clearly corresponds to the Scale of Severity of Psychopathologic Signs.[80] It became possible after a certain point to speak of the stabilization of the process: no new symptoms developed, and the clinical picture continued essentially unchanged. Arrest occurred during the second decade of the process. Duration of the stable period from initial arrest to the date of follow-up varied from 5 to 23 years (mean duration 10.0 $\pm$ 5.6 years).

We may generally assume that the development of psychosis will be

TABLE 2. TREATMENT AND LEVEL OF SOCIAL ADAPTATION (SAL) OF THE PATIENTS STUDIED

SAL Definition	Score	Treatment					Lack of Information	Total
		Without Therapy	Various Kinds, Several Times	Insulin	Insulin + Neurol.	Medic. or Electric Convulsions		
Optimal	5	17	—	10	1	—	—	28
Good	4	13	1	9	3	12	3	41
Middle	3	14	13	8	4	8	2	49
Poor	2	5	13	3	6	4	3	34
Pessimal	1	—	36	4	2	2	4	48
Total		49	63	34	16	26	12	200

accurately reflected in the dynamic alteration of the clinical picture. If a disease develops slowly, we are able to observe the orderly succession of its stages distinctly. The first symptoms to manifest themselves will be those characteristic of the less severe impairments of cerebral functions, while succeeding symptoms will correspond to increasingly severe stages of disability. This pattern was effectively maintained in the group of cases under investigation.

The last symptoms to appear in our clinical picture were those of lucid catatonia, generally associated with the most malignant course of schizophrenia. We may therefore say that we were indeed dealing with the disease in its final state, with the *result* of the schizophrenic process, variously referred to as the "outcome," the "terminal state," of the "Endzustand."[18, 22, 46, 54]

We should be careful however not to be misled by the term arrest. As noted above, vague fluctuations and periodic exacerbations were observed in certain cases. By final state we mean to imply not only those cases characterized by completely static, unchangeable pictures, but also subacute elapsing processes or "Dauerzustände."[54, 56, 74, 84] The essential point is that there is no further deterioration in the mental state of the patient. This phenomenon has been described by O. Diem[16] and more recently by A. Molokhov,[59] who reports that it is often observed among patients in their 25th to 30th year of life. Descriptions of the psychopathological syndrome that later was referred to as "terminal state" in the Simple schizophrenia could be found both in classic[6, 16, 18, 31, 38, 43, 75, 77] and modern[40, 57 59 60] psychiatric literature.

We may note here that the features characteristic of this final stage of the Simple schizophrenia resemble those found in cases of pure "Sluggish-course" form of schizophrenia (referred to in the United States as pseudoneurotic and pseudopsychopathic schizophrenia).[15] One may read descriptions of the final state of the sluggish process by modern psychiatrists who have adhered to the common distinctions between this and the Simple form.[65a, 66, 78, 86] These descriptions emphasize the relatively favorable condition of the patients; dementia is characterized as "comparatively mild," or of "moderate degree." Although "intellectually crippled," the subjects are generally ambulatory: they hold simple jobs or subsist as beggars, vagabonds, or inmates of prisons and workhouses.

In attempting to resolve taxonomic difficulties of this order, to distinguish between different psychoses or to distinguish among the clinical forms of a single psychosis, one must be careful to keep in mind the complementary criteria of course and outcome. The case must be examined in its successive states—the phases and clinical pictures of the psychosis—and the pace of its evolution must then be determined. This manner of proceeding was recommended by the founders of scientific psychiatry—G. Falret,[21] K. Kahlbaum,[35] and especially Kraepelin[42]—and has been actively defended by many of their successors in this point.[24, 41, 56, 58, 79, 80] In recent years, these dynamic criteria of course and outcome have almost superseded the static approach in which the differentiation of clinical forms is based almost exclusively upon current syndromes.[30, 33]

I. Davidovsky's interesting concept of the *pathokinesis* of disease[13, 14] testifies to a similar tendency in general pathology. This term pathokinesis, which has suggestive implications for psychiatric study, refers to the evolution of a manifest process through all of its stages in the direction of a particular pathological stereotype. (Italian psychiatrists refer to the *nosodromia*[8].) Applying this concept to the case of the Simple schizophrenia, we note that there is nothing in either the order of appearance or the rate of succession of its symptoms that permits us to distinguish it from the Sluggish-course or pseudoneurotic form.

Nevertheless, despite the basic similarity of their pathokinetic stereotypes, we believe that certain features present over the prolonged course of illness in these cases enable us to distinguish the Simple form.

1. The clinical picture was dominated by changes in personality to a greater extent than in sluggish schizophrenia.

2. The picture was dominated by negative symptoms with underlying reduction of "energy potential"[10]; positive symptoms were less developed than is typical of the "Sluggish-course" form.

3. Pseudoneurotic symptoms were comparatively monotonous: hysterical symptoms were completely absent; psychoasthenic features, derealization and depersonalization appeared only rarely.

4. Onset of the Simple schizophrenia was, as a rule, restricted within a narrow age range and corresponded to the onset of puberty. In a special comparative study[97] of two follow-up homogeneous groups, onset of illness was found to have occurred between ages 12 and 14 in 58% of 200 of the cases predominantly diagnosed as the Simple form[49]; the figure for 303 patients diagnosed as pseudoneurotic and pseudopsychopathic[78] was 23.9%. Additional note must be made of the fact that the preponderance of males was significantly greater in the first group $(3.2:1)$[49] than in the second $(1.1:1)$.[78]

5. Stabilization of the process was observed to occur after 15 to 20 years of illness, as compared to 25 to 35 years for the Sluggish form.

6. The clinical picture characteristic of the outcome of the Simple schizophrenic process were generally worse than in cases of the Pseudoneurotic form. Symptoms such as indifference, sluggishness, passivity, and decreasing productivity were more pronounced. Psychic infantilism was

more frequently and notably expressed. Social adaptation was inferior. Rudimentary catatonic symptoms typical of final states in the Simple schizophrenia were not observed in the "Sluggish-course" schizophrenia, even after a course of illness of 30 to 40 years' duration.[78]

7. Hypomania and the alternation of excessive candor and excessive timidity observed during catamnesis in typical cases of the "Sluggish-course" form were likewise absent.

DISCUSSION

Among the Simple schizophrenia's distinctive features, we consider its comparatively higher incidence among males and the correspondence between onset of illness and commencement of puberty to be of primary importance. A specific genetic overloading and specific premorbid personalities probably play a significant role, but these questions are in need of further study.

Our evidence showed the age factor to be crucial. The following considerations seem to establish the relevance of puberty to an adequate definition of the Simple schizophrenia. First, in addition to the marked coincidence between the onset of illness and puberty, the characteristic symptoms of the Simple form frequently presented themselves as exaggerations of features typical of the adolescent psychohyperexcitability, opposition to adults, and preoccupation with overvalued ideas. Second, according to the date of psychiatrists involved in the study of late schizophrenia[72, 82] the Simplex syndrome has never manifested itself in patients over 40 to 45 years old. Third, we investigated those cases (19 in a sample of 200) where a continuous course of schizophrenia, manifested in fears, sleep disorders, and other symptoms, had developed in early childhood. In these cases, resemblance to the Simple schizophrenia only became apparent in the adolescent period. At the time of follow-up, this period had been exceeded, and the sluggishness and indifference that had been observed had been replaced by clearly expressed asthenia and obsessions. Such transformations have also been described in the literature.[9, 53, 88]

These opinions about the essential features of the Simple schizophrenia were tested and evaluated in a critical analysis of epidemiological data on 1429 patients,[50] the total population of schizophrenic patients in one of the administrative districts of Moscow. The incidence of the Simple form among recorded diagnoses turned out to be only 1.5% (the lowest of any form). In 68.1% of the cases so diagnosed, onset of illness occurred between 10 and 19 years of age. The diagnosis had been assigned in 19 of the 22 cases in which duration of illness had been only 10 years or less. (It is very possible, if the illness were to endure longer, that the diagnosis would be changed from the Simple form to other forms). Investigations were focused on three kinds of personality changes: deep changes in personality with predominance of sluggishness and apathy; pseudopsychopathic changes with predominance of irritability; and pseudopsychopathic changes with predominance of schizoid features. In 181 cases, it was showed that although these types of changes had been observed in the initial state of various forms of illness, the clinical pictures were unstable.

Symptoms such as delusions with psychic automatism, hallucinations, and catatonic or hebephrenic disorders began to dominate to such a degree that it became impossible to speak of the Simple schizophrenia. Syndromes characterized by apathoabulic changes in personality were rather rare (25 cases). The picture of psychosis changed within 10 years in 81.2% of all cases, and within 20 years in all the remaining cases.

It is especially interesting to observe the correlation between the manifest psychopathology, mostly in the form of personality changes, and the sex of the patient. Patients whose illness began with changes in personality were contrasted with the rest of the sample. Debuts with prominent personality changes were present almost invariably in cases where age at onset was under 30. They were twice as frequent in males as in females. The M/F ratio was different in different age groups. It was maximal (2.4:1) only in cases with onset of illness in the second decade of life (see Table 3).

In conclusion, it is easy to see how the Simple schizophrenia has become "a sort of diagnostic wastebasket."[51] One diagnostic term has been used to describe a variety of different conditions. One of these is the initial stage of "nuclear" schizophrenia—in this case it is indeed a "shibboleth." Another is one variant in a large group of sluggish-course schizophrenias.[49] In other words, the classical Simple form—in accordance with the descriptions of Haslam and Kraepelin—is only the Simple stage of the development of the schizophrenic process. The Simple Dementia—as it was described by Diem and Bleuler—is a particular variant of the so-called sluggish-course schizophrenia. Its peculiarities are caused primarily by the age of onset.

We can confirm the existence of a special variant of schizophrenia developing over the course of several decades with predominance of mild changes in personality rather than delusion, hallucinations, and other so-called positive symptoms. But to label this variant the Simple form is misleading, since we can deduce no clear pattern of succession in the psychopathologic pictures (syndromes), such as is generally characteristic of independent forms.

An old clinical rule suggesting that the longer one interviews the patient, the more psychopathology one elicits was appropriately paraphrased

TABLE 3. CORRELATIONS OF TYPE OF DEBUT WITH THE AGE OF ONSET AND SEX (M/F = COEFFICIENT MALE/FEMALE)

Type of Debut			Onset Age						
			0–9	10–19	20–29	30–39	40–49	50+	Total
With Predominance	a	Number	18	93	32	6	2	—	151
of Personality	b	%	11.7	61.8	21.3	3.9	1.3	—	100.0
Changes	c	M/F	2.0	2.4	1.9	0.5	—	—	2.0
All Other	d	Number	30	159	178	113	57	13	550
Together	e	%	5.4	28.9	32.4	20.6	10.3	2.4	100.0
	f	M/F	1.0	1.0	0.9	0.6	0.2	0.1	0.7
Criterion t (between b and e)			2.26	7.92	2.72				
Total		Number	48	252	210	119	59	13	701
		M/F	1.3	1.4	1.0	0.6	0.2	0.1	0.9

apropos of this issue by R. White[90]: "The more carefully the history is taken, the less great are the chances that the case will be classified under the Simple form."

SUMMARY

1.   "Dementia Simplex" in its pure form as it was described by Diem[16] is quite rare. It is less malignant than is widely assumed and is, in essence, just a variant of the "sluggish-course" schizophrenia. Its clinical peculiarities are primarily determined by the onset of illness during puberty.

2.   The clinical entity commonly designated as the Simple schizophrenia may better be considered as the Simple syndrome, or Simple stage, common to various forms of schizophrenia. Intensive apathoabulic states, appearing during the adolescent period, are almost observed in the initial stage of Hebephrenia and other "nuclear" forms.

3.   In the pathogenesis of the Simple syndrome three factors are of the utmost importance: (a) sluggish course of schizophrenic process; (b) onset during puberty; (c) higher incidence in males.

ACKNOWLEDGMENTS

The author would like to express infinite gratitude to Margarita V. Ivanova, R.N., and to his former collaborators for their assistance in retrieving the data. He would also like to thank Virginia R. Hannon, Sc.D., for her valuable advice in the organization of the material and for the assistance of Ms. Erna H. Jansson.

REFERENCES

1. Aleksanyanz, R. A.: Prostaya forma shizofrenii. *Diss. Cand. Moskva,* 1956.
2. Ambrumova, A. G.: Techeniye shizofrenii po dannym otdalennogo katamnesa. *Diss. Doct., Moskva,* 1962.
3. Arieti, S.: *Amer. J. Psychother.* **13**:537–552, July 1959.
4. Arieti, S.: *Interpretation of Schizophrenia,* Basic Books, New York, 1974.
5. Bemporad, J. R. and Pinsker, H.: Schizophrenia: The manifest symptomatology. In *American Handbook of Psychiatry,* S. Arieti, (Ed.), Vol. 3. Basic Books, New York, 1974, pp. 524–550.
6. Bleuler, E.: Dementia praecox oder Gruppe der Schizophrenien. In Aschaffenburg G. *Handbuch der Psychiatrie,* Spez. Teil, 4 Abteil, 1 Hälfte, 1911.
7. Borinevich, V.: cit. by Nadzharov. In *Trudy 4 Vsesoyuz, s"ezda nevropatologov i psikhiatrov.* Moskva, 1965, pp. 119–121.
8. Callieri, B.: Personal communication.
9. Chekhova, A. N.: *Techenie shizofrenicheskogo prozessa, nachavshegosya v detskom vozraste,* Medgiz, Moskva, 1963.
10. Conrad, K.: *Die beginnende Schizophrenie,* Stuttgart, 1958.
11. Cornü, F.: *Psychiat. Neurol.* **135**(3):129–175, 1958.
12. Counts, R. M. and Regan, P. F.: *Monatschr. Psychiat. Neurol.* **127**(1): 47–60, 1954.
13. Davidovsky, I. V.: in *Bolshaya Sovetskaya Enziklopediya,* Vol. 23, Moskva, 1961, pp. 434–463.
14. Davidovsky, I. V.: *Vestnik Akademii Medizinskikh Nauk,* 9, 1964, pp. 81–86.
15. *Diagnostic and Statistical Manual of Mental Disorders,* 2nd ed., American Psychiatric Association, Washington, 1968.
16. Diem, O.: *Arch. Psychiat., Nervenkr.* **37**(1):117–187, 1903.
17. Dunaif, S. L. and Hoch, P. H.: In *Psychiatry and the Law,* Grune & Stratton, New York, 1955, pp. 169–195.
18. Edelstein, A. O.: *Iskhodnye sostoyaniya shizofrenii,* Moskva, 1938.
19. Edelstein, A. O.: In *Trudy 1 Moskovskogo Medizinskogo Instituta,* Vol. 8, Moskva, 1945, pp. 208–228.
20. Esquirol, E.: *Des maladies mentales,* Paris, 1838.
21. Falret, G. P.: *Les maladies mentales et des asiles d'aliènes,* Paris, 1864.
22. Favorina, V. N.: *O konechnykh sostoyaniyakh shizofrenii,* Diss. Doct., Moskva, 1965.
23. Fink, E.: *Allg. Zschr. Psychiat.* **37**(5):490–520, 1881.
24. Gannushkin, P. B.: *Psikhiatriya, Ee zadachi, ob'em, prepodavanie,* Moskva, 1924.
25. Gannushkin, P. B.: *Klinika psikhopatiy, ikh statika, dinamika, sistematika,* Moskva, 1933.

26. Guze, S.: In *Life History Research in Psychopathology*, Vol. 2., M. Roff, L. Robins, and M. Pollack, (Eds.), University Minnesota Press, Minneapolis, 1972, pp. 234-234.

27. Hecker, E. E.: *Arch. Pathol. Anatomie, Psychol. Klin. Med.* 52(1-3): 394-429, 1871.

28. Hecker, E. E.: *Irrenfreund*, 4-5:394-399, 1877.

29. Hoch, P. H., and Polatin, P.: *Psychiat. Quart.*, 4:248-276, 1949.

30. Holland, J.: Draft of USA/USSR Joint Classification of Schizophrenia. (In print: *Schizophrenia Bull.* (NIMH), Spring 1976.)

31. Ilberg, G.: In *Volkmann's Sammlung Klinisch. Vortr.* 224(14):1287-1308, 1898.

32. *International Classification of Diseases, 8* Revision, Vol. 1, WHO, Geneva, 1968.

33. Janzarik, W.: *Nervenarzt*, 2:58-61, 1963.

34. Kahlbaum, K. L.: *Cbl. Nervenkr.*, 7:470-474, 1884.

35. Kahlbaum, K. L.: *Allg. Z. Psychiat.* 46(4) 461-474, 1889.

36. Kant, O.: *Psychiat. Quart.*, 22(1):141-151, 1948.

37. Kasanskaya, E. V.: In *K probleme skhizofrenii*, Moskva, 1934, pp. 79-103.

38. Koch, J. L. P.: *Kurzgefasster Leitfaden der Psychiatrie*, 2 Aufl., Ravensburg, 1889.

39. Kolb, L.: *Modern Clinical Psychiatry*, 8th ed., Saunders, Philadelphia, 1973.

40. Koroleva, E. N.: In *Voprosy kliniki, patogenesa i lecheniya shizofrenii*, Vypusk 1, Moskva, 1964, pp. 72-74.

41. Korsakov, S. S.: *Kurs psikhiatrii*, Izd. 2, Moskva, 1901.

42. Kraepelin, E.: *Psikhiatriya. Uchebnik dlya vrachey i studentov*, Perevod s 5. nemez. izdaniva, Sankt-Peterburg, 1898.

43. Kraepelin, E.: *Psychiatrie: ein Lehrbuch fur Studierende und Ärzte*, 8 Aufl., Bd. 3, Teil 2, Leipzig, 1913.

44. Kraepelin, E.: *Z. Neur. Psychiat.* 62-63: 1-29, 1920.

45. Lehman, H. E.: Schizophrenia. Clinical picture. In *Comprehensive Textbook of Psychiatry*, 2nd ed., A. M. Freedman, H. I. Kaplan, and B. J. Sadoch, (Eds.), Williams and Wilkins, Baltimore 1975, pp. 890-922.

46. Leonhardt, K.: *Die defektschizophrenen Krankheitsbilder*, Leipzig, 1936.

47. Levit, V. G.: In *Tezisy dokladov respublikanskoy konferenzii po voprosam profilaktiki invalidonsti i trudoustroystva invalidov s psikhicheskimi zabolevaniyami*, Moskva, 1964, pp. 73-76.

48. Levit, V. G.: *Zh. Kors.* (*Zhurnal Neuropathol. Psikhiat. S.S. Korsakova*) 65(1):88-97, 1965.

49. Levit, V. G.: *Prostaya forma shizofrenii* (*kliniko-katamnesticheskoye issledovanie*), Diss. Doct., Moskva, 1968.

50. Levit, V. G., Petrova, E. S., and Rotshteyn, V. G.: *Zh. Kors.* 69(1):129-137, 1969.

51. Lewis, N. D. C. *Research in Dementia Praecox*, Committee on Mental Hygiene, New York, 1936.

52. Malinovskiy, P. P.: *Pomeshatel'stvo*, Sanctpeterburg, 1855.

53. Mamzeva, V. N.: *Klinika, lechenie i profilaktika vyaloprotekayushchey shizofrenii u detey*, Diss. Cand., Moskva, 1955.

54. Mayer-Gross, W.: In *Handbuch der Geisteskrankheiten* von O. Bumke, Vol. 9, Spez. Teil V., Berlin, 1932.

55. Mayer-Gross, W.: Schizophrenia. In *Clinical Psychiatry*, W. Mayer-Gross, E. Slater, M. Roth, (Eds.), London, 1955.

56. Melekhov, D. E.: *Prognoz i vosstanovleniye trudosposobnosti pri shizofrenii*, Diss. Doct., Moskva, 1960.

57. Melekhov, D. E.: *Klinicheskie osnovy prognosa trudosposobnosti pri shizofrenii*, Moskva, 1963.

58. Meyer, A.: cited by Bemproad J. R., Pinsker H., no. 5.

59. Molokhov, A. N.: *Formy shizofrenii i ikh lecheniye*, Kishinev, 1948.

60. Molokhov, A. N.: In *Klinika shizofrenii*, Kishinev, 1967, pp. 5–18.

61. Moreau de Tours, P.: *Psychologie morbide*, Paris, 1859.

62. Morel, B.: *Traite des maladies mentales*, Paris, 1860.

63. Morosov, V. M.: In *Trudy 4 Vsesoyuznogo s"ezda nevropatologov i psickiatrov*, Moskva, 1965, pp. 204–209.

64. Munoz, A., Kulak, G., Marten, S., et al.: In *Life History Research in Psychopathology*, Vol. 2., M. Roff, L. Robins, M. Pollack, (Eds.), The University of Minnesota Press, Minneapolis, 1972.

65a. Nadzharov, R. A.: *K klinike vyaloprotekayushchey shizofrenii*, Diss. Cand. Moskva, 1955.

65b. Nadzharov, R. A.: *Klinika Neblagopriyatno Tekushchey Yunosheskoy ("Yadernoy") shizophrenii.* Diss. Doct., Moskva, 1965.

66. Panteleeva, G. P.: *O vyalotekushchey shizofrenii s klinicheskimi izmeneniyami psik-hastenicheskogo tipa.*, Diss. Cand., Moskva, 1965.

67. Petrova, A. G.: *Nekotorye klinicheskiye i patofisiologicheskiye osobennosti prostoy formy shizofrenii*, Diss. Cand., Kharkov, 1963.

68. Pick, A.: *Zeitschr. Neurol. Psychiat.* **91**(8): 233–238, 1924.

69. Pinel, Ph.: *Traite médico-philosophique sur l' allienation mentale*, Paris, 1809.

70. Pogosjan, A. M.: In *Tesisy Vseros. konfer. molodykh uchenikh nevropatologov i psikhiatrov.*, Moskva, 1959, pp. 98–99.

71. *Psychiatric Glossary*, 4 ed. APA, 1975.

72. Romanova, N. G.: *Zh. Kors.* **64**(1):100–109, 1964.

73. Rousseau: *De la folie a l'epoque de la puberte*, Paris, 1857.

74. Schneider, K.: *Die Psychologie der Schizophrenen und ihre Bedeutung fur die Klinik der Schizophrenie*, Leipzig, 1930.

75. Scholz, L.: *Allg. Zeitschr. Psychiat.* **53**(5–6): 912–932, 1897.

76. Schüle, H.: *Handbuch der Geisteskrankheiten*, Leipzig, 1878.

77. Serbskiy, V. P., *Zh. Kors.* **2**(1–2):33–60, 1902.

78. Shmaonova, L. M.: *Klinika vyalotekushchey shizofrenii po dannym otdalennogo katamneza*, Diss. Doct., Moskva, 1968.

79. Snezhnevsky, A. V.: *Zh. Kors.* **60**(9):1163–1175, 1960.

80. Snezhnevsky, A. V.: *Zh. Kors.* **75**(9):1340–1345, 1975.

81. Stauder, K.: *Arch. Psychiat. Nervenkr.*, **102**:614, 1934.

82. Sternberg, E. Ya.: *Zh. Kors.* **68**(2):213–220, 1968.

83. Stone, A., Hopkins, R., Mahnke, M., et al.: *Amer. J. Psychiat.* **125**(3):61–68, 1968.

84. Ssuchareva, G. Ye.: *Zschr. Neurol. Psychiat.* **142**:302–321, 1932.

85. Tiganov, A. S.: *Febzil'naya shizofreniya,* Diss. Cand., Moskva, 1960.

86. Urakov, I. G.: *Zh. Kors.* **69**(3):243–249, 1969.

87. Vrono, M. S.: *Konechnye sostoyaniya shizofrenii s rechevoy bessvyasnostyu.,* Diss. Cand., Moskva, 1957.

88. Vrono, M. S.: *Shizofreniya u detey i podrostkov,* Moskva, Medgiz, 1971.

89. Weiner, H.: In L. Bellack *Schizophrenia,* Review of syndrome, New York, 1958.

90. White, R.: *The Abnormal Personality,* 2 ed., Ronald Press, New York, 1956.

91. Willis, T.: *De anima brutorum.,* Amsterdam, 1674.

92. Winokur, G.: In *Life History Research in Psychopathology,* Vol. 2, M. Roff, L. Robins, and M. Pollack (Eds.), University Minnesota Press, Minneapolis, 1972, pp. 235–235.

93. Wirt, R.: *ibid.,* pp. 234–234.

94. Wyrsch, J.: Schizophrenie. In *Allgemeine und spezielle Psychiatrie,* M. Reichardt, (Ed.), 4. Aufl., Basel, 1955.

95. Zelmanovitz, J.: *Proc. Roy. Soc. Med.* **46**(11):931–933, 1953.

96. Zharikov, N. M., Levit, V. G., Popova, M. S., et al.: *Zh. Kors.* **68**(5):742–749, 1968.

97. Zharikov, N. M., Liberman, Yu. I., Shmaonova, L. M., et al.: *Zh. Kors.* **73**(5):551–559, 1973.

98. Ziehen, Th.: In *XIII Congress international de medicine,* Section psychiatrie. CR Geneve- Lausanne-Paris, 1900, pp. 10–31.

99. Ziziashvili, Sh.I.: *Klinika, techenie i sudebno-psikhiatricheskaya ozenka prostoy formy shizofrenii,* Diss. Cand., Moskva, 1958.

100. Zuzulkovskaya, M. Ya. and Druzhinina, T. A.: *Zh. Kors.* **66**(2):273–280, 1966.

CHAPTER TWENTY

THE PSYCHOTHERAPEUTIC GROUP AS MEDIATOR BETWEEN INDIVIDUAL, FAMILY, AND SOCIETY

R. BATTEGAY

THE SOCIAL-HORIZONTAL AND THE
DEEP PSYCHOLOGICAL-VERTICAL PLANE

The psychotherapeutic group with its various interactions on the social-horizontal and its multiple and multidimensional transferences[25-27] on the deep psychological-motivational plane causes a high intensity of social and intrapsychic processes, as we would like to say a high "intensity of reality."[5] The involved individuals have thus the opportunity to get to know, on one side, the social laws. On the other side, they can come to terms with their infantile family or other collective situations of their childhood, because this milieu activates early group experiences in the phantasy of the participants. The reciprocal influences in the therapeutic group further the process of social learning of the members as well as the process of gaining insight. The experience the individual gains within a psychotherapeutic group can be extrapolated into society. Whereas in the classic dual analytic situation gaining insight and social learning do not happen at the same place, the therapeutic group combines the gaining of insight and the attainment of social knowledge. The therapeutic group is an environment that appeals at the same time to the pleasure principle and to the reality principle.[11, 13] The "amplifying effect" of the group on the feelings sets off conflicts from the preconscious and from the unconscious that have been repulsed until then. At the same time the intensity of reality of the interactional process brings the participants to the social reality. This milieu is thus especially appropriate to confront infantile impulses, expectations, and their corresponding fantasies with the social facts. By this, inhibitions of drives[28] that have either been caused in early childhood or by life history as well as the consecutive behavior structures may be loosened up.

In our time, people usually grow up in small families, and often in their childhood do not have the opportunity to set forth with others of their age and to have social contacts with them. The therapeutic group gives them a frame in which they can recover their lack of experience with a greater number of siblings and a gib family.[3, 23] They can also experience a microcosm having similar laws as does the outside society. A group, composed of 7 to 10 members, leads the participants from the narrowness of the small family into an enlarged world and it so facilitates the accession to the even more enlarged society.

In a group of schizophrenics we led since 1963 as slow-open group,[10] we saw that the 7 to 9 members (all at the age of 25 to 35) are very often—though in an ambiguous way—so fixed to the pathological relationship with their parents that primarily they can hardly get into contact with the group. They only report about their often ambivalent relation to their fathers and mothers. At the beginning of their participation in the group they talk almost only to the therapist and to the cotherapist, but hardly to their group companions. They are focussed on figures of authority, on whom they transfer their feelings for their parents. It even happens that they call the therapist and the cotherapist directly Father and Mother. Thus there can sometimes be seen an idealizing transference[16] to the therapist. By the fusion with the idealized object, the patients gain strength.

A 27-year-old patient, for example, who was suffering from hebephrenia, gave himself the academic title of the therapist—partly joking, partly serious—and looked proudly around, without, however, paying attention to the others' reaction.

After several weeks or months of participation the schizophrenics generally succeed in getting into contact with the other members of the group and in identifying themselves with the others (identifying transference according to Slavson[25-27]). They become involved into an atmosphere that produces fantasies of a bigger family. This process shows that schizophrenics are not primarily autistics, as *Eugen Bleuler*[7] described it. They are, on the contrary, excessively sensitive concerning manifestations of people in contact with them. They are so sensitive that they often feel too much exposed to the others, may fear the weakness of their ego-boundaries, or even the loss of their ego and then reactively retire from human contact.[17] Therefore, for patients whose ego is too weak to suffer the nearness of others in a group, the participation in a therapeutic group is contraindicated. For the others, however, who are able to maintain their individuality, the psychotherapeutic group teaches them slowly to live with their sensitivity without being afraid of the loss of their ego. The therapeutic group becomes a mediator to society for these patients.

But also with neurotic patients we can observe that therapeutic groups, on the one hand, reactivate acute unconscious conflicts in them, for example, oedipal problems, and that, on the other hand, the group confronts them with the social reality.

A 40-year-old doctor who had been in an individual analysis for quite a long time and who now participates in an analytic self-experience group, suddenly experienced the group as an overprotective, constraining, frustrating mother, and the leader as a mighty, threatening father. In his dreams, he was also occupied with these feelings. He once told the following dream he had the night before a group session: "An old acquaintance, a friend, came to see me. For some time, he had been my neighbor. He suffered from a strong ambiguity concerning the relation to his mother and father. At once, the house starts burning, and I have to jump out of the window to save me." In his associations, he said that after he had become a member of the analytic group which had already existed before, he had slipped back into a role he had played already in former times and temporarily during his individual analysis. During the weekend, he had been so sensitive and so effervescent that temporarily he had to retire from the contact with his wife and his children. Several group members asked him, on the one hand, whether he experienced the group as a re-edition of his mother, and on the other hand, whether he mistook his wife for his mother. First, the doctor tried to turn away from this theme and to talk about another subject. But finally, he was able to recognize that the group was touching an unconscious conflict. Another group member had the association that the colleague behaved as a "little prince." Some members thought that the talk was about St. Exupéry. But another colleague became excited. He reclined on his chair, suddenly covered his eyes, and said: "I am troubled, I was frightened when you were talking about the 'little prince'." It appeared that the colleague who had covered his eyes was deeply affected in consequence of his own oedipal ambiguity. He seemed to be seized by unconscious archaic fear to be blinded for being guilty because of his incest fantasies. His father originally wanted to become a priest, but then renounced to this career. He got married, but very soon had affairs with other women. This behavior was ended by a car accident in pursuance to which he had a cerebral damage and became dependent on his wife, the patient's mother. This colleague became then the only "support" of his mother. The same member suddenly said that since a quarter of an hour, he had the impression that another group member and the leader were twins. This group colleague was representing a kind of scion of the leader. Several members could identify with this saying. Indeed, the so-called twin of the leader had identified himself in a high degree with the therapist. Thereby, the therapist was reinforced and the group members became frightened of this "double father's" power.

This dream showed how the mother problem of one of the group members was reactivated by the experience of the group. The "old" mother conflict, respectively the oedipal impulses, became so acute in the group that in his dream the house started burning and he had to save himself. The group was a mediator for the reactivation of his mother conflict, and by this also of his father problem. His unconscious oedipal tendencies had until then prevented him from taking over a mature role as head of the family and as doctor. The other mentioned group members were identifying themselves brotherly with the colleague who reported his dream (sibling-transference[3]). At this moment, they experienced the leader as a strong father who was doubled by another group member and who became a threatening, potentially castrating father. Thus the group became a milieu in which a reactivation of incestuous-oedipal wishes of several members took place, which certainly had been hindering them. Not only in the therapeutic situation, but also in their daily life, the members are confronted with groups, and they are thus also exposed to a mobilization of their oedipal conflicts. The group, which is intended to be a therapeutic medium, can be of high efficiency to reactivate the conflicts that are unconsciously touched in a social situation. Like this, the therapeutic group becomes a forerunner into society for the individual.

LEARNING PROCESS

It is not only the furthering of insight by transference-, resistance-, dream-, and behavior-analysis in an analytic group, but also the process of social learning in the group which leads to a better understanding between the individual, family, and society.

There was a student of science who joined an analytic self-experience group which had already had 96 sessions. At the beginning, he always tried to overcome his fears by asking how he should correctly behave. After in several sessions he did not get the intended answer to these questions, he became slowly used to anxiety and initial silence. Later, he noticed that by this behavior the group helped him to gain step-by-step more security. He said that he began to feel more secure because he had to endure his insecurity and fear.

In another self-experience group of doctors one of the participants always tried to attract attention by directing aggressions against the other participants at the very beginning of the session. It appeared that he had developed a mother transference on the group and that he was still searching to be immediately and unconditionally accepted by his mother—that means in the sense of the transference: by the group. Mainly unconsciously, he was afraid of being considered by the whole family and especially by his mother as a failure like his father, who was not able to hold his position. For this colleague, it was not only important that he gained insight in his transference, but it was also important for him to experience that fact that he could not get into the expected contact with other people by his demonstrative-aggressive behavior. After he had again and again experienced the negative effect of his aggressive behavior on the group, he tried to find an adequate and more mature way to the members of the group. He could realize his intention only step-by-step. He had to learn a social adequate behavior by the feedbacks to his behavior.

The therapeutic and also the analytic group always have both a motivation elucidating and a behavior therapeutic effect. If a member several times gets a negative reinforcement to his behavior, he will change his behavior and will develop new patterns of behavior if he gets positive reinforcement for that. In a therapeutic group, it is therefore possible to work through unconscious conflicts. Moreover, a learning by success (operant conditioning) and a training for life in family and society are also possible.

Without having said it explicitly, we can already see from the named case reports that the group has a normative effect on the behavior and even on the ideas and feelings of the participants.[5, 9, 14, 24] In the group, there is a tendency toward an unitarian opinion. The strewing of different points of view diminishes the longer the group lasts. This may implicate dangers in nivelling the different participants to group beings. Therefore we often hear patients say that they feel manipulated by the group. But this normative effect of the group may also lead to a socially more adequate behavior.

One of the eight participants of a students' group who was in opposition toward authority began to speak to the leader, unusual in Europe, by his first name. He wanted apparently to shock not only the leader but also the very well educated other participants. He also spoke of his father in derogatory terms. He seemed to be astonished that the group did not react in the expected way. The group understood that he wanted in principle to be near the therapist and perhaps did not have the opportunity to have sufficient contact with his father after the death of his mother some years ago. He reported that he also had tension with a professor from whom he had received the task of writing a paper. In the first three to four sessions, he repeated in a demonstrative way his behavior toward the leader and verbally toward his father. But afterward, he slowly adapted himself to the atmosphere of the group and no longer behaved so provocative toward the therapist. The group had a normative effect on his behavior. But in this case, it was not a real success, because half a year later, he decided to leave the group, and it was clear that he had not worked through his deep "father" problem. Perhaps he had only made through a social learning process without an insight process. We doubt that he has learned better to accept social realities.

Group experience confronts the member with social norms, and when the member participates long enough, he will accept the group behavior perhaps even in a too pronounced way. We can say that one factor that decides whether a patient may not adapt to social relations is the time/exposure relationship. But we have seen that especially schizophrenics[4, 6] and also neurotics who are very deviant in their behavior want to realize themselves in a group and not offend the other group members. These individuals who have to go a long way because they are initially in the position of an outsider and have often the strongest desire not to remain inside the group.

In a large hospital group of 20 to 25 women we led many years ago, there was an elderly schizophrenic women who took part in the group sessions. She pretended in her delusions that all citizens of our town had a tutor. As she saw that the group did not understand or even laughed at her idea, she stopped in her statement and adapted to the integrated group behaviour. It was apparent that she did not want to be excluded by the group. It was the first time that for a long period she gave consideration to the outside reality.

In this small group of schizophrenics which was composed of seven to nine members, the copatients could not understand a hebephrenic who stated that the therapist is the Savior when he was farther from her feelings, and said that he is the devil when she felt her ego-boundaries threatened by his nearness. But when she was aware of the group reactions, she tried to adapt to the other members and to laugh with them when they made jokes of her.

The tendency toward the norm, toward convergence,[14] is striking because, as we have said, almost each participating in a group has the desire to be accepted by the group. The more the behavior of an individual is deviant, the more he feels the necessity to come to a middle in which he can be heard and be active. As we have observed in our group experiences that all persons, also schizophrenics who are very far from outside reality, feel the necessity to realize themselves with the others at least a little. In the case of a pronounced ego-weakness we have observed that the group may maintain these individuals in an outsider position. These members then suffer from being excluded from the group. Other participants try initially actively to remain outsiders because they want first to adapt to the group situation. But the defense mechanism of these individuals may go too far, and they regret then that they do not proceed in gaining contact with the group.

One doctor declared in an analytic self-experience group that he thought he will leave his position of a passive spectator with the time. But now he sees that time is running and he has not changed yet. He understood that he has to try more actively to change and to get nearer to the group.

The therapeutic group can be understood as the resultant of the vertical-motivational-deep psychological process in each individual and the horizontal-interactional-sociological process among the individuals. What we see in the group is naturally not the two named components, but the resultant composed once more by the deep-psychological and once more by the sociological facts. The therapeutic group can therefore not only be understood by analyzing transferences and resistances, but must also be seen as a process determined by sociological factors, for example, the space of the room in which the sessions take place, the number of individuals and their denseness of sitting, and the frequency of interactions. But already when we consider the number of interactions in the group, we cannot say that they are only to understand, for example, by the sitting order in the hic et nunc of the actual group situation, because we know how important the transference relations in the group activities are. But there are extreme situations possible, in which only the deep-psychological or only the sociological factor plays the decisive role, for example, when strong transference feelings are activated in the group or on the contrary when, for example, members sit in a room which is so large and they are so far from each other that it becomes difficult to interact with the other members.

THE FIVE STAGES OF GROUP PSYCHOTHERAPY

As we have stressed already, there is in the therapeutic group a deep psychological process which leads toward insight, and a sociological process toward change of behavior of the participants. Whereas in the beginning the sociological aspect, for example, because the number of contacts of the participants with each other predominates, in later phases deep psychological factors such as regression, transferences, and resistances are predominant. When these elements are worked through analytically, again the sociological aspect plays the dominant role, namely the modification of behavior toward a better social integration. Thus the therapeutic group work leads the individual on one side toward a better self-understanding and on the other side to a better social integration. The phases that can be observed in group psychotherapy can be enumerated in a detailed way as follows.

The Phase of Explorative Contact

In every therapeutic group we can observe in an initial stage that the participants during a more or less long lasting time try to find out whether they can enter into contact with the others or not and in what way they can do it.

When we began a therapeutic group of schizophrenics in 1963,[5] we observed that initially they sat along the walls of the room looking at the floor. They avoided in the beginning confronting the two leaders or the copatients. Only step-by-step, during the following sessions which took part weekly for one hour, they succeeded to enter into eye-contact with each other. After weeks, they could sit nearer to each other and communicate, first in a moderate verbal contact, then in a deeper understanding of each other. The problem of contact was always present at the beginning of the group. One patient, Mrs. J., once jumped toward one of the group leaders and bit him in his left arm so that the whole group had to help the group therapist. In the session afterward she behaved as if she were the doctor when he had to leave the room for a moment. This patient not only tried to get involved in intensive contact, but also wanted, by incorporation of the therapist, to get a total identification with him.

Regression

The patients expect generally to be lead and fed by the therapist. They enter into a regressive behavior in which they become involved also in multiple and multidimensional transference-relations[25-27] toward the leader and other members. This regression is a presupposition for these transferences, because only when the members can leave at least to a certain degree the reality-related attitude, they will be open to their unconscious conflicts. We can therefore say that also in group analysis the law is valid that is referred to in the French proverb "reculer pour mieux sauter" (going back to be better able to jump).

In a students' group led as a slow-open group,[10] some members had participated for 2 years or more. In particular one member developed first a father transference on the therapist and a sibling transference on the comembers. On the group as a whole, he transferred apparently a mother. As he always did in former times and especially also in the institute in which he earns money, he had apparently the unconscious wish to combat the father (chief) with the deep wish to be alone with the mother. We had the impression that he came only in the group to prove that the leader was impotent, and that he, in front of the "mother"-group, was potent. Only slowly by the group process did he recognize his oedipal tendencies and his corresponding regressive neurotic behavior. This regressive phase brought clear to light what he deeply wanted, whereas in the explorative contact he seemed to be only interested in knowing (intellectually) group dynamics. It appeared that all of the group had unconscious problems with their ambivalent link to mother. Nobody had stressed these conflicts before. Then all others spoke of it, for example, one female participant, who stood in a conflict with her mother, in spite of living independent of her. She could not overcome her hostile concurrence feelings toward her mother after the death of her father. Now, in the group, the conflict was activated. Before she had developed defense mechanisms and believed that she had overcome this problem. Now, in this stadium, she was confronted with this problem.

Catharsis

When the members of the group are confronted with the reality of the group and are not treated in the way they expect in their transferences, they feel frustrated and behave very often aggressively toward the leader. Often this aggression also activates other aggressive feelings against other persons on whom the patients project frustrative behavior.

One self-experience group of doctors was, after some sessions, very angry at the therapist, because he did not give them a theme to discuss. They began to ask what he was there for. Then, a member said, that the leader should pay them a honorarium because they helped him write his next book. When the therapist did not answer, they repeated the attacks. But slowly they asked themselves: "Why do we have to work for the leader? Let us start working without observing him!"

Such cathartic manifestation of the feelings liberates the participants of mostly unconscious frustrations. The aggressions against the therapist or others very often contain old feelings of shortcomings of the past, that is, transference feelings. The participants can say that they experience the leader as a father who did never answer when they had a question. And now they take revenge. But this cathartic phase does not have a long-lasting therapeutic effect. What is cathartically abreacted must be worked through, as *Freud* said:[13] "Remembering, repeating, working-through." After the patient remembers in catharsis, the working-through is necessary. By this we already are in the next phase.

Insight

In the group process, the members already get from feedbacks from others first more unconsciously, afterward more consciously, an information about their behavior. They can recognize in the group process that their transferences and the behavior resulting from it do not correspond to the *hic et nunc* of outside reality.

In a student group, one participant behaved toward the therapist in a way that it was apparent he was fixed to father figures. When he spoke, he always directed his words first to the therapist, and he did not feel at ease when the group was once obliged to gather without the leader. Once he told the following dream: He walks in a street and there speaks with a progressive girl. All of a sudden, he sees 6 men between the ages of 40 and 50. Among them, he sees the therapist, wearing a large hat. All appear to be revolutionary. He says: "Look, here is the therapist among revolutionary people." The student wanted to look at the therapist, but the therapist did not look into the patient's eyes. In the associations, he said that the six other people were the group. An other member said that apparently he had two images of the therapist: In one he saw him as very bound to tradition, and in the other, he saw him as revolutionary. A third member stated: "We know where the leader belongs, namely to the traditionals, as it is the case with orthodox Jews." The student who had the dream said that once the therapist was in an armor and once he was without it. A female student said: "If the therapist is a revolutionary man, then you are confronted with him. But if he is in an armor, then you are able to put him aside." The student who had the dream did not know where to place the therapist: Was he traditional or revolutionary? It appeared that he never knew what his father was like. His father very seldom spoke to him. But once he talked with his father. He was alone with him at home. His older brother, two years older, was away from home for a long time and the mother was on vacation. But all of a sudden, his father died in his presence from a heart attack. In the group, the student saw in the transference-relation with the therapist that he had unsatisfied desires to be confronted with a father figure which he had never been able to recognize before.

In this phase the members can get insight in transferential relations and in corresponding behaviors. But insight does not yet necessarily mean correction of patterns of behavior formerly produced by neurosis. This must be done in a next phase.

Change

A behavior that hurts the other members or that is ineffective for the member himself leads always again to negative reactions from the others, to "negative reinforcement" by the group. By this neurotic attitudes are slowly deconditioned, and trials for a new behavior lead to a conditioning of new behavior patterns step-by-step by positive reinforcements and the gratifications linked to it. The therapeutic group always acts therefore not only in an analytic sense, but also in a pedagogic way, or, in other words, as a milieu for social learning.

In a short-term group of prison guardians of various ages, who acted as group counsellors in their institutions, there was only one female psychologist. The guardians were, with this one exception, men. At the beginning, all members of the group were very much distressed and almost had a paranoid attitude. During the 3 days within which the group gathered—each day for 6 to 8 hours—the members abandoned more and more their defensive attitudes. Only the female psychologist, aged 32, intellectualized perpetually until almost the end of the second day. When she recognized the repeated rejection by the others at the end of the second day, she suddenly stopped her perpetual intellectualization and listened. But the negative reactions and feedbacks of the group lasted; it was not possible that she already came to a new behavior, but she did experience that she had to change the old patterns of her behavior if she wanted to realize herself in a social frame.

FAMILY THERAPY

If a natural life community, like, for example, the family, is taken totally into group psychotherapy, the communication patterns of its members can be observed and examined. For example, it can be seen who is living at whose costs. The members and the therapist will recognize that a pretended family balance is maintained by means of one member being made the "black sheep." Such a family is often eagerly bent on maintaining a social façade to the outside. But inside it is based on the oppression of one member who does not fit into its norms. The family therapy, as Ackerman,[1] Boszormenyi-Nagy and colleagues,[8], Kaufmann,[15] Richter,[21] and others have recommended, may undiscover such disturbed communication patterns and interfere with the family balance to enable them to live without victim. To take a family as a psychotherapeutic group is a means to helping the members to become opened on the one hand to the individual and on the other hand to society.

A hebephrenic female patient of 30 years always had to play the role of the patient in a family. The 56-year-old mother especially, who had a pycnical constitution, had a very overprotective attitude toward the "child." There was a brother who was 5 years younger than the hebephrenic patient, who was very inhibited in his behavior and was a stutterer. The father, 57, was a very clever foreman. After we had seen that the pharmaco- and psychotherapy with the hebephrenic patient could not affect resocialization and that she always remained at home without working in spite of the psychotic symptoms being milder under the treatment with major tranquilizers, we decided to take the whole family together in therapy. The mother was only ready to come after many efforts by the therapists—two male psychiatrists and one female social worker—but as the family was present as a whole, only she spoke or answered even the questions of the therapists to the patient. She stated that it would be impossible for her daughter to work outside her house. She also initially did not want herself to take a professional task. When the husband wanted to add something, she looked at her daughter and said: "Look how he speaks." And then she turned toward her husband and urged that he stop. The therapists had to interfere to enable him to speak. When the son was asked, the mother answered instead of him, so that the therapists had to protect him. It was clear that the family structure was entirely centered on the mother and that all other members were dependent on her. It was difficult to disturb this pattern of "family life." The therapists had to interfere if they wanted to help the hebephrenic patient develop. It was also opportune for the other members that the family learn to live without the daughter remaining in her role of a patient. When the mother finally said that perhaps she would like to work once again outside the house, for example, in a canteen of a factory, the therapists supported her with the thought that then the daughter could gain a greater responsibility for herself and, for example, cook for the family and in time take over a professional task. The mother agreed with this proposition, but she did not pursue this project a very long time. After some weeks, she stopped working. During the short time, our patient, the daughter, was a little more active. But the mother afterward took over again the role of a "tutor" and was not ready to come again to family therapy. Soon afterward the patient had to enter the psychiatric hospital because of an acute exacerbation of her schizophrenia.

As the example shows, it is not easy to interfere with old patterns of family communication. But without this approach, it may be in vain to work with a patient, because a family system like the one described above hinders a development of personality during psychotherapy. When family therapy succeeds, the patient may liberate himself from the old role his relatives pushed him to. Our patient relapsed into an acute phase of schizophrenia after the family therapy had to end because her mother stopped cooperating. It is not easy to reach a good therapeutic result. But if the family is ready to work with the therapists, the chance that the patient will come out of his psychotic or neurotic life pattern is much greater than without their support. Sometimes it is easier to get only one member of the family besides the patient to cowork in therapy. We have therefore for years run parallel to the therapeutic group of schizophrenics a group of relatives, but they only meet once a month. In this procedure we followed R. Schindler's[22] bifocal group psychotherapy. In the group of relatives the members often speak more of their own problems than of the difficulties of their daughters, sons, or spouses. In general they can better recognize the false attitudes of the other participants toward the patients than their attitudes. Also they may accept better a comember's remark than one of the therapist. This group is thus also group-centered. But sometimes the therapist cannot avoid being asked questions concerning the therapy and the prognosis, and in general he will correctly inform the relatives.

Among others we had a very dominant woman, mother of a female participant of our group of schizophrenics, in the relatives' group, whose daughter for years was in the psychiatric hospital, in spite of the psychosis being improved, because she did not want to take the risk of having her at home together with the very schizoid husband, father of the patient. All other group members always asked her why she did not try to take the daughter home. She became less and less sure about her formerly rigid attitude toward the daughter and after many sessions in the group asked the therapist what he thought when her daughter would enter a pension and work half a day in town, after having tried to begin professional work from the hospital. The therapist encouraged her to look for a boarding house for her daughter. In the end she found a room for her in the town. Now the patient has lived some months outside the hospital in a boarding house, works daily from 8 to 12 a.m. and gains visibly in self-confidence.

As the reported case shows, not only the patient's participation in the group of schizophrenics, but also the integration of the mother or other near relatives in a relatives' group can help to free the patients from the old role of an infirm within their social environment and lead them more to social rehabilitation.

SOCIAL DISINTEGRATIVE DEVELOPMENTS

After having discussed the social integrative effects of the therapeutic group, that is, in group psychotherapy inclusively family therapy, we can also report about other effects of the group. The members' integration in the outside society is not always furthered by their participation in an analytic or another group but can also be hindered. As Freud[12] has described it in individual analysis, there can also be the tendency in the psychotherapeutic group for its members to want to stay together for good. The limited or unlimited group analysis is a question that is important. In group analysis, the members very often go into a deep regression. This stage is essential for the development of transferences. But it is important for the therapist to recognize his *countertransferences* that may arise in this context and that may culminate in keeping the members permanently in a regressive attitude either in a dependence on him or on the group.

In a supervision group, a doctor said how glad he had been to have a therapeutic group of patients during his divorce. This had been a support to him. He thought that he had overcome this phase. But obviously, he took now this control group for his mother and also wanted this circle to stay together for good.

It is important to recognize tendencies of countertransference like those the mentioned colleague had toward the group. Whether a group will dissolve again or whether it tends to stay together "for good" depends above all on the therapist. It is of great importance that the therapist help the group members work through the conscious and the unconscious material that arises in the group as well as to gain insight in their behavior patterns that are connected with it. They have to learn gradually to move independently in a social frame as the group represents it. If a group only exists for itself, it will not lead into society. Only if there is attention paid to the fact that the involved members regain, acquire, or reinforce their independence, can a therapeutic group have a social integrative effect.

We also know group developments that are characterized by a growing narcissism of the whole group. Based on narcissistic disturbances of some members, as Kohut[16] described them, the development of a "narcissistic group self" can take place. The members get by comparison into a narcissistic fiction which prevents them from having to master reality.

A self-experience group of 9 to 10 doctors, meeting every 3 months for a weekend and working together for 10 hours, developed every time a narcissistic overestimated self-assessment. This self-assessment was of such intensity that they were uninclined to change and even developed resistances to notice the unconscious problems that caused this attitude, and they were not interested in obtaining a realistic estimation of themselves and of others to leave the group more mature. This tendency of the group was caused especially by one participant who was small physically and who always tended to compensate for his narcissistic disturbance by a "grandiose self" and an idealized mother object. Since he was brilliant in rhetoric, he was able to actualize similar tendencies in participants who did not primarily suffer from narcissistic disturbances. He also activated similar ideas of grandiosity in the group. This pattern of behavior did not help the members of the group integrate into society and be well prepared for their medical profession. It was therefore necessary that the therapist help the participants develop their own real selves and lead them to social reality. The colleague with the narcissistic disturbance realized by himself the necessity of an individual analysis and got into contact with an analyst.

Taking patients with narcissistic disturbances as defined by Kohut[16] into a group may be contraindicated not only because of the possible development of a narcissistic group self but also because these members need more affective support than they can be given in this setting, or because the other members do not get enough support because of these narcissistic participants.

If the group is structured in such a way that it does not sustain the individuality of the members but is an *exclusively we-centered* collective in the sense of a "Great Mother,"[20] it does not further the social integration. Especially in group psychotherapy with alcoholics we have often noticed their tendency to make the group be their mother. They also try to make the therapist one of them. In this case, they only want to gain pleasure, and they are not willing to bear any responsibility. If the therapist does not realize such a tendency, there is the danger of a withdrawal from reality.

Sometimes a therapeutic group seems to be active in a therapeutic sense, but it works in a very institutionalized way. The members take always the same attitude and, during a long period, the same role. From the therapeutic point of view such a group is more an institutionalized *club* than a therapeutic milieu.

We had a self-experience group of doctors coming together each quarter of a year for a weekend, for 11 years. During the first 9 years a therapeutic activity with role changes and a working through of manifold transferences took place. The last 2 years the group members were very indulgent toward each other, and they only wanted to be in an agreeable milieu. Because of countertransferences, the therapist liked to be among so protective "brothers and sisters." The self-experience group ended only after 2 more years, and at the end of the last group session all of the members including the therapist had tears in their eyes. In the meantime most of the members had already passed an individual analysis and were already themselves group analysts.

If in a group one or of several members always act out (we will not explain the difference between acting in and acting out in this chapter) the members do not always work through their conflicts, or if so, not in an adequate manner. As Neto[18, 19] states, we have learned to analyze acting if it takes place within the group, as well as verbal expression, as a manifestation in a special context. But if a single member or a group tends to permanently act out, the chance of becoming conscious and by this the furthering social integration is diminished. If the drive and affect outbursts even lead to a deformation of the group to a gang or a *"crowd in a small frame,"*[5] the possibility of conceptualization that should characterize a psychotherapeutic and especially analytic group work is not present. The danger exists that the members will withdraw from social reality.

In a hospital ward where we worked group-psychotherapeutically with all the 20 to 25 patients there happened an outburst of emotions led by a patient who was always furthered by the therapist after a copatient was transferred to another department because she had stolen. The members could not work through their affects until the leading patient was dismissed and the group process again became more quiet. It came out that the group suffered guilt feelings because of their emotions which were activated in an unrealistic way by the leading patient.

In a group in which the interactions become rare, but also in groups urging unconsciously or more consciously a high identification, corresponding to a norm, the danger exists that the members will remain in an *uncommunicative mass existence* or that they will defend themselves against too intensive group cohesion and try to avoid every communication. Theoretically we could determine a lower and a higher limit of the density of interactions. If this limit is undergone or exceeded, a social disintegration takes place.

We observe very often in group psychotherapy that the group members, just after having experienced a high cohesion through a very open discussion, again hold back their problems and keep themselves in a distance from each other for a certain time.

The group being used for psychotherapeutic purposes can represent a mediator between individual, family, and society. If attention is not paid to the fact that the group remains dynamic and engaged to the psychotherapeutic, respectively to the analytic aim, the danger exists that, seen from the therapeutic aspect, defective developments can take place.

GROUP STRUCTURE

It depends mainly on the group structure whether the therapeutic group has a social integrative effect—which does not mean the furthering of adaptation at any price, but can mean better possibilities to accomplish oneself— or whether it has a disintegrative effect.

Schematically, we can observe three kinds of structures of therapeutic groups:

The Group with Changing Roles

Only in a group with changing roles can the members develop different sides of their personalities. In an analytic group it will always be important that its structure is not fixed but changeable. It is therefore essential that a single member can temporarily grow into the role of an assistant therapist and give associations and interpretations, whereas in the dual psychotherapeutic situation only the therapist exerts this role. In such a group with changing roles, the transferences of the members to each other can also change. Therefore a great number of transferred feelings from one member to several others and to the therapist can take place. On another plane, parallel to this, transferences can come in which others are involved. A group like this will be group-centered. The leader will remain modestly in the background and will only interfere from time to time if no one else is giving an interpretation.

We do not want to say by group-centered proceedings that, as Argelander,[2] Stierlin,[29] and others have postulated, the group should be treated as a whole. In our opinion, such an aspect originates in individual psychoanalytic experience and not in the medium of group psychotherapy. In group analysis, we can never just address to the resultant from the activity of the single members. We always have to consider the different members separately, and, parallel to that, the whole group situation in which they are. Such a group-centered circle with changing roles is the best preparation for the outside society.

The Leader-Centered Group

The leader-centered group can be considered as a disadvantageous group structure for therapeutic and especially for analytic work. In such groups, there is the danger that the participants will remain in a permanent regression and that they will not develop their potentials. In such groups only one kind of transference is activated: the parent-child transference.

If a group is leader-centered, this situation usually is the result of the leader's countertransference. A group with a dominating leader will not prepare the participants for society, because in such a framework they do not learn to take their responsibilities.

The We-Group

It is our experience that certain group leaders, for reasons of counter-transference, cannot endure to exert a special therapeutic function in the group for a time. They want to be judged favourably by the group and merge more or less into the group. In such groups certainly many things can happen. But very little of the process of getting insight and of becoming conscious will take place, as there is generally nobody who furthers these processes. Such a we-group which corresponds, as we have mentioned already, to a "Great Mother"[20] will not facilitate the individual's growing into society. The members of such a group will live entirely their oral tendencies and will by no means be prepared for society.

FINAL REMARKS

The therapeutic group with its amplifying effect on feelings on the one side and its intensity of reality on the other side leads the members into a strong emotional experience, but also to real social relations. In a therapeutic group there is therefore the chance that the participants can live their social interactions consciously, being at the same time constantly confronted with their unconscious feelings that are activated in this frame. Thereupon they get the opportunity to work through old conflicts hindering their development. They also get a chance to realize as many as possible of their true inner tendencies.

SUMMARY

In the therapeutic group we observe the deep psychological-motivational-vertical and the social-horizontal plane. Besides facilitation of insight the interactional process of the therapeutic group furthers a social learning process. The transferences and resistances activated by the amplifying effect of the group are confronted with the intensity of reality given by the multiple and multidimensional interactions in the group. The therapeutic group gives the participants the possibility to meet in the same frame on the one hand the preponderantly unconscious inner conflicts, and on the other hand, outside reality. But we can also observe socially disintegrative developments in the therapeutic group, for example, the growing of group dependency, of a "grandiose group self," of a collective exclusively directed toward a "we-existence," of an institutionalized club, of a "crowd in a small frame," being fully dominated by emotions, and of a totally uncommunicative "mass existence." Three group structures are:

1. The group with changing roles. This structure only is therapeutically indicated, since only by this can the different sides of the participants' personality be developed.
2. The leader-centered group.
3. The we-group.

The last two group structures tend to provoke a longlasting regressive behavior in the participants. Thus also depending on its structure will the therapeutic group be socially integrative or disintegrative.

REFERENCES

1. Ackerman, N. W.: *The Psychodynamic of Family Life,* 5th ed., Basic Books, New York, 1960.
2. Argelander, H.: Gruppenanalyse unter Anwendung des Struktur-Modells. *Psyche,* **22**:913, 1968.
3. Battegay, R.: Geschwisterrelationen als Funktionsmuster der (therapeutischen) Gruppe. *Psychiatr. Psychosom.* **14**:251, 1966.
4. Battegay, R.: Psychotherapy of schizophrenics in small groups. *Int. J. Group Psychother.* **15**:316, 1965.
5. Battegay, R.: *Der Mensch in der Gruppe,* Vol. 1, 4th ed., 1973; Vol. 2, 4th ed., 1973; Vol. 3, 2nd ed., 1972; Hans Huber, Bern, Stuttgart, Wien.
6. Battegay, R. and Rohrbach, P.: Gruppenpsychotherapie mit Schizophrenen und deren Angehörigen. *Z. Psychother.* **16**:134, 1966.

7. Bleuler, E.: Dementia praecox oder die Gruppe der Schizophrenien. In: *Handbuch der Psychiatrie*, G. Aschaffenburg (Ed.), Deuticke, Leipzig, 1911.

8. Boszormenyi-Nagy, I. and Framo, J. L.: *Intensive Family Therapy*, Hoeber Medical Division, Harper & Row, New York, 1965.

9. Enke, H. and Ferchland, E.: Analytische Gruppenpsychotherapie und deren Soziodynamik in der psychotherapeutischen Klinik. In *Analytische Gruppenpsychotherapie*, H. G. Preuss (Ed.), Urban & Schwarzenberg, München/Berlin/Wien, 1966.

10. Foulkes, S. H.: *Therapeutic Group Analysis*, Allen & Unwin, London, 1964.

11. Freud, S.: Formulierungen über die zwei Prinzipien des psychischen Geschehens, Gesammelte Werke, Vol. 8, 229, Imago, London repr., 1955.

12. Freud, S.: *Die endliche und die unendliche Analyse, Gesammelte Werke*, Vol. 16, 57, 2. Auflage, S. Fischer, Frankfurt a.M., 1961.

13. Freud, S.: *Erinnern, Wiederholen und Ducharbeiten Gesammelte Werke*, Vol. 10, 125, 3, Auflage, S. Fischer, Frankfurt a.M., 1963.

14. Hofstätter, P. R.: *Gruppendynamik*, Rowohlt, Hamburg, 1957.

15. Kaufmann, L.: Familientherapie, Sozialpsychiatrie. *Akt. Fragen Psychiat. Neurol.* **8:**103, 1969.

16. Kohut, H.: *The Analysis of the Self, A Systematic Approach to the Psychoanalytic Treatment of Narcissistic Personality Disorders*, International Universities Press, New York, 1971.

17. Mahler, M. S.: *Symbiose und Individuum*, Klett, Stuttgart, 1972.

18. Neto, B. B.: Acting-out in psychotherapeutischen Gruppen. In *Gruppenpsychotherapie und Gruppendynamik*, Vol. 5, Heft I, S. 83, Vandenhoeck & Ruprecht, Göttingen/ Zürich, 1971.

19. Neto, B. B.: Psychotherapy with a group of deaf-mutes. In *Group Therapy 1974: An Overview*, L. R. Wolberg E. K. Schwartz (Eds.), Intercontinental Medical Book Corp., New York, 1974.

20. Neumann, E.: *Die Grosse Mutter*, Rhein-Verlag, Zürich, 1956.

21. Richter, H. E.: *Eltern, Kind und Neurose*, Rowohlt, Hamburg, 1969.

22. Schindler, R.: Ergebnisse und Erfolge der Gruppenpsychotherapie mit Schizophrenen nach den Methoden der Wiener Klinik. *Wiener Z. Nervenheilk. Grenzgeb.* **15:**250, 1858.

23. Schindler, W.: Transference and counter-transference. In *"Family Pattern" Group Psychotherapy*, Ref. International Psychotherapiekongress, Zürich 1954, *Acta Psychother.* **3:** Suppl., 345, 1955.

24. Sheril, M., In: *Gruppendynamik, Rowohlt, Hamburg 1957*, as well as in: *Hofstätter, P. R.: Einführung in die Sozialpsychologie*, P. R. Hofstätter (Ed.), Kröner, Stuttgart, 1963.

25. Slavson, S. R.: Gruppenpsychotherapie. In: *Die Psychotherapie in der Gegenwart*, E. Stern (Ed.) Rascher, Zürich, 1958.

26. Slavson, S. R.: *Analytic Group Psychotherapy*, Columbia University Press, New York, 1951.

27. Slavson, S. R.: *A Textbook in Analytic Group Psychotherapy*, International Universities Press, New York, 1964.

28. Schultz-Hencke, W.: *Der gehemmte Mensch*, Thieme Stuttgart, 2. Aufl., 1965.

29. Stierlin, H.: Gruppendynamische Prozesse I: Uebertragung und Widerstand. In: *Analytische Gruppenpsychotherapie*, H. G. Preuss (Ed.), Urban & Schwarzenberg, München/Berlin/Wien, 1966.

CHAPTER TWENTY-ONE

COMMUNICATIVE DRAWING AND PAINTING*

A. R. BODENHEIMER

I n this chapter I describe a procedure which, having been developed in cooperation with the occupational therapists of a public psychiatric department of a large general hospital, has convincingly proven itself to be an introductory method to psychotherapy (although not the exclusive psychotherapeutic procedure)—especially in cases of inapproachability to verbal or symbolistic contact. As the name indicates, it deals with communicative drawing or painting. The therapist and the patient (sometimes also the therapist and *several* patients) make contact on paper instead of facing each other directly. They deal with one and the same sheet of paper, mostly in alternate directions.

Several rules have become apparent in the course of our experience and these are to be presented here. As if by retrospect, we came upon certain results from the drawing process and from analysis of the drawing—several new insights into psychotherapy in general, insights that, it seems to me, would promote a deeper understanding of what happens during the psychotherapeutic process in general. Communicative drawing and painting (CDP) have thus contributed something like *a pictorial illustration for that which basically always occurs in psychotherapy.* This is one of the reasons why this process has become valuable for us. Actually it is not *the picture,* the finished page, which is to be considered, but *drawing,* the process itself, and with it that which happens during the therapy. The dynamic process involved much more than its results.

We are aware that to begin with many *objections* arise when there is talk of any kind of drawing therapy. First of all, we therefore want to confront this opposition, that is to say, to discuss the separate arguments which form the basis of this opposition.

OBJECTIONS TO DRAWING THERAPY

Objections are always entitled to a hearing, to approach, and to a discussion. Only when this is done and done in accordance with all the laws of dialectics, is a proper, free, unemotional understanding of the issue itself reached. It is through contradictions that we first begin to understand ourselves. This can be the case here as well.

Let us now discuss the individual opposing arguments:

1. *Drawing therapy is only a masked form of work therapy* and intended as such even if concealed and dressed up. It is meant to reprimand

* Thanks to my co-workers, the occupational therapists Zwia Gazit, Nira Kamm, Bracha Bezer, and Shulamith Samir, who are to be considered co-authors of this work, for the give and take of substantial suggestions.

and sets out to stimulate activity and by means of veiled pressure to deprive the individual and also the psychiatric patient of his right to confront himself and his world.

2. The word "drawing" has the same bad odor as that which clings to a concept like *Sentimentalization* (*Gemütsbildung*): the smell of romanticizing and of fogginess which cunningly circumvent the individual's sober confrontation with himself and the questioning of his world and also abrogates his acceptance of the natural and instinctual sphere.

3. *Drawing strays into aestheticizing,* in an often discussed Kalokagathia (actually a false interpretation of the Greek ideal.) One makes it easy for oneself by concentrating on the beautiful picture and the dangerous inference is then not far off that an individual who creates something beautiful is not only good but that he is healthy as well. One comes to the equation: beautiful = good = healthy. A fatally dangerous identification indeed!

4. *Drawing circumvents the necessity and discipline of verbalizing.* Discipline that requires the individual to so express that which moves, disturbs, or makes him happy, that it is formulated unequivocally, sharply, clearly, and honestly. This means verbalized, expressed in current, customary language—in words that are so sufficiently unequivocal that they can be answered just as unequivocally.

5. Thus drawing makes possible and even legitimizes the *avoidance of reality* and with it frees the individual from the necessity of saying yes or no.

6. Thus it *soothes the conscience of both the therapist and the patient* in a most cunning and polished way, the conscience which should have been startled and disturbed by honest psychotherapy.

7. No argument, but worth discussing, is the assertion that such therapy, such a therapy beginning that is, somehow is tied to the prior condition that the patient or even the therapist have *artistic talent.*

Before we reply in detail to these arguments which as a whole—and there is no doubt about this—are weighty, actual and reasonable, we must again stress the fact that the procedure here described does not simply consist of drawing as otherwise practiced, that it is not the familiar art therapy, not "creative activity" either individual or communal, but that here a special sort of confrontation is dealt with—a confrontation that leaves its traces on paper and from there carries over to verbal communication. The result, the work itself, is unimportant; actually only the moment of meeting on the drawing surface counts and also that which it induces. The drawing itself is important only as *a document,* just as a tape recording is of a conversation, but it has a more immediate effect.

Let us next look into the serious counterarguments:

1.   The danger certainly exists that *the result will be overestimated*: namely, in the patient's surroundings, by the family as well as by the nursing personnel. Tendencies of "Go, do something, don't sit around; then things will be easier for you" or "The poison of laziness" (verbatim re H. Simon,[16] the founder of work therapy) must be fought. That type of remark can be heard often, and one must keep it well in mind. One can counter it only by going into the *playful* character of drawing, and not only the playful, but even more so into the *reciprocal provocativeness* of it. We say on this subject later on.

Still, let us remain alert to this danger: Drawing must never be "degraded" to work. It must never get the bad odor of work.

2.   *Sentimentalization (Gemüt)*. Indeed there exists the immense danger that in place of serious self-encounter and confrontation there appear nebulous and excessively sentimental tendencies. Psychotherapy has suffered enough under such romantic befogging—and it turns out that whatever psychotherapy has had so patiently to endure was only the reflection of a general cultural and social misdevelopment.

We must be on guard here and never get so far as to lose ourselves in the fog of sentimentalizing. So when hearing such words as "joyful labor" or some such thing, beware!

In order to avoid this, we have developed different methods of communicative drawing which we will consider shortly.

3.   *Aestheticizing*. Substituting the beautiful for the serious "taking at his word" (Beim Wort nehmen—L. Binswanger[2]). Furthermore, this includes evasion into the beautiful and the ambition to encourage art rather than the less thankful and difficult confrontation with the task at hand.

Naturally in the end it is a question of psychiatric concept outside the realm of discussion: whether it was more meaningful for Docteur Gachet to recognize and encourage the genius of his patient, Van Gogh, or if it would rather have been his duty to prevent him from cutting off his ear and eventually his lifeline. As far as I am concerned, I would prefer to deprive the world of a few works of art, even if they count for the greatest, if thereby I could bring about the survival of a patient. But that in the end is a matter of concept.

Whatever it may be, in regard to the therapy to be described here, the aesthetic consideration is of the least interest. In this it differs markedly from the aims of H. Read.[13]

It is not here a matter of the alternative (actually artificial) often evoked by psychologists especially, that of beautiful versus true. It might be that we know what is beautiful, but the knowledge of what is true always evades psychotherapy. The opposite concept popular today that the ugly is truer than the beautiful is of course as difficult to prove as that which speaks volubly of the true, the good, and the beautiful. Truth, goodness, and beauty have nothing in common with each other: neither in terms of identity or supplementation, nor as mutually exclusive terms. They are categorically incompatible.

Communicative drawing avoids the situation wherein the patient always creates more beautiful and complete drawings and flatters himself with them. It thus avoids—and must avoid completely—the showing of beautiful pictures as proof of cure (as so often appears in the publications of art-therapists).

4. *Clean, clear verbalizing is suppressed and replaced by diffuse drawing.* The unequivocal by the ambiguous, the clear by the nebulous.

Yes, if only *the word* were always so unequivocal and if the word would always make an answer possible and necessary! It can also be the contrary. Whoever draws communicatively—this we have learned—can, with a line which is so long and exactly so thick, so curved or so extended, can with a line which is thus and not otherwise, involve his partner even more exactly and better than with his word.

5. *Avoidance of reality.* What is reality? This we don't know exactly. But *a white sheet of paper is a reality.* And we can say exactly what sort of reality it is. It is the model of that reality which I would like to call *decision reality.* And this is to be understood as follows. The white page comprises an endlessly large number of decisions. You can write any imaginable text on it, can develop mathematical formulas on it, can write a musical score, or can conjure up any number of imaginable pictures on it.

The page itself is not without limits, however; only the possibilities it offers are, and every line means a decision—no, *is* a decision—a decision, *one decision,* a single, decided decision. It is a commitment that excludes thousands of other implicit decisions now no longer realizeable, thus forcing a basically and theoretically immeasurable rich life to become infinitely poorer. This line, here on this sheet, removes thousands of other possible lines from the realm of possibility. But now *this* line, this line drawn here and now, is here to stay and can no longer be retracted. A spoken word can be revoked, a line cannot. ("Erasing is smearing," I learned during art class, and that is true.)

A neurotic is consistently a person who has no wish to put a stroke on paper. He can brilliantly rationalize this "virginity" of the empty page: "The greatest work of art is a clean, white page." Certainly, all possibilities remain open to this person, and not only that, the viewer can put into it everything that is in him and every viewer can project something different. But this person in front of the empty page remains in reality splendidly aloof. He has nothing to justify and nothing to explain, nothing to decide and nothing to prove, nothing to verify and nothing to regret. For that he may criticize everything: basically he can do everything better. And furthermore: facing the empty paper you never age, remain young forever, remain ever and always at the beginning, guard all your possibilities, all freedom—and in the end perish from their excess.

All this is clearer in drawing than in speech. The page full of jottings is a more real reality than an hour of chatter. It is part of the essence of drawing that it preserves itself in time, *must* preserve itself, unlike the word, which, as soon as it is spoken, absconds, can only be preserved by artificial means, and when played back on tape is mostly experienced as something strange and foreign to the speaker.

Furthermore in regard to the theme of reality, the reality of drawing is a different reality from that of speech, but not a lesser one. If the line that you draw is fixed and accentuated or even challenged in its position and meaning by the line with which I (communicatively) reply, the character of challenge and commitment determined and defined by reality can be even more distinct than in a spoken postulation. Of course "Yes" and "No" exist only indirectly in drawing (although very decisively and unequivocally by means of *crossing out,*) and that is one of the reasons why drawing induces and supplements speech, although it never replaces it.

As a further important function of speech, *questioning* can be very well formulated in drawing. How this occurs is explained later.

6. *Soothing of the therapist's conscience* by means of substituting drawing/painting for speech is possible as long as the therapist does not himself "climb into the arena." The arena is basically the page. But CDP can sometimes leave the region of the page and move onto the faces and bodies of both partners so that they paint one another. We have practiced this on numerous occasions. Well, then, if there is mutual stimulation, especially a natural sort, if there is mutual interference, then the therapist's peace of mind is finished!

7. *The argument: "drawing talent, respectively, lack of talent"* is familiar to us from other similar situations—and we know how little it is justified. I could not actually employ J. L. Moreno's claim (made during a lecture in Zurich, 1957) that actors are the least suited for psychodrama, and use it to refer to CDP stating that painters present the greatest difficulty in CDP. On the other hand, it cannot be said that CDP is easier with painters. But this is true: it is *more difficult* to practice with *graphic artists.* The members of this profession are so drilled in stylizing, so vexed by the abandonment of their own personal strokes and in addition so precisely trained for quick effect, that they actually shy away from the spontaneity of CDP. And yet it is an impressive experience and representative of what

psychotherapy can achieve to see how members of the graphic profession (who comparatively often suffer from behavior disorders) display a relaxation and the recapture of originality in a series of pictures.

THEORETICAL FOUNDATION

To what extent theoretical deliberations gave us the courage to proceed with CDP and, conversely, to what extent these were stimulated by CDP need not be discussed here. Theory helps—this much must be said for it—to better understand what has been undertaken and to then continue with it and develop it.

We can take the following theoretical considerations as a basis for CDP:

1. *The subdivision of the relation into its direct and indirect, sive medial form.* This is to be understood as follows:

The relationship between two partners can basically be played out in two different ways, that is, according to two possibilities:

a. As *direct relationship,* which is to say that both partners are directly related to each other. Nothing interferes between them; what happens between them comes about directly: they speak to each other and listen to each other, glance at each other, and look at each other. Therefore they are solely related to each other by means of themselves. Direct relationship can be of different degrees of closeness and therefore of variable challenge—*it is, however, always of utmost intensity.*

b. As *indirect medial relationship*; this means, the partners are not directly related to each other but are related by virtue of a third, an intermediary. We call this the *medium* (which is regrettably necessary for reasons of logic unless we want to create a neologism; the fact that the concept "medium" is commonly given a different, a parapsychological meaning which has nothing to do with the present discussion, is an unhappy coincidence.)

Examples for the direct relationship are to be found in Figure 1. The partners relate without a mediating third instance, directly—and correspondingly intensely—to each other.

Figure 2, on the contrary, offers examples of an indirect, that is, medial, relationship. As we see, the partners can relate to each other by means of looking at a tree or speaking to a third person, by the mediation of this medium. Basically a relationship exists even when, as seen in Figure 2c, a membrane is stretched between both partners so that they do not touch each other, cannot even see each other, and are connected only by the medium.

Medial relationship exists, for example, when the partners look at something, eat, or also *draw* together.

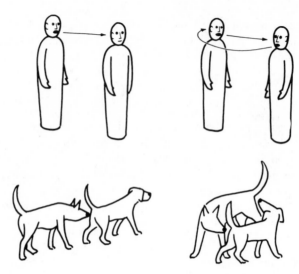

Figure 1

The relationship engendered by *speech* is *not* as unequivocal and clearly direct a relationship as one might suppose. Speech tends to become autonomous; it contains a coercion for the partners to understand each other *regarding that which is spoken, regarding the language,* and *regarding that which was meant at the* time (all of which become a certain sort of medium.)*

Whatever the comparison between these two types of relationship, the direct and the medial, the direct is always of the most pronounced intensity. It *so* intensively relates the partners to one another that the relationship can only be maintained for a very short period and with the ensuing exhaustion the direct relationship is abandoned. How long this direct, highly intensive relationship tends to last can be very exactly stated. The duration of this intensive direct relationship has a name, and it offers the basis for this measure of time: this short span during which one individual can with his eyes look into the eyes of another is called, in German, the *Augenblick* (glance). This is the duration of one intensive visual relationship. Once the Augenblick is over, at least one of the two partners diverts his glance from the glance of the other, or both partners do this, and they together look at a third person, object, or both, which then constitute a medial tie. The same

---

* These statements are taken in short summary from the author's *Versuch uber die Elemente der Beziehung.* From this book Figures 1 to 3 are also taken. With kind permission of Messrs. Schwabe Co., Publishers, Basle, Switzerland.

goes for the duration in which two partners are intensively and directly related *manually*—that is, the time of a mutually compatible and equivalent act of the hands as in the handshake of a greeting. The time span is exactly ascertainable and is called *maintenant* in French (which means "holding the hand"). If the valued reader wishes to know how long this very intensive, and in its intensity quickly exhausting, direct relationship can be kept up, let him try in the bus tomorrow to keep looking a stranger in the eyes, or try to discover how long during a greeting he can keep another's hand in his own. Then again, better not try it. . . .

Figure 3*a* and *b* shows the direct and visual relationship in its intensity.

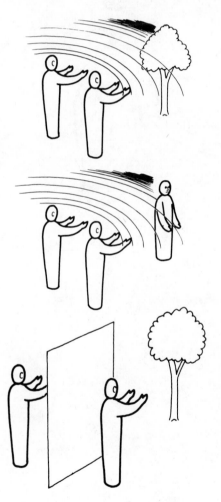

Figure 2

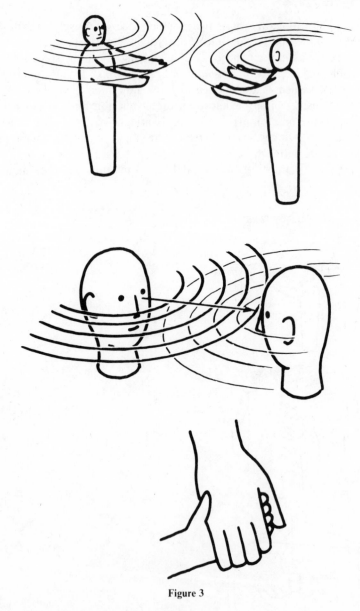

Figure 3

Figure 3c shows what happens when the intensive manual relationship of the handclasp (*maintenant*) is over: Then one partner *leads* the other *with* the hand *by* the hand.

In regard to the meaning of both these forms of relationship for psychotherapy, it is now time to consider to what extent, when, and for how

long a direct relationship in its intensity is to be established or supported
and when, in which phase or situation of therapy, an indirect relationship is
more suitable. *CDP is a form of indirect relationship* which is unforced and
gives clear evidence of what happens in the course of its practice. It is
genuine and guards the necessary distance missing from other possible
indirect relationships such as eating together. Other forms of medial relationship are too distant, as for instance the mutual visual contemplation of
an object.

As for music, mutual listening is too indifferent and leaves each partner too much
to his own personal experiences, whereas music played together, unless by two very
practiced jazz musicians, is too much confined to the given notes or otherwise
results in cacophony. At least so it seems to me, but then perhaps I understand too
little about music therapy.

When the medium is an empty page and two colored pencils, the medial
relationship can be kept well under control, can be steered, and can be
measured out finely so that the therapist, when he finds the time to be suitable, can at any moment go over to a direct verbal relationship.

2. *The difference between equal and unequal relationship.* There is
much talk about symmetrical and asymmetrical relationship in
psychotherapy. This much is clear: In verbal therapy true, not only alleged,
symmetry can hardly be established. In the end a symmetrical relationship
remains a challenge which basically cannot be fulfilled. In the verbal connex
it always happens that one remains who knows what it is about while the
other does not. Even if both speak language, the same language, there is no
symmetry.

But even when the knowledge of the knowing partner does not become
apparent (which only seldom happens) it still remains true that in verbal
interrelationships only one of the two has the right and the freedom to *question* and to a questioning challenge. In this relationship-gradation of ques-
tion/answer the inequality is very marked, more clearly than in externals
such as whether the patient, who is the client, lies down, or whether he sits
up as does the therapist.

In CDP equality is possible, and the precondition to its establishment and
maintenance is given. Both participants meet on the same surface and face
each other with the same tools; they can each influence the other (according
to principles that are soon to be described).

3. *Earnest-taking (das Ernstnehmen).* This is primarily evidence as well
as the true nature of a really equal relationship both in nature and value.
The meaning of earnest-taking in this sense is something completely defined
and clear-cut. It is to *enter into* that which the other says or does and to
enter in the same language and to *do in the same manner.*

Earnest-taking is therefore not serious application to someone or something and not earnest occupation with someone or something. I can concern myself earnestly with a patient's psychosis, I can seek to understand the symbolisms, and I can make a thorough search for the right medicine to remove this psychosis integrally—all this does not mean earnest-taking.

In other words, I do not yet take a person in earnest when I am "occupied with his delusion." I begin to take him earnestly only when I answer *to* the delusion *by means of* delusion; when I reply *to* a depressive condition *with* depressive condition.

What is possible for cases of paranoid behavior and also with depression becomes unimaginable—impossible to accomplish and unfruitful for cases of mutism or stupor. One cannot reply stuporously to stupor and in fact should not, because it only extends the deadly silence.

And yet one must find some ground on which earnest-taking, now understood as dialogue in the same language, becomes possible. If this language does not emerge from the conduct of the partner or if it does not directly become possible through the translation of his conduct, the therapist must *create* it—this common language spoken in the same way by both. And here CDP often offers a good solution.

4. *The address (Anrede) in both of its possible basic forms understood as statement*, assertion *(Behauptung) or as message, appeal (Anruf).*

Many of the most elementary errors in psychotherapeutic concepts and in the face of psychotherapy emanate from the fact that addresses of psychotherapists regarding their own field or made to their patients regarding their findings and inquiries are taken to be statements or are understood to be such by others. As if they were to say: This (which I now say) *is* so—this person, this situation, and so on.

Asserting facts is not the specific jargon in which the psychotherapist speaks to his patient.

But *what then* does the psychotherapist do when, facing a patient or his surroundings, he formulates a sentence? He creates an *impulse,* an *appeal;* he delivers a message. He gives an E-vocation. This is to say: The statement is not made—and was not meant—with the intention of transmitting a fact. (The classic example of the transmission of fact is the sentence "The hammer is heavy" from Heidegger's "Being and Time." Here there is nothing to expect and nothing to explain. The hammer is heavy and there the matter rests. The only thing that can follow is the gritty order, "Too heavy. The other hammer!") The psychotherapeutic way of address is elementarily different: No opinion is expressed. None of that. Remarks in the realm of psychotherapeutics are made with the sole intention of *stirring the addressee* or *awakening response.*

How the answers are formed and what they say is unimportant inasmuch as it is insignificant whether the answers that were evoked are affirmative or negative. Negation is even better than affirmation. This is so because a person can with his "No" decisively find himself and better confirm his uniqueness and special identity than with "Yes."

It is the current order of the day to pass over and forget or ignore this particular of the psychotherapeutically intentioned remark and this lies behind most if not all the misunderstandings regarding psychotherapy and also behind most if not all the founding of new psychotherapeutic schools that claim to deliver a new "concept of man" or "understanding of man"— as if that were the task of psychotherapy.

It is not necessary to go into further detail about this here; but it was appropriate to at least refer to this theoretical basis of psychotherapeutics because then more can be understood paradigmatically of what *the stroke* of the therapist-sketcher indicates and stimulates, and also what *the word* of the therapist needs to and should accomplish: *to stimulate and address*. The difference between right and wrong address (equally in word as in stroke) is given solely in this: an address is right if it stimulates and if it promotes and challenges; an address is considered wrong if it evokes either nothing or at most a pale agreement.

This must become completely clear: *The answer "No" is not a proof of wrong address—on the contrary, it proves that there has been stimulation and that the stimulation has taken effect.* "No" is, I repeat, mostly proof of greater correctness (Richtigkeit) than is the answer "Yes." We speak only of right and wrong or false respectively; talk of true and untrue, truth and untruth, transcends the realm of psychotherapeutics and should therefore be omitted. The word "truth" has no place in psychotherapeutics.

From here on we understand the task of CDP in the framework of the following concept: *The stroke is understood as address.* It is not a statement. It does not say, "This is how it is"—it says, "Take this up and make something out of it." *What* the partner wants to do with it is up to him. In this respect the difference between the psychotherapeutic consulting room in which CDP is practiced and art school should become very clear. The teacher instructs the student in how he can make statements through his art. In my opinion the artists sometimes get lost on the wrong path: They want to *address* rather than make statements. This, I believe, is where Kitsch and snobbery begin (and this is, as far as I see, the only acceptable paraphrasing of Kitsch.)

Salvador Dali is very pleased with himself in the role of addressor. I am consciously overstepping my competence as doctor and am entering the cherished preserves of art connoisseurs by calling Dalis art Kitsch or better still, snobbery, no matter how talented he might be in his craft and in the exact calculation of effect. But let us leave that. Let us return to the theme: the addressing function of the statement in the realm of psychotherapeutics.

How now do we come to this addressing, how can we stimulate this "make-something-out-of-it" by means of CDP? This question occupies us from now on.

THE PRINCIPLES OF CDP—CDP AS
PARADIGM OF PSYCHOTHERAPY

Five principles lie at the root of CDP: The first principle embraces the triad: accompaniment—amplification—disturbing. The second principle may be embraced under the concept of giving Gestalt. These are followed third by address, fourth by the principle of indication, and fifth by interpretation.

The first principle, *accompaniment—amplification—disturbing,* CDP can be practiced in three ways:

1. *Accompaniment.* As schematically exhibited in Figure 4*b* a form, a ductus, a "thought," here reproduced as a circle in 4*a*—not by chance as a circle, by the way, as for the ancients it was the absolute complete form—is picked up, taken over, and *continued in the same sense.*

One can translate this process in many ways, as for instance: "We are going together in the same direction" or "I understand you." Translation is not necessary; this is the point: it can be understood without translation. The mutuality is self-understood as mutual thinking, feeling, acting, experiencing.

Such accompaniment has a most basic meaning. One might say it makes life together possible in the first place. It is not productive, however, not in itself and not as a challenge. It is the paradigm of rest, this mutual accompanying movement.

It does not suffice because it brings nothing new. In order for something new to be brought in, other motifs are necessary as shown by CDP.

2. *Amplification.* This is illustrated in Figure 4*c*. Figures 4*c*1 and *c*2 show that different degrees of amplification are possible: its extent is considered by the partner in proportion to each situation.

With the principle of amplification it is not only that the given is extended and not simply is a distance covered together, here something is *taken over, but then productively extended.*

A thought (circle) is given. But the circle does not only stimulate another circle; it does not simply say "I know what you mean and how you mean it," or not only "We understand each other," but it says more and can actually say several things. It can say, "Look here at all these potentials that are in your statement—maybe more than you yourself know or thought

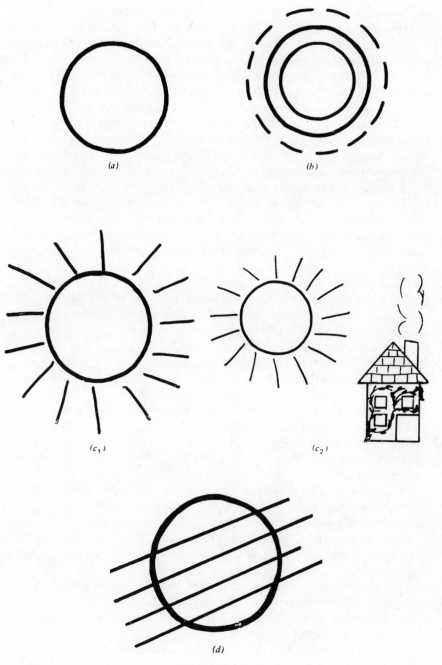

(a) *(b)* *(c₁)* *(c₂)* *(d)*

Figure 4

or intended or wanted." A question of concept will remain even if one wants to formulate it a second way—"That which I make out of the suggestion (you transmitted to me), this sun, this house, is in you unconsciously—it is in your artistic expression and consequently also inside yourself." Now this is exactly what becomes so beautifully obvious by means of CDP: How senseless and superfluous are discussions regarding such statements (as the second made here), and how little is to be gained from discussions of whether a circle is "unconsciously" to be understood a priori as a sun or if one prefers to say "A circle is not a sun—a circle is a circle and simply a circle and nothing but a circle and that is all there is to that." I have always considered such discussions that fill libraries of psychological and psychotherapeutic literature to be superfluous because they misunderstand the very principle of psychotherapy. And whoever cannot accept this in itself, may discover it in CDP: *Everything is only that and always only that, which we make of it.* The more productive this making of it, the better—this is what is worth discussing, not that which is "intrinsically" within the subject.

One can therefore say, "Look at all the things that are in your statement, in your representation, all the things you potentially have to say." Or one can formulate it differently, "Look what your statement tells *me*; how it stimulates *me*—and then reciprocally again, in that I add mine to yours, how *you* are stimulated to proceed."

In this way you have move and countermove, reciprocally productive and rich and reciprocally fruitful: the circle becomes a sun, in the sun there is a house. . . .

But just as there is little in psychotherapy (and in life), so can and may (4*b*) accompaniment and (4*c*) amplification be all there is to CDP. To make it whole what must be added is what in the philosophical dimension of H. L. Goldschmidt is called "Freedom to Contradict." [9] We here call it by a shorter and coarser name:

3. *Disturbing.* This is graphically interpreted by Figure 4*d*. Here there is a circle—and then there is someone who tranquilly draws his circles, his self-enclosed figures. "Noli perturbare circulos meos," is what the self-absorbed commander of Syracuse asked for some 2000 years ago. But that he was not prepared to allow himself to be disturbed in his circles is what cost him his life.

What it is all about is learning, without metaphysics, to disturb circles and allow one's own circles to be disturbed—without killing or getting killed. Disturbing as stimulation belongs to the program of psychotherapy just as accompaniment and amplification.

Disturbing (Stören) is possible always only as *challenge,* but not as destruction (*Zer*-stören). If I, as illustrated in Figure 4*d* cross through the circle, energetically, clearly, and with emphasis, if I do not move onward, but make a countermove, I do not make the circle invisible, and it is not destroyed: on the contrary, it is accentuated in its individuality, its meaning, its "circleness." The circle "understands itself" as circle much sooner and better if it is set off by the straight lines that are drawn through it.

It is with contradiction that the statement is realized, it is only from antithesis that synthesis emerges. This leads to the second principle of CDP.

THE 2ND PRINCIPLE: GIVING GESTALT

Destruction does not achieve the truth it intended. One cannot by destruction achieve invisibility. This law is valid at least in the realm of psychology. And we can make this very clear with CDP.

As an example, let us take some image; let us say the word and situation "psychosis" as exemplified in Figure 5. Let someone try to take this "drawing" represented in this ductus to be read as "psychosis" and try to so disturb it that finally the whole picture and its message are destroyed: It does not succeed. No matter how intensively one works at it, how destructively one crosses it out—the picture "psychosis" (I leave it to the fantasy of the reader to replace the word with the image of house and sun) cannot be obliterated! On the contrary, from behind those bars it emerges even more challengingly, it activates even more keenly the necessity to discover what was covered up here. The "psychosis" cries out through the barriers.

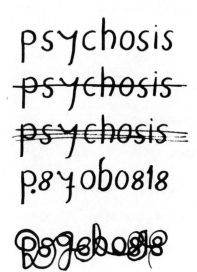

Figure 5

And yet there is a possibility, a process for "overcoming" the content and statement of a picture, a destiny, or a situation—not to make it invisible, but to "solve" and thereby "neutralize" it.

This succeeds not through destruction, but through giving Gestalt.

The principle of giving Gestalt is amazingly simple: It consists of continuing along with the ductus, *the same* ductus that contains and determines the message of the picture. How it happens is made clear in Figure 5. It is much more difficult to grasp with words. One must try it this way: No matter how contradictory it might sound to the ears of philosophers, I can transcend the "psychosis" and all it implies, states, and means only if I remain in the realm of immanence. This means if I like-mindedly and *productively continue* that which lives in and speaks through the "psychosis."

There are no limits for this process, neither to the extent nor to the manner of its configuration. This is what makes it so significant and so interesting. And namely: *It can restructure something destructively experienced* (such as that which is collectively understood as "psychosis") *into something productive.*

THE 3RD PRINCIPLE: ADDRESS (ANREDE)

It is possible to address one another in signs and strokes also, not only in words. Address means: *to evoke an answer.*

We speak of address intentionally and not of an impulse. When we say "impulse," it all too easily calls forth the image of an almost forced reaction. If one wishes to induce a reflex—no matter whether a spinal reflex or a conditioned reflex—one sets up an impulse, and the whole arc of reflexes comes into play.

This is not the case with address: Here uncounted answers are possible and conceiveable, not the least of them the "nonanswer." Also this counts as an answer, as a very real, meaningful, and vital answer.

How the answer turns out very much depends on the nature of the address. Here again in the way in which the address is formulated, CDP gives us in its obvious illustrativeness and amazing reductivity an impressive picture of that which can happen in psychotherapy and in relationship in general as well as what is possible in them.

Figure 6 shows us what essentially are the possible forms of address. In Figure 6a, the *circle* illustrates (and at the same time means) the self-enclosed statement: It is so. I am informing you of it. Meant as address, this statement has little power to stimulate. One must simply accept a closed, "round" statement. Finished, that is how it is. If you say so—and say it *this way*—well, then that is how it is. In Figure 6b, the energetic

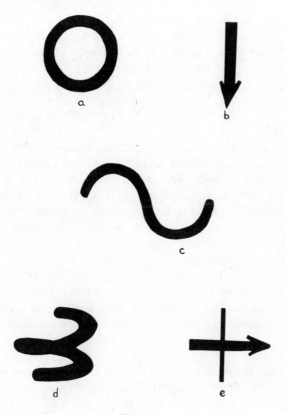

Figure 6

stroke (directed toward the partner) has an unusually strong character of challenge. This is said, said to *you*. In and of itself the stroke says nothing as yet and it has little meaning. The partner must give it meaning. The stroke waits for that. In Figure 6c, the *waving line* runs notably without beginning and without end. It *opens up possibilities* and does it while preserving freedom. It is a proposition. Much can begin this way; more still can be made of it. In Figure 6d, the reclining Gamma is paradigm of an *opened figure*. It appears as a challenge to answer, as illustration of *the question*. More, actually, than the question mark, the symbol of the question in a written text. What have you got to say to that? In Figure 6e, the *line across* a drawn line is the negation expression. The patient has drawn the first line; now comes the "No." But implicit in this already is that it can be seen differently, as an upsetting. Now go and choose.

These are several proposals of address or reply; only a few and yet enough to show how many possibilities for challenge are given. Also there are enough to make evident how exact consideration should be given as to *how* in every individual case and in each phase of treatment the challenge should be given.

THE 4TH PRINCIPLE: INDICATION

Here we deal with a remarkable circumstance about which we can hardly wonder enough. It once became clear to me as a personal experience in a most disconcerting manner. This is what happened. I had received a very beautiful wristwatch as a present and wore it happily from the start while receiving patients. But on this day several of my patients were very angry. They were all convinced that I was bored with them. And why? Because I constantly looked at my watch. It was difficult for me to convince them that *I was not looking at the time but that I was looking at my beautiful new watch.* I looked at it, enjoyed the looks of it, and yet the time it indicated was of no interest to me—I did not even recognize the time.

But in this special case it was necessary that an indicator lose or surrender its indicating function and return to being an object—a condition such as the spontaneous experience of a watch as a piece of jewelry, even if it indicates time.

Whatever we can read, we can look with effort only. *The indicator function blots out the picture image* (this difference seems more substantial to me than the observe-and-effect image of von Uexküll[17]). I can see Chinese lettering as pictures, for the simple reason that I cannot read them. But for the same reason I find it difficult to look at a word constructed of Latin script without reading it.

So it is with drawing: We always ask for the content and the meaning and forgo our capacity and the possibility of seeing the picture, not as finished representation ("this is so") but simply as the combination of actions (strokes) that produced it and fill up the space.

How and by what means can this ability be won, or better still: how can it be won back? The answer is: by means of CDP, by drawing together, not by looking at pictures. Here the stepping behind the content of the picture to its appearance becomes unnatural and unspontaneous. I might almost say that it becomes something inadmissible. All this changes when one allows oneself to be addressed directly by the statement itself and continues with it in its own language. When watchmakers create a timepiece, the schism between regarding the watch as jewelry and regarding it as an indicator of time disappears by itself.

THE 5TH PRINCIPLE: INTERPRETATION

So much has been said and written about interpretation that one hardly knows where to set the limit. Particularly the German schools of theologists and philosophers have taught us to differentiate between exegetics and hermeneutics, between understanding, explanation, and comprehension.

We make it simpler for ourselves. Here and now we call interpretation *making one thing out of another.* To make the unconscious conscious is only a single special case of that achievement that we call interpretation.

To make one thing out of another thing can be expressed even more exactly, namely, *to lead from one system into another system.* For example, to make *audible* harmonious melodies from *written* notes, from visible signs. It is this way of giving a new meaning that makes a work of art out of the interpretation of a score. More is written in the notes than can be heard.

In the special case of CDP, interpretation means to take that which was drawn or painted together *after* it is finished and mutually (this is important, *always together*) look at it; and finally in common to put that which was previously *drawn* together and viewed together into *language*; in other words, to translate from the motor-induced and visibly portrayed and expressed in signs into language that which was said in those signs found on the paper.

We interpret our own actions, both patient and therapist. As stimulation for this work of interpretation we take that which previously, when alternately stimulating each other, we ourselves had put on paper. *We thus interpret ourselves.* We interpret in another dimension that which we had previously communicated to each other by means of signs. Now words are stimulated in place of spontaneous strokes.

This self-interpretation has a fundamentally insight-provoking component. That is the reason why I much prefer the interpretation of drawings which came into being during CDP to projective tests. The patient can much more easily accept and observe what he himself has produced than that which he is obliged to read from strange ink blots or photographs or obscure images.

That which interpretation gains from communicative drawing in both freedom of approach and impetus toward interpretation more than compensates for the inaccuracy that is due to the fact that these drawings cannot be standardized in advance.

From the psychotherapeutic viewpoint the use of standardized testing procedures is mostly undesirable because appended to it is a "superior knowledge (Herrschaftswissen)" (in the sense of Scheler[15]) which for its part disturbs the psychotherapeutic contact considerably—this superior knowledge that knows exactly, for instance, what the animal percentage or the reactions to color in the Rorschach test indicate. Nothing is left to the person examined but to accept what the tester knows about him. The tester is right; he is right a priori. What can the experience and understanding of a single person undergoing tests amount to in the face of the knowledge, the hard superior knowledge, which has been gained from the experience of so many thousands of test protocols and has been proven over and over again?

Communal interpretation of communally created drawings is in itself a psychotherapeutically effective act, and as such allows itself to become part of psychotherapy as a matter of course as transition from drawing to verbal contact.

Then it is acceptable, often even very helpful, if the therapist in his stimulation toward verbal expression regarding the communally drawn picture diverges from the concrete contents (if such were created at all) and calls attention to elements in the picture which mostly would not reveal themselves to the drawing patient, for example, *space-distribution* and *space-filling*. We now interpret what it is we see regarding the freedom of both sketchers to exploit the expanse of a white page. Whether, for instance, we freely move across the whole expanse, whether we exceed it altogether and let the strokes reach beyond the paper or if, on the contrary, the game of communicative drawing is played out tightly in the center of the page.

Then the stroke itself is of interest: How is the stroke formed? How long, how thick, how confident, how strong in pressure did it come out? How has the character of the stroke changed in the course of communicative drawing?

Most essential of all is the question: *How is the communication of the drawing being accomplished?* How do both partners answer each other, to what extent do they take each other up? To which extent do they complement each other? Which principles of CDP are more effective? What is the reaction to amplification? What is caused by disturbing? Does it paralyze or stimulate? To which degree? Who stimulates whom; who disturbs whom?

And at the very end comes the interpretation of contents, of the pictures as objects, a mutual discussion regarding what was actually drawn. This is the least important.

This procedure has the advantage of being to a large extent independent of both theoretical elements and the belief that there are premises "in themselves" that build up the personality. After all it is conceivable that someone come tomorrow and explain that all concepts regarding the conscious and unconscious are nonsense because they cannot be proven. It may be quite difficult to find something substantial with which to counter this argument. But it is quite obvious to the drawer that the manner in which he fills up space is less conscious than the rigor, length, and strength of the stroke and this again less conscious than the object that he draws. With this "the unconscious" expressed in the manner in which the stylus crosses the page is more convincingly unconscious than a symbol that has been drawn on the page. This manner of expressing the unconscious in symbols can be "learned" much more quickly and easily by for instance occupying oneself with psychological literature—than the self-movement on the surface of the page.

Mutual examination of the pictures drawn during CDP can disclose a number of things and supplement much. Its undertaking is, however, not always indicated. It is often better to leave the pages aside without any subsequent interpretation. Interpretation, no matter how free and self-understood it might seem during the course of therapy, often carries with it the danger that the spontaneity and the worryless freedom of CDP might suffer. It is valid for the interpretative task related to CDP, as for anything that, there is neither a simple correct nor an unequivocally wrong method of procedure. It is in the first place a matter of *timing*: that moment in which the pictures are taken in hand—or perhaps taken in hand *again* (perhaps for the second or third time) and this point of time can often be arrived at only several weeks after having drawn together. Perhaps it never arrives. Then the pictures remain uninterpreted—and are for that reason no less effective than if they had been considered interpretatively.

CONDITIONS FOR THE PRACTICE OF CDP

Who can include this type of psychotherapy into his store of treatments? The answer is: everyone who has mastered the basis of psychotherapeutics.

It is necessary to note that when the basis of psychotherapeutics is mentioned it is not the knowledge of psychotherapy which is the issue, but rather the equanimity of the confrontation with another person. A more important basic requirement for CDP than one's own didactic psychoanalysis (no matter how desirable this might be) is a friendly relationship within the therapeutic community.

Moreover I would like to emphasize: *CDP is psychotherapy*. It is just as important and should be taken just as seriously and it can be just as helpful within its limits; but it can also be just as harmful if carried out incorrectly and awkwardly, accompanied by inept remarks or practiced in a false framework, just as any other type of psychotherapy, namely the usual verbal therapy.

We have worked with our entire personnel, doctors, psychologists, social workers, and nurses. Mostly we have worked with occupational therapists, and I must emphasize that these young women, who have generally little psychological sophistication but show much spontanaeiety, freshness, and capacity for contact, have proven to be the most suitable therapists.

A prerequisite for the practice of such therapy is an approach valid for all psychotherapeutics which I would like to call (very much simplified) *controlled spontaneity*. To know how much impulse or stimulation to give or receive, to deliberate the extent and way in which to answer a patient's comment (i.e., to accompany, amplify, disturb, or—and this is also a reply—to pass it by altogether) so that he will be led onward without being overtaken and so that at the decisive moment he can be addressed regarding the representation or begins to speak himself is what must constantly be considered.

If the patient speaks about his experiences during CDP, or if he, perhaps previously mutistic, begins speaking at all only in the process of CDP, this can signify the moment when the doctor or psychologist is drawn into the conversation. This must happen with the utmost caution and restraint. The doctor or psychologist must avoid leaping into the midst of a freshly developing wellspring with highly intelligent interpretations full of reference to symbols or indications regarding the representation. In that case the whole impulse of the proceeding engendered by emphasizing the spontaneous and talking in a still wordless language—which even at the start of verbal contact must not be allowed to turn into an inept naming of terms— will be demolished.

For the therapeutic team to be informed of what happens during drawing therapy, weekly sessions are held in which we discuss the pictures and the dynamics of their creation, the aspect of results, the sequence of presentation—in the realm of a single picture as well as in the sequence of pictures—also the relationship between CDP and clinical developments, the relationship between CDP and concurrent verbal psychotherapy, and the relevant questions regarding the change of therapeutic methods. We discover what happened up to the time that the picture came into being; what sort of stimulation was used by the therapist or which intentional movements were undertaken by the patient. This is most important, because it determines the activity of the therapist both qualitatively and in the extent of his activity.

MAIN INDICATIONS FOR CDP

Of all the many possibilities for the employment of CDP, it is most highly indicated in two types of disturbances:

1. Cases of *mutism, stupor,* or authentic *muteness* (the latter referring to cases of aphasia, peripheral neurological illnesses, also after surgical operation of the vocal apparatus).

2. Even more important and also more decisive for the success of this therapy are those numerous cases that (actually only when proceeding from the purely auditive) connote "the opposite of muteness": patients who *talk and talk*—not gossip, but talk about their conflict and their need. But *the* need of such patients derives from the fact that their talk always leaves them lonely. One can respond to words only with words, yet even the silence of the partner provokes further talk, because *talk means fear of silence.*

It is extremely difficult to approach the ductus of talk with talk. This can be done only with CDP.

METHODOLOGY

CDP is practiced in pairs and without previous verbal explanation. This is important. Drawing should speak for itself from the start. It should be *the* method of communication. One should leave to the stroke itself, and to the white page as such, its provocative character. Types of remark such as "we want to draw a bit" take from the process that element of earnestness which it deserves and turns CDP into an expression of embarassment or fear of silence. This must never happen to CDP.

If CDP does not evolve by itself, then perhaps it was not indicated or not initiated at the right time, and then it should not be undertaken. But the start of CDP can be simplified if one observes that the words spoken presently would perhaps be better confided on paper. The surprise effect of this is very welcome and fortifies the readiness for free graphic revelation. Often also the confrontation succeeds, which in this case is the patient's ability and readiness to act aggressively or challengingly, sooner and easier on paper than in awkward words.

At this point one could give very exact instructions on how to proceed. That would give everything an impressive scientific appearance. Instead, we will leave that be. Whoever has psychotherapeutic understanding must transfer it to the special conditions of CDP (whoever does not have it will not be helped by such instructions anyway). For that reason it makes little sense at this point to go into extensive explanations of the basic conditions of psychotherapeutics.

To give an example, one of the basic requirements of all types of psychotherapy is to give consideration to the type and number of possibilities one offers each time. That is demonstrated in the process of CDP as in psychotherapy throughout, since CDP is an altogether obvious illustration for that which happens during psychotherapy generally; here it appears in very simple externals, for instance, the size of the paper—a large sheet has an altogether different effect, i.e., a more inviting, but also more fearsome because more oppressive aspect of challenge than a smaller sheet.

Colors. What more need be said about the meaning of colors, their stimulating but also shocking effect, after the experience and knowledge gained from the Rorschach test? It is recommended that the therapist keep his own same color throughout the course of CDP. Later one can then read off exactly what happened during the drawing dialogue, and what sort of stimulation and answers were given by the therapist. That is a great help in understanding the dynamics under which this therapy proceeded. For monochrome drawings, I often and gladly take the pencil and give the patient a ball point or felt pen, or the reverse, depending on whose initiative is to be considered more weighty.

As said, the course of the procedure needs to be suited to the situation. If the patient is sufficiently activated to begin himself, then this is always preferable. If, on the contrary, the therapist must start, he must consider the patient's readiness to reply when deciding whether it is preferable to start with a clear stroke that separates and cuts and to which a clearly continuing but counterplaying reply is possible, or if a closed figure, or a provocative hook shape or a cloudy, vague picture should be offered.

Naturally one must always be inspired and think of something new. But is this not necessary throughout psychotherapy? For instance, on the day when I wrote this, I was called for a consultation. It was a matter of initiating contact with a prisoner who showed a stuporous reaction to detention. He was a person born deaf and blind in one eye. The stupor was surmountable without drawing therapy. If one spoke in the inarticulate language of the patient, dialogue could be established. But several basic questions remained to be cleared up. This did not seem possible by means of conversation. The patient dodged the attempt at drawing by explaining that he had never learned to write and did not know how to draw either. I found a tattoo on his upper arm, however, with his name and a few of the common tattoo marks. And so I began to copy these tattoos and wrote first his name and mine next to it and then drew the emblem. From here on, the way was open to an intensive drawing and verbal communication. In careful doses partly through CDP and partly in conversation, the background of the actual stupor condition could be examined. Needless to say I will under no condition reveal the facts regarding the crime that were entrusted to me by the patient. CDP as lie detector—that is a repulsive thought!

A FEW PRACTICAL EXAMPLES

We are in possession of a series of over 100 treatments. Every choice made here is arbitrary and more a matter of chance due to the simple possibility of photomechanical reproduction of the pictures themselves drawn during

CDP (the expressiveness of the pictures) than a matter of consideration for the breadth of the indicator spectrum.

CASE 1. The *first series* represented here is that of CDP practiced with a child. The boy is 4 years and 9 months old, and mutistic. He makes sounds only occasionally. Examination followed the request of the Phoniatric Department of Tel Hashomer Hospital, in the presence of the speech therapist in charge who could not make progress by the usual means of speech therapy.

I disregard attempts to open verbal or phonetic communication. That has been done already and in such situations one must start afresh, newly, and differently. I combine movement 1 on Figure 7 with a suitable tune. The child replies with his tune in movement 2, which I, through accompaniment, lead to an end. The same happens in movement 3: the child initiates the spiral movement, and I continue the movement while singing along and onward. The same continues throughout phase 4. A transition from the provocative to the indicative (5) occasions no reply. The child remains with his

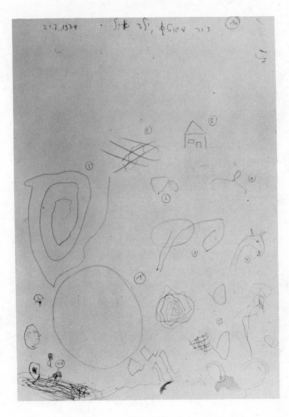

Figure 7

monotonous movements (6). Only crossing out, that is, a disturbing gesture, leads to a freer confrontation. From 7 onward CDP becomes freer. That becomes clearer in Figures 8 and 9. In Figure 9 there is a breakthrough of the spatial enclosure. That is the moment when we leave the paper for the person, that is, *the transfer from medial to direct relationship.* I paint the child's face, and I need hardly mention how happily the child accepts my invitation. Singing along we cover each other with war paint. Had I not been wearing a brand new pair of pants that day this could have gone on; but it was good that at the moment in which my clothing was about to be painted I turned to a rhythmic hand-clapping. In this situation the mother who had been sitting there in a quiet depressed mood could be very naturally drawn into this children's game. Now she joined in with us by clapping and chatting along and, as I withdrew from the circle, she continued alone with the child, apparently, according to her, for the first time.

Only at this juncture was the point reached where conversation with the mother was possible on a natural basis. It is beyond the task of this presentation for us to illustrate all

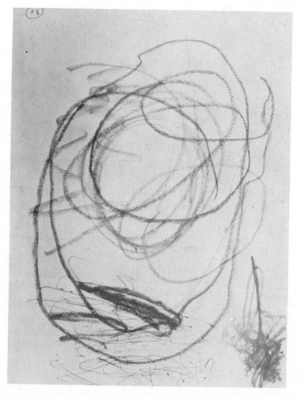

Figure 8

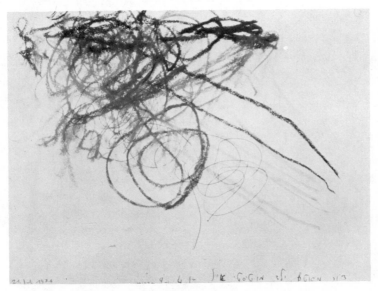

Figure 9

that was behind the mutistic development which a child, fearful of the world, developed as an ever-tightening circle. The communal game produced a relaxed atmosphere which was good for the mother as well; it also prevented the emergence of a latent distancing and mutual rejection which unhappily often occur between therapists and the mothers of their patients.

CASE 2.   A young, educated, and refined man lies in heaviest stupor (without bodily injury) in bed like a log in a worrisome condition: he does not move or speak and shows no noticeable reaction even toward familiar people in his surroundings; also he neither eats, sleeps, nor urinates. Twenty-four hours after admission the therapist draws this chaos in deep red on a large sheet (Figure 10). Thereupon the patient tries to follow the line just as chaotically. But then, decisively, he surrounds the borderless, disordered chaos with a belt of canons or tanks. Now he begins to speak, to repeat his experiences. Then the anuria dissolves; the patient eats. Slowly the amnesia diminishes, partly during CDP, partly during conversation. Twelve days later the patient could be discharged from the hospital.

This therapy could of course also have been handled differently, with high doses of neuroleptic drugs or by means of narcoanalysis. If I prefer CDP it is not only because it seems less violent, but mainly because it makes for *a more specific approach* to the very nature of the disturbance and its causes in a therapeutic situation which encourages equality from the start.

The reader might find the report of this case hard to believe. It even

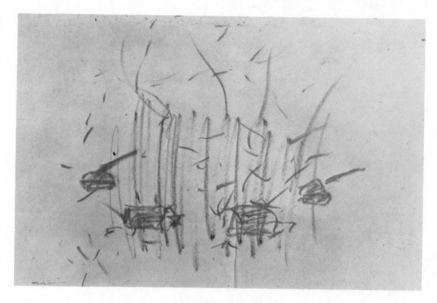

Figure 10

seems so to me. Had I not lived through it, not seen it, not followed up on it, as it happened, I would not believe it myself!

CASE 3. A well-known excellent artist has been for several years in a serious creativity-and-relationship crisis. There is no visible advancement in conversation. The drawing begun by the patient (Figure 11) indicates both his talent and his neurosis. The doctor disturbs him profoundly with a reference to the sexual background of the neurosis heretofore only hinted at. (Not all the pictures of the series can be represented here.) The next picture, initiated by the author, allows the aggressive tendencies which up to now were never permitted relevation to arise in the patient (Figure 12), and the last picture of the series (Figure 13) shows, more in the distribution of space than in the stroke, what can happen during about half an hour of CDP.

This is, I repeat again, in itself not sufficient therapy. But it is an introduction and a beginning and, above all, a means toward the patient's confrontation with himself and his surroundings which is difficult to achieve by other means.

CASE 4. Born deaf, single woman is now 36 years old. Immigrated to a small town in Northern Galilee with her parents from a North African country, she could not be educated either in Africa or in Israel and thus never learned to speak nor to write. She never took up relations outside her large patriarchally cohesive family. She is, as seldom encountered, completely mute and voiceless, although her vocal and articulative

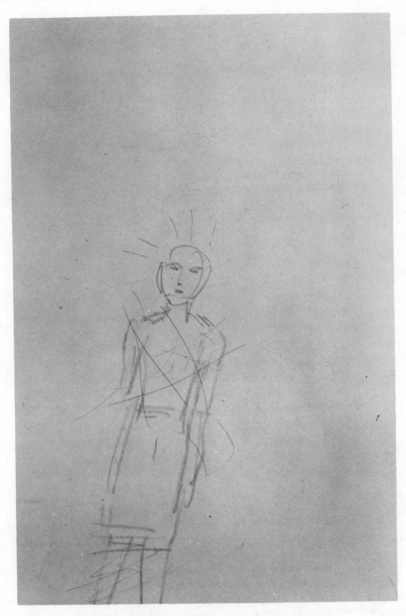

Figure 11

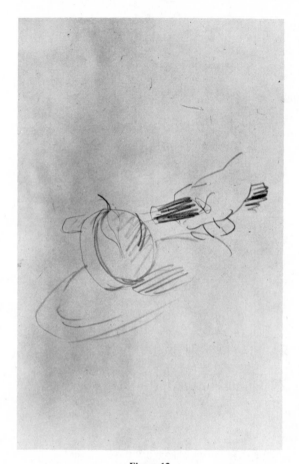

Figure 12

apparatus is fully developed, and her hidden intelligence—this I feel after 25 years of experience with the deaf—is concealed and only awaits development.

This complete spiritual and social seclusion continued until a short time ago when the father died at a very old age. The mother is also old and weak, and the family worries about what will happen when the mother dies. It seems as if the sister senses some of this: recently she has been restless and sometimes—this is new—aggressive.

Now she sits before me as if absent, her eyes turned toward her lap or to the distance. An immediate start toward indirect relations, drawing for instance, did not seem indicated. Here one must consider carefully. She might not answer, and then the chance of later participation is diminished. To touch would be especially out of place because it is too intimate, too frightening, and all too unfamiliar. I begin to move my lips as if speaking to her and look at her while I am doing so. I am doing as "the others," as all the people

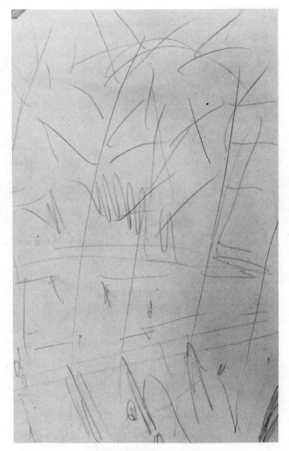

Figure 13

who communicate with each other, who not only *inform each other of something,* but *impart themselves to others.* And she begins to join in with my mute speech movements. We conduct a mute dialogue which contains all the essential characteristics of conversation: it unites, it maintains the moment (*Augenblick*), it is without commitment, other than to the preservation of the connection.

And so we remain for about 2 minutes. Then I take a sheet of paper. The patient reacts to my circle by adding a body and legs. Then she draws the same to the left of this figure. After I add face and hat to her figure, she adds the same to the first figure. Two little men have been drawn (Figure 14). The following drawing comes in a more relaxed, independent manner (Figure 15), and as I (Figure 16) sketch a face, she copies it, only—truly shattering—with four ears—this drawn by a 36-year-old woman, born deaf. She who has never heard and has never let anyone hear her sees people as having two pairs

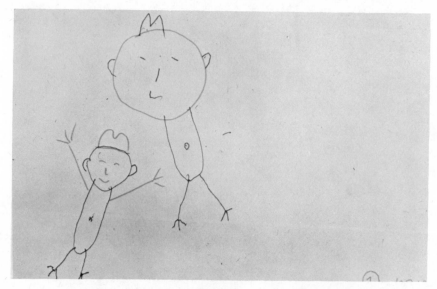

Figure 14

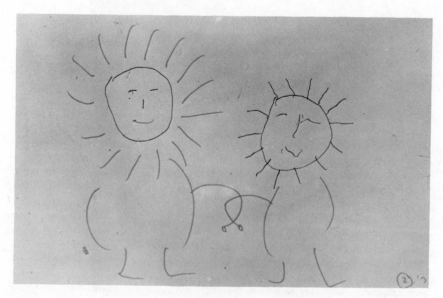

Figure 15

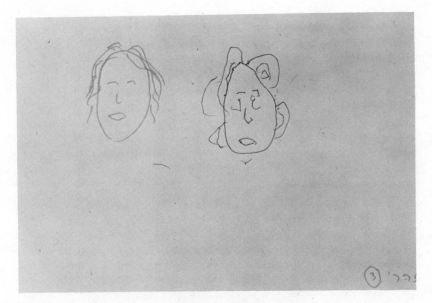

Figure 16

of ears! Now I put my open hand near hers and she takes it, cautiously but definitely into hers. Before she leaves, we make the last try in CDP; we scribble on a sheet of paper (Figure 17). I do not remember who started, she or I, as it is not very important. What is written on it is neither Hebrew nor Arabic nor Latin lettering. And yet it is a correspondence. The beginning of a relationship or its record after a seclusion of over three and a half decades.

CASE 5.   One should actually finish with a brilliant success. I will deny myself this satisfaction. It is not a matter of straining after effect, but a matter of promoting understanding. This last case is an almost 40-year-old man suffering from a psychogenic paralysis of both legs for over 3 years following an automobile accident (he was formerly a truck driver). Three years of exhaustive verbal psychotherapy have allowed all conflicts, both the evident and those arrived at during therapy, to come to the surface, but the man remains glued to his crutches.

Upon admission the pride of this patient is obvious: he cannot and never will forgive himself so much as to admit—I can walk. Another way must be found. I advise the occupational therapist to paint together with him, but separate from the other patients, *with the feet*. The idea behind this is simple: he will not admit walking to himself and to others but perhaps his feet can successfully be mobilized through this detour.

The whole matter starts very promisingly; there is drawing, and the patient accepts the challenge and impressive pictures emerge. Figures 18 and 19 prove it. During CDP-treatment serious incidents occur: twice epilepsy simulating attacks take place, both times

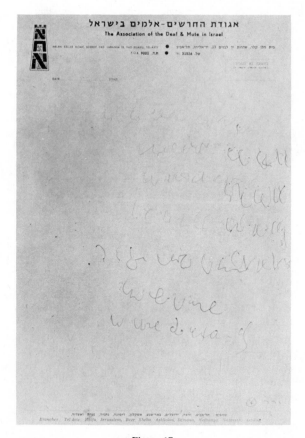

Figure 17

followed by a sort of terminal sleep. And 3 months after, having become fully impotent following the accident, this man comes to a continuously painful hours-long priapism which finally must be alleviated by means of a urological emergency operation (by-pass). These episodes are worrisome and possibly dangerous, yet they do present the hope that we are on the right track especially because of the concentrated dynamics which point to the underlying tension—in grotesque contrast to the flaccid paralysis which had been maintained for years.

Finally one day the patient draws the upper part of his body (Figure 20). He leaves the poor lame lower part aside. And following this he states, "I will not walk, you can do what you like and *I do not want to walk*." And with that he leaves the department.

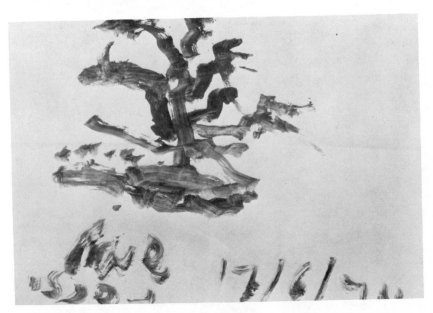

Figure 18

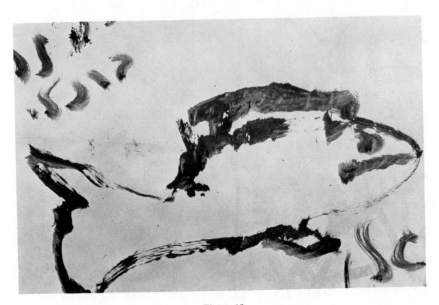

Figure 19

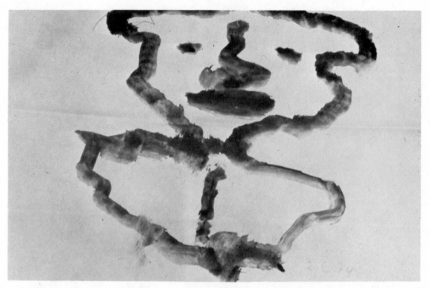

Figure 20

SUMMARY COMMENTS

CDP is a method for initiating psychotherapy, a method that makes possible treatment in cases that are otherwise refractory to psychotherapy.

In addition, CDP is a model of what happens during psychotherapy and what is at all possible in *every* type of psychotherapy. Namely:

1. *Psychotherapy can be practiced:*

a. *In a direct or an indirect (medial) form.* Both partners can meet directly or they can relate through mediation, in this special case through communal drawing.

b. *As equal or unequal relation,* in a manner in which both partners are in equal related positions or that one then emerges as the leader while the other follows.

2. *The condition for psychotherapy is given:*

a. *In taking in earnest (Ernstnehmen).* This is understood not as a morally generalizing prerequisite, but simply and clearly as *speaking the same language;* as traffic in the same jargon. If this does not happen by itself, it must be brought about.

b. In this that the declaration of the therapist be understood and used as *message and appeal (Anruf)* and not as statement *(Behauptung)*.

3. *Five principles are applicable during psychotherapy:*

a. *The principle: accompaniment—amplification—disturbance.* These three types of answers or continuations of declarations present the total of the actually possible reactions. To my knowledge, there are no other types of reaction.

b. *The principle: giving Gestalt.* Understood here is the productive continuation of a thought, an idea, a ductus, while preserving its immanent basic tendency. Only by preserving this immanence does the idea allow itself to be transcended, not by the counterpoise of an adverse tendency.

c. *The principle: address.* This is the way one partner evokes his counterpart's answer or tries to answer the latter's challenge.

d. *The principle: indication.* This means considering a matter as both a combination of tendencies filling a space and as a whole made of traces sketched in this space, thus overcoming the one-track inquiry for meaning.

e. *The principle: interpretation.* This principle is understood simply as: *Making one thing out of another,* whereby a matter is changed by being transthought or transinterpreted into another system.

Drawing has long been practiced in psychotherapy, and many authors have dealt with the psychology of drawing and painting. The experience gained by my co-workers and myself during the course of our work with CDP has shown us, however, that if one really wishes to understand and advance, one must always begin on one's own initiative. One certainly does not need, as is the present fashion, from the sheer joy of one's discovery to consider one's experience as an epochal discovery comparable to Freud's *Interpretation of Dreams.* As concerns us, we have simply come to understand some matters in a new way and for that reason are presenting them here.

ACKNOWLEDGMENT

I wish to thank Mrs. Hella Kace, Tel-Aviv, who has been untiring in arranging and improving the English manuscript.

REFERENCES

1. Binder, H.: *Die Helldunkeldeutungen im psychodiagnostischen Experiment von Rorschach,* Schweiz. Arch. Neur. Psych., Vol. 30, 1933, pp. 1–67, 233–286,

2. Binswanger, L.: *Grundformen und Erkenntnis menschlichen Daseins,* 2nd ed., Niehans, Zürich, 1953.

3. Bodenheimer, A. R.: *Versuch über die Elemente der Beziehung,* Schwabe, Basel/Stuttgart, 1967.

4. Bodenheimer, A. R.: *Die psychotherapeutische Beziehung mit dem gehörlosen Kinde,* Praxis Kinderpsychol., Vol. 17, 1968 ed., pp. 87–97.

5. Bodenheimer, A. R.: *Doris: The Story of a Disfigured Deaf Child,* Wayne State University Press, Detroit, 1974.

6. Bodenheimer, A. R.: *Die Handschuhe von Stefan Zweig. Ueber den Sinn von Deutungen und über deren Gerechtfertigssein,* Zeitschrift Psychosomat. Med. Psychoanalyse, Vol. 20, 1974 ed., pp. 177–192.

7. Bodenheimer, A. R.: *Guernica. Oder über die Grenzen der Kunst und der Psychologie,* to be published.

8. Furrer, W.: *Objektivierung des Unbewussten,* Huber, Bern/Stuttgart/Wien, 1969.

9. Goldschmidt, H. L.: Freiheit für den Widerspruch. *Inform. Phil.* **1:**3–4, 1973.

10. Hegel, G. W. F.: *Wissenschaft der Logik,* Vol. 1 and 2, Meiner, Hamburg, 1967 (1812).

11. Heidegger, M.: *Sein und Zeit,* 7th ed., Niemeyer, Tübingen, 1953.

12. Landau, E.: *Psychologie der Kreativität,* 2nd ed., Reinhardt, München/Basel, 1971.

13. Read, H.: *Education Through Art,* German translation: *Erziehung durch Kunst,* Droemer-Knaur, München/Zurich, 1968.

14. Rorschach, H.: *Psychodiagnostik,* 6th ed., Huber, Bern, 1948.

15. Scheler, M.: *Die Formen des Wissens und die Bildung* (1925). In *Philosophische Weltanschauung,* 3rd. ed., Francke, Berne, 1968.

16. Simon, H.: *Aktivere Krankenbehandlung in der Irrenanstalt,* De Gruyter, Düsseldorf, 1929.

17. von Uexküll, J.: *Streifzüge durch die Umwelten von Tieren und Menschen* (1929), Rowohlt, Reinbek, 1956.

CHAPTER TWENTY-TWO

RECENT ADVANCES IN RESIDENTIAL
AND DAY-CARE TREATMENT
OF NEUROTIC PATIENTS:
CONCEPT OF INTEGRATED PSYCHOTHERAPY*

FERDINAND KNOBLOCH, M.D., AND JIRINA KNOBLOCH, M.D.

. . . I don't believe that increased understanding of the processes involved in this dyadic relationship (individual psychotherapy) will greatly affect practice in the future. If significant breakthroughs in therapy are to come, I believe they will be through methods that mobilize group forces to involve the whole person, or direct approaches to the nervous system through psychological, pharmacological or neurophysiological interventions.

Jerome D. Frank[8]

Moving from one socioeconomic system and culture to another—from the Czechoslovak Socialist Republic to the United States and Canada—and being able to observe in a somewhat detached way psychiatry in both systems, we were vividly struck by the old truth: that institutional structure (in a broad sociological meaning) powerfully influences the activity of professionals, molds their views, rewards them for conforming, and inhibits or even punishes innovative attempts. In the field of neuroses, we all tend to take institutionalized patterns of care for granted. And yet, if observed in its totality, relatively little is done to alleviate the suffering of neurotics and its social implications. The treatment of neurotics—either as outpatients (mostly in individual psychotherapy in private offices or clinics) or as inpatients—is either not very efficient, or is very time-consuming, or both. Consequently, many neurotics wander from one psychiatrist to another for years, or from one encounter group to another.

The following anecdote gives a hint of what we have in mind in speaking about patterns of care being dependent on institutional structure, and a variety of examples could be easily added from other countries. After World War II there was a struggle in Czechoslovakia between neurologists and psychiatrists over who should treat neurotics. Since Pavlov was an ideologically acknowledged authority who defined neuroses as "disorders of higher nervous activity," and neurologists were felt to be experts on "nervous activity," their claim for the treatment of neuroses was strong. However, when medicine was socialized, neurologists lost their private practices that were mainly comprised of neurotics; they lost interest in such patients and began to refer them to psychiatrists. And so a "scientific" conflict was solved by an institutional change, automatically affecting the involvement of professionals.

Deep economic, social, and political changes in Czechoslovakia after 1948 were associated with an increase of patients seeking help for neurotic

* We would especially like to extend our thanks for numerous comments to Drs. J. E. Miles and J. C. A. Morrant. We also appreciate comments of the following: J. Billing, J. Cumming, M.D., J. Lazerson, M.A., M. H. Miller, M.D., F. Perry, R.N., and R. Remick, M.D.

symptoms. The newly born socialized medicine, with its free treatment accessible for all, faced the problem: How can psychotherapy of neuroses be rendered more efficient, less time-consuming, and less demanding of professionals, so that it can be available to all those who could benefit? This question was not spelled out by the organizers of medicine, who at first tried to close their eyes and minimize the problem of neurotics and dreaded their costs of treatment. However, statistics soon persuaded them that neuroses could not be ignored. For example, in the 1960s more than 1% of all employed men in Czechoslovakia each year were certified by a doctor as disabled for work for almost a month because of the condition diagnosed as psychoneurosis, and 2½% of women, for a somewhat shorter period.

We were among those who felt the social demand. The possibilities of unified medicine were a challenge to us, and we designed and realized a unified system of psychotherapy, which could be used as a model of efficiency and economy across the country.

When we arrived in the United States in 1968, most of the psychiatrists that we met did not show much interest in the problem of efficiency and economy of treatment. Institutional pressures were missing. Some of our psychoanalytic friends, saturated with well-to-do patients, were even inclined to regard such a problem as a symptom of a restless, impatient psychotherapist. But what surprised us most was the fragmentation in the field of psychotherapy. We were struck by the rigidity of boundaries between professions (psychiatrists, social workers, counsellors), institutions (private practice, clinic, private, or state hospital), and schools of thought (psychoanalysis, Gestalt, transactional analysis, family and group therapy) and so on. Each therapist sees the patient in his specialized way. Thus the same person may ponder about his childhood with one therapist, go with his wife to a marital counsellor, and attend family meetings arranged by the therapist of his 15-year-old daughter. One psychotherapist refuses to see another member of the family; another refuses to see the patient if he does not bring his whole family. Some psychotherapists and many encounter leaders live in the pre-Freudian era as far as their knowledge of transference and resistance is concerned. On the other hand, many psychoanalysts declare, without blushing, that they know nothing about group and family therapy, have never seen a psychodrama, and have no opinion about any of them.

Institutional structure supports this fragmentation. It is, of course, typical of the health care in the United States as a whole which many regard as being in "critical condition"[15] and ripe for radical change. However, it seems to us that in no other field of medicine is the organizational fragmentation projected into theory to such a degree as in psychotherapy. Each psychotherapeutic method seems to have its own "theory." One well-known professor of psychiatry complained that the residents, using different methods of psychotherapy, were unable to switch easily from one "model" to another, for example, from psychoanalytic model to family model. The trouble is not with the residents: they are waiting for an integrated conceptual model (they rightly guess a mature theory of psychotherapy cannot be expected at the present stage of knowledge). We agree with Fenichel[7] that there are many ways to treat neuroses, but there should be only one way to understand them. Since we find that the methodological reasons for seeking a theoretical unity are not obvious to many psychotherapists, let us draw a parallel. Suppose that there are three drugs for combating hyperthyroidism and that the explanation of their actions leads to three different theories of thyroid functioning. There is no field of scientific endeavor that would leave it at that: the attempts would not cease until a theoretical unity was established. Only in the field of psychotherapy can each method have its own "theory."

Freud was aware that psychoanalytic treatment is not a possible solution for the vast problem of neuroses and suggested to "alloy the pure gold of psychoanalysis with copper of direct suggestion." However, something more is needed today, an integration—not superficial eclecticism—of experiences dispersed over the whole fragmented field of psychotherapy, including psychoanalysis, behavior therapies, and encounter techniques.

SYSTEM OF INTEGRATED PSYCHOTHERAPY

Accepting the challenge of a model center for the treatment of neuroses in Prague in 1948, we at first considered ambulatory treatment. We were influenced by our psychoanalytic training and the discouraging experience of traditional residential treatment. We believed that neurotics should only be treated as ambulatory patients, remaining in the same environment where their coping capacities failed. Thus we put our efforts into finding ways of treating many neurotics through psychoanalytically oriented individual and group psychotherapy. However, the results did not satisfy us, and the number of patients was growing. We realized that we were not succeeding, as Frank puts it, "to mobilize group forces to involve the whole person."[8] Finally, through trial and error, we established the Residential Center in Lobec and later a Day Center. We were inspired by Makarenko's community for adolescents in Russia in the 1920s which we knew about from his book[30] and from N. Ekk's film, and by our visit to M. Jones' Center in Sutton in 1948.

We built up three interrelated units with the same staff at the Charles University in Prague in 1951, namely a Clinic, a Residential Center in the countryside, soon to be transferred to Lobec, and later a Day Center in Prague. We offered treatment to neurotics referred by district psychiatrists to patients who had not responded to treatment. We were free in choosing the patients for treatment and were not limited in time. Our self-imposed aim was to examine the problem of how to treat neurotics more efficiently and economically.

The transition of a patient from one unit to another was easy; usually, however, a patient started as an outpatient for a short time (receiving individual, group, or family therapy, or a combination of these). If more extensive treatment was necessary, he was advised to go to Lobec or the Day Center. Later, he could continue as an outpatient if necessary. This procedure was in agreement with the requirements that (a) no therapeutic method is used before a less time-consuming one is fully tried; (b) each step is a screening procedure testing motivation for the next step; (c) an improved patient can stop at any step, according to his motivation; and (d) one step did not preclude the use of the next step, for example, going through Lobec did not interfere, in our experience, with a patient continuing in postresidential intensive individual psychotherapy. In such a system, individual therapy of long duration as a first step is highly uneconomical. In the first months of treatment a proper combination of group methods can be superior diagnostically and therapeutically and in most cases is all that is needed.

The Residential Center in Lobec was not only a successful treatment modality, but also gave us a new perspective on psychotherapy in general. The insights and techniques developed there infiltrated all other forms of treatment, including psychoanalytic therapy. And the comparison of treatment modalities helped us to develop the conceptual framework which influenced in turn our clinical work. What we call "integrated psychotherapy"—and we are aware, of course, that it is more a program than an accomplishment—is a system of interlocking treatment modalities tied together by a conceptual framework. At the end of this chapter, due to lack of space, we only list our leading ideas.

Before describing the therapeutic community for neurotics in Lobec and Haney, we summarize our observations about treatment of neurotics in hospitals.

TRADITIONAL RESIDENTIAL TREATMENT OF NEUROTICS

When we asked administrators in State Hospitals in the United States about their numbers of nonpsychotic, particularly neurotic, patients, the answer was usually that the numbers were negligible. However, we discovered that this was not so. There were many neurotics and personality disorders—their percentage seemed to us at least as great as described in Hollingshead and Redlich's study.[13] According to Hollingshead and Redlich, of their sample of treated neurotics, 13.2% were in hospitals and of that number 9.8% were in state hospitals. They conclude:

> Hospitalized neurotic patients are in the minority of cases in all classes, but the lower the class the higher the percentage who are hospitalized. . . .
> . . . the class V neurotics are either clinic patients or they have been committed to the State Hospital. Those treated in the clinics tend to drop out of treatment shortly after they begin, but the neurotics in the state hospital tend to be retained in hospital indefinitely.

In Vancouver, Canada, neurotics represented 18% to 36% of psychiatric inpatients, not including the state hospital.[6] In one hospital, the average duration of stay was 20 days, despite a sufficient network of day-care facilities.

In the wards of American state hospitals, the nonpsychotic patients are mixed with severely disturbed patients. Such a mixing benefits neither group. The nonpsychotic patients often gladly accept the relaxed norms ˙geared to the most disturbed patients. In one state hospital nonpsychotic patients rarely came to community meetings, as they were busy begging for money at the entrance. It was difficult to say which played the greater part, such patients demoralizing the ward, or the ward demoralizing such patients.

In any case, they contributed to the ward becoming "social slums," which demoralized patients and staff. We often witnessed talented and enthusiastic nurses who became apathetic because of organizational deficiences they could do nothing about. The community meetings in some American institutions, with a mixed population of acute psychotics, neurotics, and psychopaths, often seemed to us a grotesque ritual. Valuable time is spent each day for 1 hour or so, in a more-or-less leaderless group, with patients and staff leaving more depressed than when they came.

Sometimes we heard mental health professionals reasoning that it could be undemocratic to separate patients, yet it is not undemocratic to have special wards for patients with cardiac and renal disorders if the homogenization is convenient for more efficient treatment. Again, it has to be remembered that mixed ward applies in the United States to poor patients, as affluent neurotic patients do not go to State Hospitals and are often not placed in private hospitals together with psychotic patients. Another reaction toward separation of patients is a dislike of "diagnostic pigeon-holing."

However, we are not interested in diagnostic labels per se, but in homogenizing groups so that a social structure can be designed which maximizes therapeutic results with the minimum of staff. Fortunately, voices have been raised recently against the thoughtless application of the therapeutic community concept to psychotic patients.[12, 34]

It might seem that in our view all difficulties would be resolved by simple separation of psychotic and nonpsychotic patients, but this is not so. Homogenization is only one of many conditions, as shown in examples from Czechoslovakia where, generally, separation of the psychotic and neurotic wards exists.

From patients admitted to all psychiatric inpatient facilities in Czechoslovakia in 1 year,[33] 13% were schizophrenics and about 36% were neurotics. From these neurotics, 32% were readmissions—about 16% once, 6% twice, and so on; and from these readmitted neurotics, about 30% had not been out of the psychiatric hospital for more than 3 months! These figures of the outcome of inpatient treatment of neurotics are unimpressive and make one wonder whether the return of a patient is not unwittingly supported. Having had the opportunity to follow up many of these patients, we believe that this is the case.

In Czechoslovakia, wards for nonpsychotic patients are mainly occupied by neurotics. Generally the rules are few, such as being punctual for meals and for psychiatric interviews, asking permission for overnight and weekend passes. The participation in groups and other activities, such as occupational therapy and sports, is mostly voluntary. The patients apparently like this form of treatment, since about 44% of patients diagnosed as neurotics, and about 33% diagnosed as personality disorders, have a duration of stay between 1 and 3 months. The treatment is, as with all medical treatment, free of charge.

Although an homogenous ward, composed of neurotics, gives better opportunities to work with the patients as a group, as opposed to heterogenic wards of American state hospitals, it is not in itself sufficiently advantageous to make such an environment useful. As one neurotic inpatient, who held an important position in industry, said: "I found that nobody, including myself, is immune against demoralization, if one is put into a situation of not having to do anything and to be without any obligation and responsibility. . . ." In the first years of our career, inspired by having an opportunity to observe M. Jones' Rehabilitation Center in 1948, we tried to change such a ward in a university setting into a therapeutic community, but only with limited success, since one ward cannot be easily changed, because of its connections with the hospital as a whole. We concluded that admitting neurotics to hospital, accept in cases of suicidal risk, is not only of little value, but that in many cases it is harmful. It often helps the patient escape from his problems, and we become his allies. A long-term stay in the hospital creates new situations in the lives of the patients which are potentially harmful to their marriage, profession, or studies.

There are other settings in Czechoslovakia for the treatment of neurotics who are equally ineffective—the nationalized sanatoriums and spas. The Czechoslovak spas were famous all over Europe, and had been for centuries, for treatment of almost any disease including neuroses, with a reputation of miraculous cures. Many kings, noblemen, and artists, such as Beethoven, Goethe, and Chekhov, went through them. When spas were socialized, the idea was that this wonder treatment, which only a few could afford in the past, would be offered to all working people. The experience of a typical patient exemplifies the therapeutic limitation of this treatment.

A woman from Prague, with neurotic complaints closely connected to her marriage, a connection that she later became aware of, lost her headache a few days after arriving at the spa, but it started again in the train on her way back to Prague and to her unresolved marital problems. This expensive treatment—including voluntary individual or group psychotherapy with a psychiatrist, recreational therapy, massages, and mineral baths—is of little therapeutic value, although in this case the hospital environment could not be blamed for it. There was an attempt by the Department of Psychiatry, Charles University, Prague, in which we both participated, to structure the program for neurotics in a spa by establishing a therapeutic community. This attempt was partially successful—it was apparent that the ecology of a spa could be more favorable than that of a hospital, if used in an untraditional way with the special effort of knowledgeable and dedicated staff. Still, this was not worth the effort, as it was similar to the treatment of neurotics in hospitals.

We therefore built up the triad mentioned—Clinic, Lobec, and Day Care. Here we are going to describe the Residential Center in Lobec only.

THE THERAPEUTIC COMMUNITY OF
THE RESIDENTIAL CENTER IN LOBEC

Together with the Clinic in Prague, we established a residential Neurosis Center in the country in 1951. It was soon transferred to the State Farm in Lobec, a small village 65 km from Prague, Czechoslovakia. The treatment was continuously changed and refined until the authors left the country (1968 and 1970). It is still in existence.

There were 25 to 30 neurotic patients and 2 social therapists living in the Center. Since the right choice of the social therapists is essential for the success, we characterize them. Both therapists were women, who had not formal psychiatric training and had never worked in a psychiatric institution before. They were both healthy, middle-aged women, capable of working with the patients in the fields and forests, intelligent, well aware of their limitations in knowledge, and experienced in organizing groups of people. They were fond of people, trusting but not naive, had a high frustration tolerance and a gift of inoffensive humor which dissolved tense situations. They both possessed a natural mental health talent. A male social therapist, with a university diploma who had received 4-years psychoanalysis and had a respectable knowledge of Western psychiatric literature, was employed temporarily but was a failure. Psychiatrists (the authors or residents), a psychologist, or social worker from our staff in Prague, came for the whole weekend, but later with the increased experience of the social therapists came only half a day each week.

The patients, led by elected foremen, work 6 hours a day for the State Farm. This is not occupational therapy, but genuine work in the fields, gardens, and woods. The group as a whole is responsible for a certain amount of work every day, planned by the State Farm. Since the patients are city people, unaccustomed to farm work, and sometimes the work has to be done under harsh climatic conditions, this situation is often a test of individual stress tolerance and attitude toward a group task. The patients also have to take care of the cleaning of the building, the heating, laundering, and so on. The life conditions are primitive compared to their lives at home—it is somewhat like life in a camp.

Most of the afternoons and evenings are spent in group activities, using both verbal and action techniques including sports, dances, social games, and group psychotherapy. Actually, there is no rigid line between psychotherapy and all the other activities. All activity is regarded as potentially useful to elucidate aspects of a patient's behavior and as being the vehicle for changing it.

Problems and conflicts in the community are of central interest to the patients ("here and now"), but they reflect a spectrum of situations from the outside ("there and now") and from the patient's past ("there and then"). Conflicts that emerge in work between two patients, one of them a foreman, raise some of the difficulties they both had in their jobs for years. Is one bossy as the foreman? Does he or she do all the work himself or herself because they are inhibited in giving orders? Is the other avoiding duties or unable to accept orders?

Several women are irritated by a man in precisely the same way as his wife is—as she later reveals. A young man has the same difficulties with an older man in the group, as with his father.

An episode that led to transference analysis, stretched over several weeks, might exemplify the process. During his work, a young man became angry with the female social therapist, because of a misunderstanding, he felt unjustly criticized for not working enough. He abandoned his tools and ran away from the field. In the evening we asked the community to reproduce the event psychodramatically. The patient acted his own role (but other patients imitated him later during the discussion); the social therapist was represented by an older and tolerant female patient A. In the discussion, another female patient E, expressed her own unfavourable attitude toward the recalcitrant young man. It appeared that they had some prior conflicts which resembled the conflicts she had with her son. She also reminded the patient of his mother who actually was a difficult person and had mistreated and frustrated him. Three other women, B, C, and D, showed a disposition to play a maternal role toward him and a spectrum of attitudes emerged—from the accepting attitude of A to the rejecting attitude of E. In the following weeks, the boy's relationship to his mother was worked through, and he became aware that getting angry with the social therapist in the field was unjustified and was caused by transferring the relationship from his mother to the therapist.

The presence of other women A–E helped him to see that not all women in authority are like his mother. And when several weeks later he enacted a dream in a psychodrama, he chose the social therapist as his ideal mother. He embraced her crying. Further development showed that he went through a successful corrective experience which he scarcely could have achieved in psychoanalytic treatment in such a short time.

While the patients are in Lobec, significant persons—spouses, parents, friends, co-workers, even bosses, at the invitation of the patient—come to a group in Prague. There are sometimes joint groups with significant persons and social therapists on weekends in Lobec, which is the only time that visits from Prague are possible. After the patients return to Prague, they have group meetings, both by themselves and jointly with their significant persons.

Those who continued in treatment in outpatient psychotherapy (psychoanalysis, group, or family therapy), after Lobec in our Clinic in Prague, were substantially more advanced than those who were treated for a corresponding time without Lobec. Lobec significantly shortened the total treatment time. Also, the decision to take a patient into a time-consuming individual therapy was much easier for us, since the stay in Lobec gave a more thorough picture of the patient's personality and motivation for treatment than any alternative we knew. As a matter of fact, it often happened that the patients in Lobec were able to say more in group about a patient after a week than psychiatrists knew about him after 3 months of inpatient treatment in the psychiatric university hospital.

When lecturing in North America, we often heard the objection that Lobec could not be established on this continent, as the patients would not want to work and live in a more primitive environment than that to which they are accustomed. This is not so, as was shown in the "Haney Project" in British Columbia, Canada. The first author established a therapeutic community for 4 months in the University of British Columbia Forestry Camp at Haney, and a Day Center. In a research project, conducted together with Dr. G. Reith and Dr. J. E. Miles, three comparable groups of neurotics were treated in the Haney Camp and the Day Center, and as psychiatric inpatients of the Health Sciences Center, University of British Columbia. An extensive battery of tests, both of questionnaire type and behavior ratings, were used. The outcome was most favorable (statistically highly significant) in the Camp, second best in the Day Center, whereas there were only a few indices of improvement (and none of them statistically significant) in inpatients.[23] The same order of the three institutions was found in a 2-year follow-up study.[36] The costs were in reversed order: Inpatient treatment (100%), Day Center (32%), and Haney Camp (16%). It may be remarked that the cost of 1 day in the Day Center is less than a 1-hour session with a psychiatrist.

In agreement with our findings were those of Caine and Smail.[4] They compared two groups of chronic neurotics in a hospital, one being treated in therapeutic community and the other by more conventional methods. They found significantly decreased scores on both symptom and personality measures for the therapeutic community group, which was not present in the comparative treatment sample.

In summary, we started with a negative attitude to any residential treatment, but gradually we were compelled to qualify it. Although we spent most of our professional time as psychiatrists in outpatient intensive psychotherapy, the most visible results in 6 weeks were achieved in Lobec, where we spent only one half day a week and where most of the work was done by two devoted and talented women without formal training—and by the patients themselves. True, some of the patients needed further treatment and many others could have profited from further treatment, if it had been available, but the large majority did not regard further treatment as necessary. J. Linhart, a district psychiatrist in Prague, referring patients to our care, concluded in his study that those who went through Lobec turned to him much less for further help and if they did, they demanded drug treatment less often and generally asked for less medical attention.[26]

BASIC CONDITIONS FOR INTENSIVE TREATMENT
IN A THERAPEUTIC COMMUNITY FOR NEUROTICS

The Residential Center in Lobec and Haney are therapeutic communities of a special sort. That is, they satisfy the conditions for therapeutic communities as formulated by M. Jones[14] and Rapoport,[35] but they have additional features that make them a particular modality of intensive psychotherapy for neurotics. To give a simple example, the upper limit for therapeutic community according to M. Jones[14] is 100 patients; the complex program of our therapeutic community cannot be accomplished with more than 30 patients. We shall not deal here with all kinds of possible psychiatric units which have been recently called "therapeutic communities" without any resemblance to M. Jones' Center, nor with the often justified criticism of them.[12, 34]

We now formulate basic conditions of this special therapeutic community; however, the description of therapeutic and administrative techniques to secure them is beyond the scope of this article. The basic conditions concern (1) rewards and costs; (2) group goals, norms, contract; (3) shared leadership; (4) closed socioecological system; (5) similarities to and differences from natural groups.

Condition 1—Rewards and Costs

The rewards and costs that the patient receives have to be contingent on his behavior in such a way that the motivation for therapeutic change of himself and others is maximized. We regard this condition (the rudiment of which is Freud's "abstinence rule") as basic for all psychotherapy, but there are special pitfalls in applying it successfully to residential treatment. As in all psychotherapy aiming at personality changes, dealing with resistances successfully is essential. The patient is divided in his motivation—wanting to get well, yet trying to avoid costs (anxiety, sad memories, awareness of decisional, and postdecisional conflict). Being in a group of people with a similar dilemma, nothing is easier than to form coalitions of resistance, unless special organization makes it both difficult and clear to the patient what his resistances are. In traditional hospitals, whether in America or Czechoslovakia, the patient can disappear in a labyrinth of social relations without responsibility, can spice his dull life in hospital by acting-out (skipping appointments and meetings, being late from passes, drinking, starting to smoke excessively, engaging in sexual adventures, playing one therapist against another or at least creating misunderstandings which never can be disentangled, and so on). An enthusiastic young therapist may try hard for 1 hour a day to understand a patient but his efforts, although heroic, are futile because he cannot offer competitive rewards—the patient could lose many small pleasures by becoming open. And besides, being open would be disloyal to his peers.

The rewards and costs in therapeutic community are more subtle than in token economy systems. They are mainly social in character, such as receiving social approval-disapproval, being included in or excluded from the group, being respected and trusted with power, and so on. All these rewards-costs come not only from therapists, but also from other patients.

In formulating this condition, "maximizing" is meant relative to present limited knowledge. There cannot be any doubt that better knowledge in the future will lead to more precise and effective reward-cost systems. The help of a computer may be necessary because of the complexity of social interactions.

Condition 2—Group Goals, Norms, Contract

Therapeutic community admits a patient who is willing and able to make a contract in which he confirms his desire to pursue group goals (elimination of symptoms and the modification of every patients' personality) and to follow the program and norms. In a well-organized community, the patients support each other in satisfying this condition. This condition cannot be satisfied when psychotic patients are admitted who cannot (or it appears they cannot, or it would take too long to find out) make the contract. One community with different norms for different categories of patients is a very uneconomical procedure and both sides lose. The neurotics do not receive the intensive pressure that they need in psychotherapy. And a schizophrenic in a neurotic community with high morale suffers by being pressed to do what he probably cannot do.

Nothing enhances the cohesiveness of a group more than a difficult group task, which the group accepts and is in the process of mastering.

In Lobec the main task was, of course, therapeutic improvement of everybody. But the group tasks of the program—such as physical work on the farm which had to be finished during a certain period—were also effective agents for producing cohesiveness and morale. During a longer period of heavy rain or snow storms, which made work outside impossible, morale and therapeutic results dropped and acting-out increased. Later, when we could use the gym to play basketball and other competitive games the situation improved. Artificial goals such as competitive games, if accepted and stressful enough, served well as agents for enhancing cohesiveness and morale.

The norms should reflect real life—and they should not be too few or too many. Some norms are unproblematic, that is, cannot be changed by vote and are formulated by the therapists beforehand. They are kept to a minimum and reflect the theoretical views of the therapists and the conditions under which they are willing to operate. For example, such an unproblematic norm is that each patient is expected to participate in all parts of the program.

The patient's attitude toward the norms of the therapeutic community reflects closely the patient's attitude to social norms in his life, his ethical profile. He shows it through transgressions, following norms slavishly, guilt feelings, overanxiousness, watching transgressions of others, or trying to be group executioner, and so on. We agree with Arieti[1] that psychiatric treatment must consider man's ethical dimension and that it is often ignored by psychotherapists. We do not know of a better opportunity in psychotherapy to study a patient's moral values than a therapeutic community. Sometimes a patient discovers through the group process that change of his moral values would make life easier and happier for him.

Condition 3—Leadership

The more the patient, pursuing therapeutic goals, shares leadership with the therapists, the more effective the therapy becomes. There are good reasons for this in any group. K. Lewin[25] stated that group members assimilate more easily the views, values, and criticisms of a peer than those of a leader. Makarenko, the Russian forefather of therapeutic community, gives an account of a boy in the reeducational community of delinquent adolescents who systematically avoided work, but who changed radically after he became responsible for the work of others.[30] Without the shared leadership, the therapists in Lobec could achieve only a fragment of what is achieved.

One other advantage for shared leadership is that it leads to shifting of transferences. Therapists functioning as the sole leader concentrate strong ambivalent transference reactions, and this must be avoided. It would not only be extremely strenuous for them, but they would have difficulties, being also the administrative leaders, to disentangle the transferred and realistic elements in their interactions. Their transference analyses would be at best unconvincing and at worst onesided and incorrect. When patients share leadership, a considerable amount of ambivalent transference reactions can be shifted to the patients themselves. It took us years to elaborate this strategy in Lobec, and initially the social therapists did not like it. But they soon experienced great relief, since it was taxing to be the target of transferences from 25 to 30 patients. For example, the patients act as committee members and foremen in deciding about sanctions for breaking rules, the committee of patients make suggestions, and the staff members have one vote like everybody else. When the unwinding of transference reactions goes on toward other patients, the therapists may contribute more as objective participant observers. Also, the therapeutic spectrum is enlarged, since the choice of certain patients as new transference targets is of therapeutic interest.

Although under the conditions described, the role of therapists becomes more restricted, its quality increases. Executive leadership is shifted to the patients themselves, whereas the therapists can concentrate more on their expert leadership—serving as resource persons to the committee and foremen.

Condition 4—A Closed Socioecological System

The Therapeutic Community is a relatively closed socioecological system of a small group, with defined spatiotemporal boundaries, and the patients have only limited and regulated contacts with persons outside the system. This gives the group a unique opportunity to identify the maladaptive interpersonal circuits as these run uninterrupted inside the system, and to use group resources and pressures for therapeutic change. What is the function of the closed system? To a certain degree, the closed system is typical of various kinds of intensive psychotherapy. In classical psychoanalysis, the two-person system of the patient and the analyst is closed for an hour, during which time a third person may not enter. Moreover, through psychoanalytic techniques, and avoidance of extratreatment contacts between the two participants, creation and continuity of a separate world (in a certain sense) are formed. The closed system of a group in intensive group psychotherapy, that is stability of membership, is regarded as desirable by many group psychotherapists. In extended group meetings (like weekend groups and marathons), the effect and intensity would dissipate if visitors came to the meetings or the participants left to meet outside persons. The closed system is essential in Synanon and similar types of treatment for drug addicts: leaving the system, at least for the first few months, would increase the risk of repetitive pathological behavior (taking drugs) and jeopardize a change in behavior. Another form of strict closed system of treatment is the Morita therapy which seems to be reasonably successful in Japan.

Besides the therapeutic settings mentioned, there are of course also nontherapeutic closed systems, like wards in old-fashioned psychiatric hospitals, prisons, and special "brainwashing" prisons. A therapeutic closed system differs from them, such that in a therapeutic closed system, *all* five conditions must be satisfied. Also, the patient stays in the system for a relatively short duration (4 to 6 weeks in Lobec).

Let us imagine that a patient in the community suddenly becomes depressed, feels hopeless, anxious, angry, and gets a headache. There are, typically, four stages in the recognition of the origin of the symptom. In the first stage, the patient does not know how the symptom came about. In the second stage, he admits that it is a reaction to the behavior of some members of the group. In the third stage, it usually turns out that their behavior was a reaction to his behavior, and so the patient has an opportunity to see just how he contributes to his own misery. If everything goes well, the patient reaches the fourth stage: through analysis of resistance and transference, through corrective experience (with emotional and cognitive aspects), and with the support and pressure of the group he changes his self-defeating behavior. From the state where he felt helpless and things "happened" to him, he reaches the state where he understands that his behavior is a link in the causal network of the group system: he begins to understand what he does to others and why they react to him as they do.

If the community was *not* a closed system and the patient could interact with outside persons, his vicious circles would run outside the system where they would be difficult to trace, except through his biased report. Also, the group pressures for change would be considerably diminished as he could obtain rewards for his neurotic needs outside the group.

A patient may come believing everybody hates him, and the group shows him in detail how he manages to achieve this. Or a girl may break down because of repeated disillusionments in love with unsuitable partners, and in the community it becomes apparent that she is doing everything to become attached to a patient who is similar, and as she later recognizes, unsuitable in the same way. Another man complains of being "overworked" because of the tasks an inconsiderate boss imposes on him, but the next week as a member of the patients' committee he begins to invent new duties and regulations which exhaust him as well as the others. In the closed system of the community a patient cannot escape the consequences of his behavior and cannot easily escape seeing what he is doing, since at the same time he is dependent on the group for his rewards and costs and he is under strong group pressure to change. Instead of feeling that he is a defenseless victim of outside forces, he discovers that he is co-creator of his own destiny, a more important *causal* factor in his life than he believed.

The persistence of maladaptive behavior, despite the apparent lack of rewards, is a phenomenon of central importance in neurosis. It has been described in different theoretical frameworks by Freud ("repetition compulsion," "neurosis of destiny"), by H. Schultz-Henke[37] ("the vicious circle of neurosis," perhaps the first interpersonal explanation of neurotic repetition), and by O. H. Mowrer,[31] ("neurotic paradox"). In many instances, the hidden rewards of interpersonal vicious circles can be identified in therapeutic community.

The size of the group is important, with the upper limit of 30 patients. Up to that size, it can be regarded as a small social group. Due to intensive interactions, each patient knows the others well and forms a pattern of relationship typical for him. A group smaller than 20 is not sufficiently stable, a group larger than 30 is difficult to survey.

Condition 5—Similarities and Differences from Natural Groups

It is essential that there are similarities to natural groups in some respects, and differences in others. Therapeutic community is a *model* of natural groups. It imitates their broad range of functions such as group tasks, norms, distribution of roles, and opportunities for sharing leadership. Living closely together and sharing group tasks is a source of satisfaction and enjoyment, safety, and feeling of belonging; but, as in real life, it creates stress and frustration and gives each patient the opportunity to initiate his characteristic neurotic behavior. Quasi-familial and quasi-professional relations develop, since every patient is likely to find complementary roles resembling those of father, mother, siblings, boss, spouse, girlfriend, or boyfriend, and every complementary role is likely to be represented by several patients.

The importance of *work* as a group task must be stressed, since with a few exceptions—like that of Maxwell Jones[14] and J. Cumming and E. Cumming[5]—an emphasis on the importance of work is lacking. Is a patient bossy as a foreman? Does another foreman do all the work himself because he is too inhibited to give orders? Is somebody skillful at avoiding his duties? These are some topics for the afternoon group meetings.

Work in Lobec helped many patients restore their self-confidence which they lost in their jobs or studies, although their tasks in Lobec were quite dissimilar from both. Many housewives who wanted to work outside home but lacked confidence to seek employment started work after Lobec. We had a similar experience in the Haney Camp. Here, the words of Konrad Lorenz come to mind: "Self-esteem depends largely upon successes which one achieves in overcoming obstacles." The opportunity to overcome various obstacles, sometimes with support and urging of the group is, in Lobec, extensive. Since the obstacles have similarities with situations in real life, the confidence is more likely to generalize to real life than that ephemeral self-confidence which often emerges in encounter group or verbal psychotherapy.

Differences from real life are also essential. The only aim of therapeutic community is therapeutic change, and the patient's behavior no longer has consequences other than therapeutic. Unlike in real life, nobody is fired for criticizing the foreman or being angry with the therapist. The group is flexible, stabilization of relationships is counteracted, and a change of relationships often takes place from one day to another. A patient can try out a variety of different ways of relating to others.

What gives a patient this freedom to experiment? One important ingredient is the extensive use of play and fantasy. The group switches easily from serious problems to jokes, from reality to fantasy; tears are compensated for by laughter. This is intensified by special techniques such as psychodrama, psychogymnastics,[21] dramatic, pantomimic and imagination exercises, and indoor and outdoor games. The aim is to provide each patient with "surplus reality", imaginary situations in which his idiosyncratic solutions can be identified in detail, and where he can find and try out different solutions, situations from his personal history can be revived, and he may go through the corrective experience of receiving support and care from the group which he missed in his past. Finally, by creating 'surplus reality' the patient may face situations he will likely meet in the future which are not readily available in the life of therapeutic community.

A therapeutic community such as Lobec becomes to many patients a model of familial, professional, and other groups. There is a tremendous difference, for example, between the supervisory function in the patient's profession and his function as a foreman in Lobec, and yet the reaction is similar. The following example is typical of this. A director of a large factory in Prague and government consultant in international economic transactions came to Lobec with the leading symptom of severe insomnia. After arrival his sleep improved considerably, but after his election to chairman of the community his symptom reappeared as severely as before. What happened? A subgroup of patients broke the rules and pressed him not to reveal this to the group and especially not to the therapists, and he was torn by the conflict between solidarity with the patients and loyalty to the therapeutic principles and the therapists. This conflict was basically the same as the conflict which was the immediate cause of his insomnia before he came for treatment: he experienced a conflict between loyalty to the ministry of industry with its excessive demands, and solidarity with the workers. Although there is a tremendous difference between the two situations, and the importance of being chairman is negligible compared with his function as director, the similarity is sufficient to elicit similar reactions.

DAY CENTER AND OTHER PARTIAL THERAPEUTIC COMMUNITIES

The reader may ask: Why should I be interested in the therapeutic community described, when I never intend to work in such a setting? There are several answers to that.

1. First, if our analysis is correct, residential treatment of neurotic and other nonpsychotic patients has to move in the direction indicated. (Although we avoid dealing here with psychotic patients, from our own experience, from one outcome study[32] and from "camping therapy,"[29] we believe that many psychotic patients would profit if living and working in somewhat differently organized centers, which could be established as small units even on the grounds of a state hospital. We saw some impressive examples in Poland and the United States.)

In countries where there is a shortage of psychiatrists, therapeutic communities can become an important part of psychiatric treatment; the work of Nigerian psychiatrist Asuni about "psychiatric villages"[2] points in the same direction. A knowledgeable psychiatrist can train endogenous workers as social therapists—their personalities and capability, not their formal education, is what matters primarily. This does not mean that such a community would be a second-rate substitute; the community itself has healing power that the therapists need not necessarily understand theoretically.

In the Canadian study mentioned, both the Forestry Camp and the Day Center were improvized, with the same clinical supervisor and comparable (partly identical) staff, not fully trained for this kind of work. Yet the results were significantly better in the camp and day center than in the hospital, and the results in the camp were significantly better than in the day center. There is a range from fairly simple communities with limited goals, to sophisticated ones with the best psychotherapeutic treatment available. Lobec went through the whole range.

If a developing country sends doctors for psychiatric training to a developed country, and they return and treat a small number of affluent patient, the reasons may not only be the obvious ones. They have perhaps not learned to do anything else, such as organizing a therapeutic community. It was especially striking for us when we, as visiting professors, lectured in Cuba in 1963. Many psychiatrist we met were trained in the United States, but they were not able at that time, despite their enthusiastic attitude to the socialized health care, to organize efficient therapeutic communities or group psychotherapy.

2. The Residential Center is excellent for *training* purposes. When we were asked by the Polish Ministry of Health to train some Polish psychiatrists and psychologists in psychotherapy, we started by taking them in the

role of patients to Lobec. This is also how we trained each new member of our Prague and Lobec staff-residents, nurses, and social workers; they usually claimed it later as the most useful part of their professional training. Once in a while, we closed Lobec for patients and replaced them by psychiatrists and other professionals from different institutions across Czechoslovakia, as a training opportunity.

3. Another reason why we think this form of therapeutic community deserves attention is a *theoretical* one. All diagnostic and therapeutic components of psychotherapy can be found there—desensitization of fears, shaping of behavior by rewards and costs, change of cognitive maps, analysis of resistance, and transference with corrective experience (correcting social misperceptions, recapitulation of childhood situations, and a change of role relationships—changes both emotional and cognitive), a broad opportunity to actualize one's conflicts in a model situation, learning of social skills, assertiveness, leadership, and so on. True, some other therapies give a better opportunity to deal in concentrated form with one or another component (e.g., psychoanalysis with the development of transference focused on one person), but those not familiar with this form of treatment will no doubt underrate what can be achieved in 6 weeks in all components mentioned. Some of the patients need further therapy, and we know that a further stay in Lobec at our present stage of knowledge would be unlikely to change their condition, whereas intensive individual psychotherapy may.

4. But the fourth and most important answer is that closed therapeutic community offers directives on how to organize more difficult forms of treatment such as Day Center. Apparently, it is often not realized that the Day Center poses special theoretical and practical questions. We scarcely saw any other psychiatric institution where so much money was wasted as in some United States day centers. Often, the centers suffered from an abundance of staff, interfering with co-ordinated treatment, and because of the relaxed norms, the attendance of patients was unpredictable and there were sometimes more staff members than patients. Again, mixing of patients, with different capacities to enter a therapeutic contract, is demoralizing. Very likely, a neurotic arriving 2 hours late should be dealt with differently than a schizophrenic patient. But it is difficult to establish different norms in the same group.

At the University of British Columbia, the first author, with co-workers, established two day centers, one for neurotics and personality disorders, and the other one for psychotic and postpsychotic patients, usually on psychotropic drugs. The neurotic patients have a separate house ("Day House") with a garden, and they are responsible for looking after house and garden. They work on different projects, on some of them earning money for the patients' fund. The next bigger projects are a greenhouse, building a hut in the forest, and so on. Besides their own activities, the patients meet one night together with their Significant Persons—spouses, parents, friends, or bosses if they wish. This joint families' technique, developed by the second author in Prague in the early 1950s is complementary to dealing with marital family problems in the group of patients, without relatives. In that group, the marital and family problems are reconstructed and solutions psychodramatically simulated (*simulated family*) or partly emerge, because the patient uses the same interpersonal techniques toward other patients (*quasi-family*) as in his family. (To foster the development of "quasi-family", the group is divided into three "second-chance families.") In the Significant Persons Group, the problems of real families are *amplified*: as the real family interacts in front of the group, other patients come and "amplify" the roles of the family members (psychodramatic "doubling"). We find this combined method of dealing with family relations as superior to sole family therapy, both in efficiency and economy. Inviting the real families helps the group compare the patient's often distorted perception about his relatives and helps him to generalize to real life what he learned in the Day House. In the motivational system of relatives, approval of the group is introduced as a factor; and amplification of the relatives' unexpressed needs speeds up the problem-solving process in their family.

Again, as in residential community, the number of patients and staff is essential. Whereas the upper number of patients in residential community is 30, in the Day Center it is about 20. There should be, as much as possible, only full-time staff members. The interrelationships among patients and staff members of therapeutic community are complicated enough: to keep up sufficient communication and co-ordinate strategy with part-time members would require more time than the treatment and it would still not counteract all disadvantages. And so an unnecessary increase of the number of staff may be a sufficient factor to make the therapeutic community ineffective.

We regard the knowledge of Therapeutic Community as the best background for group treatments, where the closed system exists for a short time only—such as Night Centers with evening activities, weekend workshops, or group therapy of several hours. The therapeutic potential of a group of motivated people being together and being open seems to be great and sometimes produces surprising changes without much expert knowledge. Some of our patients with previous individual therapy (or training psychotherapy in the case of a psychiatrist) told us about crucial experiences not from their therapy, but from encounter workshops which they visited years ago. They did not mention the influence of leaders, but people who were with them. We do not want to discuss here the extremely heterogenous encounter movement—its merits, its risks, and so on. But we want to stress that under favorable conditions through "group forces" beneficial effects may result which are not so easily achieved in the usual ambulatory individual or group treatment.

Principles of therapeutic community described can be applied in educational and preventive work—recreational camps for adolescents, children, marital couples (e.g., in Czechoslovakia summer camps for the families of treated ex-alcoholics) and in training of professional and endogenous workers for community mental health work.

An essential part of the success of the therapeutic community goes to the patients themselves. As we said elsewhere,[17] professionally supervised use of patients may well be a solution to many problems of mental health. Their capacity for empathy, support, and help can be called the atomic energy of future psychiatry, but proper techniques for its control must be elaborated further.

TOWARD A THEORY OF INTEGRATED PSYCHOTHERAPY

Although our conclusions are, we hope, plausible enough, it would likely be more so if we could present them in the conceptual framework of integrated psychotherapy. This framework could not have been formulated on an empirical basis of individual therapy alone—therapeutic community and family therapy contributed significantly. But this framework, once formulated, influenced in turn our psychotherapeutic technology and tied together all forms of therapy. Only leading statements will be enumerated, but without attempting to justify them. (This has been done particularly in Refs. 18 and 19 and will be presented in detail in a forthcoming book, *Integrated Psychotherapy*.)

1. The obstacles in integrating psychotherapy are not only in the present lack of knowledge, but also in conceptual pitfalls. Particularly, there are pseudodichotomies, such as causal-finalistic, determinism-freedom of will, intrapsychic-interpersonal, cognitive-emotional, behavioral-phenomenal, behavioristic-humanistic, and so on. They give rise to opposing views which can be, we believe, eliminated by logical analysis of concepts. So far, they keep a wall between behavioral and psychodynamic schools. For example, many psychoanalysts would agree with behavior therapists as voiced by C. M. Franks and G. T. Wilson, stating that in their opinion, "the profound philosophical differences between the behavioral and psychodynamic schools . . . can never lead to the emergence of philosophical unity between the two schools of thought."[10] We disagree. Of course, one serious conceptual obstacle for behavioral schools is "intrapsychic dimension" of

dynamic schools. However, we believe that it can be shown[19] that the concept of "intrapsychic" belongs to a linguistic framework that has alternatives compatible with present behavior theories such as social learning theory in formulation of Bandura.[3] The conceptual clarification will help people who stand on different sides of the fence to join forces in attacking the serious unresolved empirical problems.

2. Even in studying an individual, a group in which he operates is, according to our view, the minimum system where uninterrupted interpersonal circuits can be followed. The conceptual framework or small group structure and processes, including social learning, forms sufficient basis for psychotherapy if extended as follows.

3. An imaginary group, a product of social experience, accompanies an individual even if alone. We call this a Group Schema and apply to it the concepts of real groups. The Group Schema functions as a "cognitive map," it is used in thinking as a model for social training and problem-solving, and it provides vicarious satisfactions and can replace reality in fantasy, as is most vividly seen in day dreams, dreams, and hallucinations. The imaginary feedback from Group Schema persons can sometimes outweigh that coming from real persons. We believe to have shown that intrapsychic processes can be conceived mainly as interpersonal processes in fantasy—a solution suggested by H. S. Sullivan, but one which is not sufficiently warranted by him.

4. The hypotheses about the Group Schema of a patient can be tested, particularly with the help of action techniques such as psychodrama and psychogymnastics.[21] The same techniques can be instrumental in fostering corrective experience (in both of its aspects, cognitive and emotional) either in relation to transference persons, or directly to imagined significant persons from the past.[20]

5. The central task of psychotherapy is to change "Group Schema" (in J. Frank's language, "assumptive world"[9]). Group situation—be it therapeutic community or individual psychotherapy (once called by Freud "Group of Two") becomes a group model that gives the patient an opportunity to handle it as his Group Schema. Therapeutic community is especially suited to make the patient's social misperceptions and related "vicious circles" manifest and gives impetus to their change.

6. Possible contribution of ethology to the theory of psychotherapy was discussed by us elsewhere.[20] For example, the therapeutic use of abreaction seems to have parallels in "stimulus therapy"[27] of animals which, because of deficient rearing in a zoo, are not able to release certain species-specific action patterns. This may turn out to be one of the "direct approaches to the nervous system through psychological interventions" envisaged by Frank—with strictly circumscribed but definite place in the process of psychotherapy.

REFERENCES

1. Arieti, S.: Psychiatric controversy: Man's ethical dimension. *Amer. J. Psychiat.* **13**:39-42, 1975.

2. Asuni, T.: Community development and public health by-product of social psychiatry in Nigeria. *West African Med. J.* **13**:151-154, 1964.

3. Bandura, A.: *Social Learning Theory,* General Learning Corporation, U.S.A., 1971.

4. Caine, T. M. and Smail, D. J.: *The Treatment of Mental Illness,* University of London Press, London, 1969.

5. Cumming, J. and Cumming, E.: *Ego & Milieu,* Atherton Press, Chicago, 1962.

6. Cumming, J.: Personal communication, 1975.

7. Fenichel, O.: *The Psychoanalytic Theory of Neurosis,* Norton, New York, 1945.

8. Frank, J. D.: Common features account of effectiveness. *Int. J. Psychiat.* **7**:122-127, 1969.

9. Frank, J. D.: *Persuasion and Healing* (revised edition), The Johns Hopkins University Press, Baltimore & London, 1973.

10. Franks, C. M. and Wilson, G. T. (Eds.): *Annual Review of Behavior Therapy—Theory and Practice,* Bruner/Mazel, New York, 1974.

11. Glasscote, R. M., Kraft, A. M., Glassman, S. M., and Jepson, W. W. (Eds.): *Partial Hospitalization for the Mentally Ill,* American Psychiatric Association, Washington, D.C., 1969.

12. Herz, M. I.: The therapeutic community. *Hosp. Community Psychiat.* **23**:17-20, 1972.

13. Hollingshead, A. B. and Redlich, F. C.: *Social Class and Mental Illness,* Wiley, New York, 1958.

14. Jones, M.: *Social Psychiatry in Practice,* Penguin Books, England, 1968.

15. Kennedy, E. M.: *In Critical Condition: The Crisis of America's Health Care,* Simon & Schuster, Canada, 1972.

16. Knobloch, F.: The Diagnostic and Therapeutic Community as Part of a Psychotherapeutic System. In *Proceedings, Second International Congress of Group Psychotherapy,* Stockvis, B. (Ed.), Basel & New York, S. Karger, 1959, pp. 331-340.

17. Knobloch, F.: The system of group-centered psychotherapy for neurotics in Czechoslovakia. *Amer. J. Psychiat.* **124**:113-117, 1968.

18. Knobloch, F.: Toward a conceptual framework of group-centered psychotherapy. In *New Directions in Mental Health,* Grune & Stratton, U.S.A., 1968.

19. Knobloch, F.: Toward a theoretical integration of psychotherapies. *Contemp. Psychoanal.* **10**:209-218, 1974.

20. Knobloch, F.: Towards an integrated theory of curative factors in psychoanalysis, family and group therapy. In *Proceedings of the Psychoanalytic Forum,* Zurich, 1974. (In print)

21. Knobloch, F. and Knobloch, J.: Psychogymnastik. In *Psychotherapie—Korperdynamik,* Petzold, H., (Ed.), Junfermann, Paderborn, 1974.

22. Knobloch, F. and Knobloch, J.: From family therapy to integrated psychotherapy. *Proc. V World Congr. Psychiat.,* Mexico, 1971, Excerpta Medica, Amsterdam.

23. Knobloch, F., Reith, G., and Miles, J. E.: The therapeutic community as a treatment for neurotics. Presented at The Twenty-third Annual Meeting of the Canadian Psychiatric Association, Vancouver, 1973.

24. Knobloch, J. and Knobloch, F.: Family psychotherapy. In *Aspects of Mental Health in Europe,* Buckle, D. (Ed.), Public Health Paper No. 28, World Health Organization, Geneva, 1964.

25. Lewin, K.: *Resolving Social Conflicts,* Harper Row, New York, 1948.

26. Linhart, J.: Neurotic patients in a district psychiatric clinic. Paper presented at a Seminar, Charles University Psychiatric Clinic, Prague, 1965.

27. Lorenz, K.: Preface. In Schulze, H., *Das Prinzip Handeln in der Psychotherapie,* F. Enke, Stuttgart, 1971.

28. Lorenz, K. and Leyhausen, P.: *Motivation of Human and Animal Behavior: An Ethological View,* Nostrand Reinhold, New York, 1973.

29. Lowry, T. P.: *Camping Therapy,* Ch. C. Thomas, Springfield, 1974.

30. Makarenko, A. S.: *The Road to Life,* Oriole Editions, New York, 1973 (reprint of 1951).

31. Mowrer, O. H.: Learning theory and the neurotic paradox. *Amer. J. Orthopsychiat.* **18:**571–610, 1948.

32. Myers, K. and Clark, D. H.: Results in a therapeutic community. *Brit. J. Psychiat.* **120:**51–58, 1972.

33. Psychiatric Care in 1966. Health Statistics of Czechoslovak Socialist Republic, Institute of Health Statistics, Prague, 1967.

34. Putten, Van I.: Milieu Therapy: contraindications? *Arch. Gen. Psychiat.* **29:**640–643, 1973.

35. Rapoport, R.: *Community as Doctor,* Tavistock, London, 1960.

36. Reith, G., Knobloch, F., and Miles, J. E.: One and two year follow-up of psychiatric inpatients, day care and therapeutic community treatment. Paper presented at the Twenty-fourth Annual Meeting of the Canadian Psychiatric Association, Ottawa, 1974.

37. Schultz-Hencke, H.: *Der Gehemmte Mensch,* G. Tieme, Leipzig, 1942, pp. 72–73.